FIRST AID FOR THE®

Obstetrics & Gynecology Clerkship

Third Edition

MATTHEW S. KAUFMAN, MD
Assistant Professor, Albert Einstein College of Medicine
Department of Hematology
North Shore–Long Island Jewish Medical Center
New Hyde Park, New York

JEANÉ SIMMONS HOLMES, MD, FACOG
Co-Director of Academic Curriculum
Obstetrics and Gynecology Residency Program
The Methodist Hospital-Houston
Assistant OB/GYN Clerkship Director at St. Joseph Medical Center
Department of Obstetrics and Gynecology
Assistant Professor, Weill Cornell Medical College
Houston, Texas

PRITI P. SCHACHEL, MD, FACOG
Co-Director of Academic Curriculum
The Methodist Hospital-Houston
Obstetrics and Gynecology Residency Program
Assistant Professor, Weill Cornell Medical College
Houston, Texas

LATHA G. STEAD, MD, MS, FACEP
Chief, Division of Clinical Research
Professor of Emergency Medicine
University of Florida College of Medicine at Gainesville
Adjunct Professor of Emergency Medicine
Mayo Clinic, College of Medicine
Rochester, Minnesota
Editor-in-Chief, *International Journal of Emergency Medicine*

McGraw Hill Medical

New York / Chicago / San Francisco / Lisbon / London / Madrid / Mexico City
Milan / New Delhi / San Juan / Seoul / Singapore / Sydney / Toronto

First Aid for the® Obstetrics & Gynecology Clerkship, Third Edition

1 2 3 4 5 6 7 8 9 0 QDB/QDB 14 13 12 11 10

ISBN 978-0-07-163419-9
MHID 0-07-163419-3

Notice

Medicine is an ever-changing science. As new research and clinical experience broaden our knowledge, changes in treatment and drug therapy are required. The authors and the publisher of this work have checked with sources believed to be reliable in their efforts to provide information that is complete and generally in accord with the standards accepted at the time of publication. However, in view of the possibility of human error or changes in medical sciences, neither the authors nor the publisher nor any other party who has been involved in the preparation or publication of this work warrants that the information contained herein is in every respect accurate or complete, and they disclaim all responsibility for any errors or omissions or for the results obtained from use of the information contained in this work. Readers are encouraged to confirm the information contained herein with other sources. For example and in particular, readers are advised to check the product information sheet included in the package of each drug they plan to administer to be certain that the information contained in this work is accurate and that changes have not been made in the recommended dose or in the contraindications for administration. This recommendation is of particular importance in connection with new or infrequently used drugs.

This book was set in Electra LH by Rainbow Graphics.
The editor was Catherine A. Johnson.
The production supervisor was Catherine Saggese.
Project management was provided by Rainbow Graphics.
Quad/Graphics was the printer and binder.

This book is printed on acid-free paper.

Library of Congress Cataloging-in-Publication Data

First aid for the obstetrics & gynecology clerkship / [edited by]
Matthew S. Kaufman, Latha G. Stead.—3rd ed.
   p. ; cm.
  Includes index.
  ISBN 978-0-07-163419-9 (pbk. : alk. paper)
   1. Obstetrics—Study and teaching (Graduate) 2. Gynecology—Study and teaching (Graduate) 3. Clinical medicine—Study and teaching (Graduate)
I. Kaufman, Matthew S. II. Stead, Latha G.
  [DNLM: 1. Clinical Clerkship. 2. Obstetrics. 3. Gynecology. WQ 18]
RG141.F45 2010
618.076—dc22

                                          2010037133

International Edition ISBN 978-0-07-174277-1; MHID 0-07-174277-8.
Copyright © 2011. Exclusive rights by The McGraw-Hill Companies, Inc., for manufacture and export. This book cannot be re-exported from the country to which it is consigned by McGraw-Hill. The International Edition is not available in North America.

CONTRIBUTORS

MARQUITA D. ANDERSON
Class of 2010
University of Texas Medical School at Houston
Houston, Texas
16/Infertility
23/Pelvic Masses

MARTINA T. AYAD
Class of 2010
University of Texas Medical School at Houston
Houston, Texas
14/Menstruation
15/Premenstrual Syndrome/Premenstrual Dysphoric
*   Disorder*
17/Amenorrhea
18/Hyperandrogenism
19/Hyperprolactemia and Galactorrhea
20/Abnormal Uterine Bleeding

LAUREN K. BANKS
Class of 2010
University of Texas Medical School at Houston
Houston, Texas
8/Obstetrical Complications of Pregnancy

ARIELLE L. CAPERS
Class of 2010
University of Texas Medical Branch at Galveston
Galveston, Texas
6/Postpartum

LAUREN P. GIBSON
Class of 2010
University of Texas Medical School at Houston
Houston, Texas
7/Medical Conditions in Pregnancy
9/Infections in Pregnancy

TRACILYN HALL, MD
Resident
The Methodist Hospital-Houston
Obstetrics and Gynecology Residency Program
Houston, Texas
31/Sexually Transmitted Infections/Vaginitis

MAE KATHLEEN HAYES
Class of 2010
University of Texas Medical School at Houston
Houston, Texas
5/Intrapartum

JAMIE G. HERNANDEZ
Class of 2010
University of Texas Medical School at Houston
Houston, Texas
13/Contraception and Sterilization

CATHLEEN G. HOFFMAN
Class of 2010
University of Texas Medical School at Houston
Houston, Texas
Section I: How to Succeed in the Obstetrics and
*   Gynecology Clerkship*

CHRISTOPHER A. HOLLWEG, MPH
Class of 2011
St. George's University School of Medicine
Granada
Minicases and Vignettes

ROXANNA A. IRANI, PhD
Class of 2011
University of Texas Medical School at Houston
Houston, Texas
4/Antepartum
11/Abortions and Fetal Death

CHARLIE C. KILPATRICK, MD
Assistant Professor
Department of Obstetrics, Gynecology and Reproduc-
   tive Sciences
Lyndon Baines Johnson Hospital
University of Texas Health Science Center at Houston
Houston, Texas
10/Twin Gestation
32/Breast Disease

VANESSA M. LOPEZ
Class of 2010
University of Texas Medical School at Houston
Houston, Texas
21/Pelvic Pain
22/Endometriosis/Adenomyosis

MARGARET MARKHAM
Class of 2010
University of Texas Medical School at Houston
Houston, Texas
24/Cervical Dysplasia
25/Cervical Cancer

LYNDA E. MBAH
Class of 2010
University of Texas Medical School at Houston
Houston, Texas
11/Abortions and Fetal Death
12/Ectopic Pregnancy

KATHERINE M. NELSON
Class of 2010
University of Texas Medical School at Houston
Houston, Texas
36/Menopause
37/Pelvic Relaxation
38/Urinary Incontinence

BRIDGETTE J. PARISH, MD
Resident
The Methodist Hospital-Houston
Obstetrics and Gynecology Residency Program
Houston, Texas
30/Gestational Trophoblastic Disease

MICHAEL L. PIRICS, MD
Resident
The Methodist Hospital-Houston
Obstetrics and Gynecology Residency Program
Houston, Texas
33/Women's Health Maintenance
34/Female Sexuality
35/Ethics

GAVIN P. PUTHOFF
Class of 2010
University of Texas Medical School at Houston
Houston, Texas
26/Endometrial Hyperplasia and Endometrial Cancer
27/Ovarian Cancer and Fallopian Tube Cancer

JENNY VAN WINKLE, MD
Resident
The Methodist Hospital-Houston
Obstetrics and Gynecology Residency Program
Houston, Texas
28/Vulvar Dysplasia, Vulvar Cancer, and Vaginal Cancer
29/Vulvar Disorders

GERILYNN S. VINE
Class of 2010
University of Texas Medical School at Houston
Houston, Texas
3/Physiology of Pregnancy

CRISTINA M. WALLACE
Class of 2010
University of Texas Medical School at Houston
Houston, Texas
1/Normal Anatomy
2/Diagnosis of Pregnancy

STUDENT REVIEWERS

SILKE HEINISCH
Class of 2010
Temple University School of Medicine
Philadelphia, Pennsylvania

FRANK SANTORO
Class of 2009
University of Connecticut School of Medicine
Farmington, Connecticut

CONTENTS

SECTION IV: CLASSIFIED   375

INTRODUCTION

This clinical study aid was designed in the tradition of the *First Aid* series of books, formatted in the same way as the other titles in this series. Topics are listed by bold headings to the left, while the "meat" of the topic comprises the middle column. The outside margins contain mnemonics, diagrams, summary or warning statements, "pearls," and other memory aids. These are further classified as "exam tip" noted by the ⬛ symbol, "ward tip" noted by the 🩺 symbol, and "typical scenario" noted by the 🧍 symbol.

The content of this book is based on the American Professors of Gynecology and Obstetrics (APGO) and the American College of Obstetricians and Gynecologists (ACOG) recommendations for the OB/GYN curriculum for third-year medical students. Each of the chapters contain the major topics central to the practice of obstetrics and gynecology and closely parallel APGO's medical student learning objectives. This book also targets the obstetrics and gynecology content on the USMLE Step 2 examination.

The OB/GYN clerkship can be an exciting hands-on experience. You will get to deliver babies, assist in surgeries, and see patients in the clinic setting. You will find that rather than simply preparing you for the success on the clerkship exam, this book will also help guide you in the clinical diagnosis and treatment of the many interesting problems you will see during your obstetrics and gynecology rotation.

ACKNOWLEDGMENTS

We would like to thank the following faculty for their help in the preparation of the third edition of this book:

Eugene C. Toy, MD
The John S. Dunn Senior Academic Chair and Program Director
Obstetrics-Gynecology Residency
The Methodist Hospital
Houston, Texas

Patti Jayne Ross, MD
Clerkship Director
Department of Obstetrics and Gynecology
The University of Texas–Houston Medical School
Houston, Texas

HOW TO CONTRIBUTE

To continue to produce a high-yield review source for the obstetrics and gynecology clerkship, you are invited to submit any suggestions or correction. Please send us your suggestions for:

- New facts, mnemonics, diagrams, and illustrations
- Low-yield facts to remove

For each entry incorporated into the next edition, you will receive personal acknowledgment. Diagrams, tables, partial entries, updates, corrections, and study hints are also appreciated, and significant contributions will be compensated at the discretion of the authors. Also let us know about material in this edition that you feel is low yield and should be deleted. You are also welcome to send general comments and feedback, although due to the volume of e-mails, we may not be able to respond to each of these.

The preferred way to submit entries, suggestions, or corrections is via electronic mail. Please include name, address, school affiliation, phone number, and e-mail address (if different from the address of origin). If there are multiple entries, please consolidate into a single e-mail or file attachment. Please send submissions to:

firstaidclerkships@gmail.com

Otherwise, please send entries, neatly written or typed or on disk (Microsoft Word) to:

Catherine A. Johnson
Senior Editor
McGraw-Hill Medical
1221 Avenue of the Americas, 45th Floor
New York, NY 10020

All entries become property of the authors and are subject to editing and reviewing. Please verify all data and spellings carefully. In the event that similar or duplicate entries are received, only the first entry received will be used. Include a reference to a standard textbook to facilitate verification of the fact. Please follow the style, punctuation, and format of this edition if possible.

How to Succeed in the Obstetrics & Gynecology Clerkship

Be on Time

Most OB/GYN teams begin rounding between 5 and 7 AM. If you are expected to "pre-round," you should give yourself at least 10 minutes per patient that you are following to see the patient and learn about the events that occurred overnight. Like all working professionals, you will face occasional obstacles to punctuality, but make sure this is infrequent. When you first start a rotation, try to show up at least 15 minutes early until you get the routine figured out.

Dress in a Professional Manner

Even if the resident wears scrubs and the attending wears stiletto heels, you must dress in a professional, conservative manner. Wear a *short* white coat over your clothes unless discouraged (as in pediatrics). Recommended attire (professional vs. scrubs) can vary based on rotation, so it is a question that should be addressed to the team on the first day of the rotation.

> **Men** should wear long pants, with cuffs covering the ankle, dress shoes, a long-sleeved collared shirt, and a tie. No jeans, no sneakers, no short-sleeved shirts. Facial hair should be well groomed.
>
> **Women** should wear long pants or knee-length skirt, and a top with a modest neckline. No jeans, no sneakers, no heels greater than 1½ inches, no open-toed shoes.
>
> **Both men and women** may wear scrubs occasionally, during overnight call or in the operating room or birthing ward. You never know what to expect on labor and delivery, so as a general guideline, always keep a spare pair of scrubs available on your hospital-issued scrub card.

Act in a Pleasant Manner

The rotation is often difficult, stressful, and tiring. You will have a smoother experience if you are nice to be around. Be friendly and try to learn everyone's name. If you do not understand or disagree with a treatment plan or diagnosis, do not "challenge." Instead, say, "I'm sorry, I don't quite understand, could you please explain? ..."

Be aware of your demeanor and reactions. It is always good to approach each rotation with an open mind, but there will be times when you are bored or just not in the mood. Try to look interested to attendings and residents. When someone is trying to teach you something, be respectful and look grateful, not tortured.

A crucial aspect of being a good doctor is to always treat patients professionally and with respect, which is good to be aware of starting at the student level. Your relationship with patients is also used to assess your performance in all clerkships. Thus, having a good rapport with your patients is usually noted by attendings and residents, which will be reflected on positively in final evaluations. However, if a resident or attending spots you being impolite or unprofessional, it will damage your grade and evaluation quicker than any dumb answer on rounds ever could. Also, be nice to the nurses—really nice! If they like you, they can make your life a lot easier and make you look good in front of the residents and attendings.

2

Be Aware of the Hierarchy

The way in which this will affect you will vary from hospital to hospital and team to team, but it is always present to some degree. In general, address your questions regarding ward functioning to interns or residents when the attending isn't present. Address your medical questions to attendings; make an effort to be somewhat informed on your subject prior to asking. But please don't ask a question just to transparently show off what you know. It's annoying to everyone. Show off by seeming interested and asking real questions that you have when they come up.

Don't be afraid to ask questions, but be conscious of the time and number of questions asked during rounds so that everyone can finish their work and go home at a reasonable time. Remember, you are usually not the only one who doesn't know, and as a medical student, you are often able to ask questions that the residents should know, which gives the attending the opportunity to teach the students, with the secondary benefit of reviewing for the residents.

Address Patients and Staff in a Respectful Way

Address patients as Sir or Ma'am, or Mr., Mrs., or Miss. Don't address patients as "honey," "sweetie," and the like. Although you may feel that these names are friendly, patients may think you have forgotten their name, that you are being inappropriately familiar, or both. Address all physicians as "doctor," unless told otherwise. While your resident may tell you to call them by their first name, remember to maintain professionalism on rounds and when working with patients by still referring to the resident as "doctor."

Be Helpful to Your Residents

Being helpful involves taking responsibility for patients that you've been assigned to, and even for some that you haven't. If you've been assigned to a patient, know everything there is to know about her, her history, test results, details about her medical problems, and prognosis. Keep your interns or residents informed of new developments that they might not be aware of, and ask them for any updates as well.

If you have the opportunity to make a resident look good, take it. If some new complication comes up with a patient, tell the resident about it before the attending gets a chance to grill the resident on it. Don't hesitate to give credit to a resident for some great teaching in front of an attending. These things make the resident's life easier; he or she will be grateful, and the rewards will come your way.

After rounds, assess what needs to be done on your patients and take ownership of their care by finding out the necessary information or making the appropriate phone calls to follow up what was discussed on rounds. Volunteer to do things that will help out. So what if you have to run to the lab to follow up on a stat H&H? It helps everybody out, and it is appreciated. Observe and anticipate. If a resident is always hunting around for some tape to do a dressing change whenever you round on a particular patient, get some tape ahead of time.

Respect Patients' Rights

1. All patients have the right to have their personal medical information kept private. This means do not discuss the patient's information with family members without that patient's consent, and do not discuss any patient in hallways, elevators, or cafeterias.
2. All patients have the right to refuse treatment. This means they can refuse treatment by a specific individual (you, the medical student) or of a specific type (Pap smear). Patients can even refuse lifesaving treatment. The only exceptions to this rule are a patient who is deemed to not have the capacity to make decisions or understand situations—in which case a health care proxy should be sought—or a patient who is suicidal or homicidal.
3. All patients should be informed of the right to seek advance directives on admission. This is often done by the admissions staff, in a booklet. If your patient is chronically ill or has a life-threatening illness, address the subject of advance directives with the assistance of your attending.

Volunteer More

Be self-propelled. Volunteer to help with a procedure or a difficult task. Volunteer to give a talk on a topic of your choice. Ask your resident about the length and timing of the talk. When you present a learning issue to the team, give your fellow students a heads-up beforehand—they will appreciate the heads-up on what is going to be discussed as well as having the opportunity to prepare a topic. Volunteer to take additional patients. Volunteer to stay late. The more unpleasant the task, the better.

Be a Team Player

Help other medical students with their tasks; teach them information you have learned. Support your supervising intern or resident whenever possible. Never steal the spotlight, steal a procedure, or make a fellow medical student look bad. Don't complain—no matter how hard you have worked or how many hours you have been at the hospital, your residents have done more.

Be Honest

If you don't understand, don't know, or didn't do it, make sure you always say that. Never say or document information that is false (eg, don't say "bowel sounds normal" when you did not listen).

Keep Patient Information Handy

Use a clipboard, notebook, or index cards to keep patient information, including a miniature history and physical, labs, and test results at hand.

Present Patient Information in an Organized Manner

Here is a template for the "bullet" presentation:

This is a **[age]**-year-old **[ethnicity]** female with a history of **[major history such as abdominal surgery, pertinent OB/GYN history]** who presented on **[date]** with **[major symptoms, such as pelvic pain, fever]**, and was found to have **[working diagnosis]**. **[Tests done]** showed **[results]**. Yesterday the patient **[state important changes, new plan, new tests, new medications]**. This morning the patient feels **[state the patient's words]**, and the physical exam is significant for **[state major findings]**. Plan is **[state plan]**.

The newly admitted patient generally deserves a longer presentation following the complete history and physical format (see below).

Some patients have extensive histories. The whole history can and probably should be present in the admission note, but in ward presentation it is often too much to absorb. In these cases, it will be very much appreciated by your team if you can generate a good summary that maintains an accurate picture of the patient. This usually takes some thought, but it's worth it.

Document Information in an Organized Manner

A complete medical student initial history and physical is neat, legible, organized, and usually two to three pages long (see page 7).

HOW TO ORGANIZE YOUR LEARNING

The main advantage to doing the OB/GYN clerkship is that you get to see patients. The patient is the key to learning and the source of most satisfaction and frustration on the wards. One enormously helpful tip is to try to skim this book before starting your rotation. Starting OB/GYN can make you feel like you're in a foreign land, and all that studying the first 2 years doesn't help much. You have to start from scratch in some ways, and it will help enormously if you can skim through this book before you start. Get some of the terminology straight, get some of the major points down, and it won't seem so strange.

Select Your Study Material

We recommend:

- This review book, *First Aid for the® Obstetrics & Gynecology Clerkship*, 3rd edition.
- A full-text online journal database, such as *www.mdconsult.com* (subscription is $99/year for students).
- A small pocket reference book to look up lab values, clinical pathways, and the like, such as *Maxwell Quick Medical Reference* (ISBN 0964519119, $7).
- A small book to look up drugs, such as *Pocket Pharmacopoeia* (Tarascon Publishers, $8).

As You See Patients, Note Their Major Symptoms and Diagnosis for Review

Your reading on the symptom-based topics above should be done with a specific patient in mind. For example, if a postmenopausal patient comes to the office with increasing abdominal girth and is thought to have ovarian cancer, read about ovarian cancer in the review book that night.

Prepare a Talk on a Topic

You may be asked to give a small talk once or twice during your rotation. If not, you should volunteer! Feel free to choose a topic that is on your list; however, realize that this may be considered dull by the people who hear the lecture. The ideal topic is slightly uncommon but not rare. To prepare a talk on a topic, read about it in a major textbook and a review article not more than 2 years old, and then search online or in the library for recent developments or changes in treatment.

HOW TO PREPARE FOR THE CLINICAL CLERKSHIP AND USMLE STEP 2 EXAM

If you have read about your core illnesses and core symptoms, you will know a great deal about medicine. To study for the clerkship exam, we recommend:

2–3 weeks before exam: Read this entire review book, taking notes.
10 days before exam: Read the notes you took during the rotation on your core content list and the corresponding review book sections.
5 days before exam: Read this entire review book, concentrating on lists and mnemonics.
2 days before exam: Exercise, eat well, skim the book, and go to bed early.
1 day before exam: Exercise, eat well, review your notes and the mnemonics, and go to bed on time. Do not have any caffeine after 2 P.M.

Other helpful studying strategies include:

Study With Friends

Group studying can be very helpful. Other people may point out areas that you have not studied enough and may help you focus on the goal. If you tend to get distracted by other people in the room, limit this to less than half of your study time.

Study in a Bright Room

Find the room in your house or in your library that has the best, brightest light. This will help prevent you from falling asleep. If you don't have a bright light, get a halogen desk lamp or a light that simulates sunlight (not a tanning lamp).

Eat Light, Balanced Meals

Make sure your meals are balanced, with lean protein, fruits and vegetables, and fiber. A high-sugar, high-carbohydrate meal will give you an initial burst of energy for 1–2 hours, but then you'll drop.

Take Practice Exams

The point of practice exams is not so much the content that is contained in the questions but the training of sitting still for 3 hours and trying to pick the best answer for each and every question. You can also use practice questions to assess where the gaps in your studying are in order to guide your future studying.

Tips for Answering Questions

All questions are intended to have one best answer. When answering questions, follow these guidelines:

Read the answers first. For all questions longer than two sentences, reading the answers first can help you sift through the question for the key information.

Look for the words "EXCEPT," "MOST," "LEAST," "NOT," "BEST," "WORST," "TRUE," "FALSE," "CORRECT," "INCORRECT," "ALWAYS," and "NEVER." If you find one of these words, circle or underline it for later comparison with the answer.

Evaluate each answer as being either true or false. Example:

Which of the following is *least* likely to be associated with pelvic pain?
A. endometriosis **T**
B. ectopic pregnancy **T**
C. ovarian cancer **F**
D. ovarian torsion **T**

By comparing the question, noting LEAST, to the answers, "C" is the best answer.

TERMINOLOGY

G (gravidity) 3 = total number of pregnancies, including normal and abnormal intrauterine pregnancies, abortions, ectopic pregnancies, and hydatidiform moles. (*Remember, if patient was pregnant with twins,* **G** = 1.)

P (parity) 3 = number of deliveries > 500 g or > 20 weeks gestation, stillborn (dead) or alive. (*Remember, if patient was pregnant with twins,* **P** = 1.)

Ab (abortus) 0 = number of pregnancies that were lost before the 20th gestational week or in which the fetus weighs < 500 g.

LC (living children) 3 = number of successful pregnancy outcomes. (*Remember, if patient was pregnant with twins,* **LC** = 2.)

Or use the "TPAL" system if it is used at your medical school:

T = number of **Term** deliveries (3)
P = number of **Preterm** deliveries (0)
A = number of **Abortions** (0)
L = number of **Living children** (3)

MS3 H&P
Date
Time
Estimated gestational age (EGA): $38^5/_7$ weeks
Last menstrual period (LMP): First day of LMP
Estimated date of confinement: Due date (*specify how it was determined*) by LMP or by ____ wk US
Chief complaint (CC): Uterine contractions (UCs) q 7 min since 0100
History of present illness (HPI): 25 yo Hispanic female, G3P2002, $38^5/_7$ weeks GA, dated by LMP (10/13/09) and consistent with US at 10 weeks GA, who presented to L&D with CC of uterine contractions q 7 min. She reports that fetal movement is present, denies leakage of fluid, vaginal bleeding, headaches, visual changes, or right upper quadrant pain. Prenatal care (PNC) at Montefiore Hospital (12 visits, first visit at 7 wks GA), uterine size = to dates, prenatal BP range 100–126/64–83. Problem list includes h/o + group B *Streptococcus* (GBS) and a +PPD with subsequent negative chest x-ray in 5/06. Pt admitted in early active labor with a vaginal exam (VE) 4/90/–2.

Past Obstetric History
1) '02 NSVD @ term, girl, wt 3700 g, St. Joseph's Hospital
No complications during pregnancy, delivery, and puerperium
No developmental problems in childhood
2) '04 NSVD @ term, boy, wt 3900 g, St. Joseph's Hospital
Postpartum hemorrhage, atonic uterus, syntometrine given and hemorrhage resolved
No developmental problems in childhood

Past Gynecological History
13 yo/28 days/regular (age at first menstrual cycle/how often/regular or irregular)
No significant history of PID, intermenstrual bleeding, dyspareunia, postcoital bleed
Last pap smear: 3/4/09—normal, no h/o abnormal Pap smear
Last mammogram:
Contraception: None
Blood group: O–, anti D prophylaxis given at 30 weeks GA
Allergies: NKDA
Medications: PNV, Fe
Past Medical Hx: H/o asthma (asymptomatic × 7 yrs), UTI × 1 @ 30 wks s/p Macrobid 100 mg × 7 d, neg PPD with subsequent neg CXR (5/06)
Surgical Hx: Negative
Social Hx: Denies h/o alcohol, smoking, drug abuse. Feels safe at home
Family Hx: Mother—DM II, father—HTN
ROS: Bilateral low back pain. Denies chest pain, shortness of breath, nausea, vomiting, fever, chills

PE
General appearance: Alert and oriented (A&O), no acute distress (NAD)
Vital signs: T, BP, P, R
HEENT: No scleral icterus, pale conjunctiva
Neck: Thyroid midline, no masses, no lymphadenopathy (LAD)

A good way to elicit information about complications in previous pregnancies is to ask if the baby went home from the hospital with mom.

Lungs: CTA bilaterally
Back: No CVA tenderness
Heart: II/VI SEM
Breasts: No masses, symmetric
Abdomen: Gravid, nontender
Fundal height: 36 cm
Estimated fetal weight (EFW): 3500 g by Leopold's
Presentation: Vertex
Extremities: Mild lower extremity edema, nonpitting, 2+ DTRs
Pelvis: Adequate
Sterile speculum exam (SSE)? (Nitrazine?, Ferning?, Pooling?); membranes intact
Sterile Vaginal Exam (SVE): 4 cm/90%/–2 (dilatation/effacement/station)
US (L&D): Vertex presentation confirmed, anterior placenta, AFI = 13.2
Fetal monitor: Baseline FHR = 150, accelerations present, no decelerations, moderate variability. Toco = UCs q 5 min

Assessment

25 yo G3P2002 @ $38^5/_7$ weeks GA presented with regular painful contractions.

1. Early active labor.
2. Group B strep +
3. H/o + PPD with subsequent – CXR 5/06
4. H/o UTI @ 30 wks GA, s/p Rx—resolved
5. H/o asthma—stable × 7 yrs, no meds

Plan

1. Admit to L&D
2. NPO except ice chips
3. H&H, RPR, HIV, HBsAg and hold clot tube
4. D5 LR @ 125 cc/hr
5. Penicillin 5 million units IV load, then 2.5 million units IV q 4 hr *(for GBS)*
6. External fetal monitors (EFMs)
7. Epidural when patient desires

SAMPLE DELIVERY NOTE

Always date, time, and sign your notes.

25 yo G3 now P3003 s/p spontaneous vaginal delivery (SVD) of viable male infant over a second-degree perineal laceration @ 12:35 P.M. Infant was bulb suctioned on the perineum. Nuchal cord × 1 was reduced. The infant was delivered with gentle downward traction. The cord was doubly clamped and cut; the infant was handed to the awaiting nurse. Cord blood and arterial pH was obtained. The placenta was delivered spontaneously, intact, with 3-vessel cord. No vaginal or cervical lacerations were noted. The second-degree laceration was repaired with 3-0 vicryl in layers using local anesthesia. Rectal exam was with in normal limits. EBL = 450 cc. Apgars 8 & 9, wt 3654 g. Mom and baby stable.

SAMPLE POSTPARTUM NOTE

S: Pt ambulating, voiding, tolerating a regular diet. Denies preeclampsia symptoms

O: T_{max}: 99.1 $T_{current}$: 98.6 BP:128/70 (117–130/58–76) HR: 86 (76–100) RR: 18

Heart: RRR, no murmurs/rubs/gallops

Lungs: CTA bilaterally

Breasts: Nonengorged, colostrum expressed bilaterally

Fundus: Firm, mildly tender to palpation, 1 fingerbreadth below umbilicus

Lochia: Moderate amount, rubra

Perineum: Intact, no edema

Extremities: No edema, nontender

Postpartum Hgb: 9.7

VDRL: NR, HIV neg, HBsAG neg

A: S/p SVD, PP day # 1—progressing well, afebrile, stable

P: Continue postpartum care

SAMPLE POST-NSVD DISCHARGE ORDERS

1. D/c pt home
2. Pelvic rest × 6 weeks
3. Postpartum check in 4–6 weeks
4. D/c meds:
   a. $FeSO_4$ 325 mg, 1 tab PO TID, #90 (For Hgb < 10; opinions vary on when to give Iron supplementation postpartum)
   b. Colace 100 mg, 1 tab PO BID PRN no bowel movement, #60 (A side effect of Iron supplementation is constipation)
   c. Ibuprofen 600 mg, 1 tab PO q 4 hours, PRN pain, #60

SAMPLE POST-CESAREAN SECTION NOTE

S: Pt c/o abdominal pain, passing flatus, minimal ambulation. Denies preeclampsia symptoms. Foley in place.

O: T_{max}: 99.1 $T_{current}$: 98.6 BP: 128/70 (117–130/58–76) HR: 86 (76–100) RR: 18

I&O (urinary intake and output): Last 8 hr = 750/695

Heart: RRR without murmurs

Lungs: CTA bilaterally

Breasts: Nonengorged, no colostrum expressed

Fundus: Firm, tender to palpation, 1 fingerbreadth above umbilicus; normal abdominal bowel sounds (NABS)

Incision: Without erythema/edema; C/D/I (clean/dry/intact)

Lochia: Scant, rubra

Extremities: 1 + pitting edema bilateral LEs, nontender
Postpartum Hgb: 11
VDRL: NR, HIV neg, HBsAG neg

A: S/p primary low-transverse c/s for arrest of descent, POD # 1– afebrile, + flatus, stable

P: 1. D/c Foley
2. Strict I&O—Call HO if UO < 120 cc/4 hr
3. Clear liquid diet
4. Heplock IV once patient tolerates clears
5. Ambulate qid
6. Incentive spirometry 10 × hr
7. Tylenol #3, 2 tabs PO q 4 hr PRN pain

Reporting about flatus and bowel movements is important after a C-section. These are less relevant after an NSVD.

SAMPLE DISCHARGE ORDERS POST–CESAREAN SECTION

1. D/c patient home
2. Pelvic rest × 4 weeks
3. Incision check in 1 week
4. Discharge meds:
   a. Tylenol #3, 2 tabs PO q 4 hr PRN pain, #30
   b. Ibuprofen 600 mg, 1 tab PO q 4 hr, PRN pain, #60
   c. Colace 100 mg, 1 tab PO bid, #60

High-Yield Facts in Obstetrics

Reproductive Anatomy

An adequate knowledge of the normal female anatomy is essential in obstetrics and gynecology. Each time a physician delivers a baby or performs a gynecologic surgery, he or she must be well versed in anatomy of the region. This chapter will discuss the major structures of the pelvis. The major blood supply to the pelvis is from the **internal iliac artery (hypogastric artery)** and its branches. The lymphatics drain to the inguinal, pelvic, or para-aortic lymph nodes. The major parasympathetic innervation is via **S2, S3, S4,** which forms the pudendal nerve. The major sympathetic innervation is via the aortic plexus, which gives rise to the **internal iliac plexus.**

A 30-year-old female presents to the emergency room with a lump in the vulva and acute onset of pain for 2 days. The pain has gradually ↑ and she is unable to sit. She reports no fever, chills, nausea, or vomiting. She has no medical conditions and takes no medications. On exam, the right labia majora is noted to be swollen. A 4 × 4-cm fluctuant tender mass is palpated at the 8 o'clock position; no drainage is noted. What is the most likely diagnosis? What is the best treatment?

Answer: Bartholin's gland abscess. The best treatment is incision and drainage followed by marsupialization, packing, or placement of Word catheter. Can consider broad-spectrum antibiotics. If an older patient with recurrent Bartholin's abscess or cysts, consider adenocarcinoma and take a biopsy.

The vulva consists of all structures visible externally from the pubis to perineum. It includes: The labia majora, labia minora, mons pubis, clitoris, vestibule of the vagina, vestibular bulb, and the greater vestibular glands (see Figure 1-1). The vestibule itself contains the urethal opening, vaginal opening, bilateral Bartholin gland ducts, and bilateral Skene's (paraurethral) glands.

- **Clitoris:** Homologue of the male penis. Composed of a glans, a corpora, and two crura. Rarely exceeds 2 cm in length, and normal diameter is 1.5 cm.
- **Bartholin glands:** Located at 4 o'clock and 8 o'clock of the vaginal orifice and are typically nonpalpable. They function in secreting mucous to provide vaginal lubrication and are homologous to the bulbourethral glands in males.
- **Skene's glands:** Ducts of these glands open on either side of the urethral orifice.

Blood Supply

From branches of the external and internal pudendal arteries, which are subdivisions of the hypogastric artery (internal iliac).

Lymph

Medial group of superficial inguinal nodes.

Bartholin gland blockage
Causes a cyst or abscess.
Most often:
Cysts: Asymptomatic.
Abscesses: Painful.

Posterior Branch
Iliolumbar
Lateral sacral
Superior Gluteal

Anterior Branch
Inferior Gluteal
Middle rectal
Obturator
Inf. vesical art
Internal pudendal
Umbilical
w/o Uterine/Deferential art.

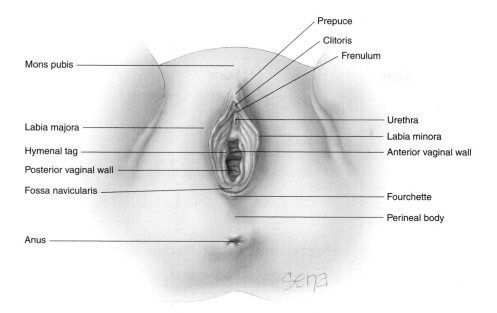

Mons pubis

Labia majora

Hymenal tag

Posterior vaginal wall

Fossa navicularis

Anus

Prepuce

Clitoris

Frenulum

Urethra

Labia minora

Anterior vaginal wall

Fourchette

Perineal body

FIGURE 1-1. External female genitalia.

(Reproduced, with permission, from Cunningham FG, Leveno KJ, Bloom SL, et al. *Williams Obstetrics*, 23rd ed. New York: McGraw-Hill, 2010: Fig. 2-2.)

Nerve Supply

Pudendal branches:

- **Anterior parts of vulva:** Ilioinguinal nerves and the genital branch of the genitofemoral nerves.
- **Posterior parts:** Perineal nerves and posterior cutaneous nerves of the thigh.

A pudendal block can provide pain relief at the time of a vaginal delivery.

VAGINA

The vagina is a tubular, muscular structure that extends from the vulva to the cervix. Exteriorly, the vaginal orifice is located anterior to the perineum and posterior the urethra.

Blood Supply

- **Hypogastric artery (anastomotic network):**
- **Vaginal branch of the uterine artery** is the primary supply to the vagina.
- **Middle rectal and inferior vaginal branches of the hypogastric artery** (internal iliac artery) are secondary blood supplies.
- Anastomoses with cervical arteries.

Nerve Supply

- **Hypogastric plexus:** Sympathetic innervation.
- **Pelvic nerve:** Parasympathetic innervation.

The cervix is actually a part of the uterus. It is the specialized narrow inferior portion of the uterus that is at the apex of the vagina.

Components

The cervix can be further subdivided into:

- **Portio vaginalis:** Portion of the cervix projecting into the vagina.
- **External os:** Lowermost opening of the cervix into the vagina.
- **Ectocervix:** Portion of the cervix exterior to the external os.
- **Endocervical canal:** Passageway between the external os and the uterine cavity.
- **Internal os:** Uppermost opening of the cervix into the uterine cavity.

Cervical Epithelium

A 36-year-old G3P3 woman presents to the office for a follow-up visit. Her most recent Pap smear was abnormal, showing a low-grade squamous intraepithelial lesion (LSIL). The colposcopic biopsy shows cervical intraepithelial neoplasia II. She undergoes a loop electroexcision procedure. What portion of the cervix must be completely excised to ensure proper treatment?

Answer: The transformation zone should be completely excised because that is where the majority of cervical cancers arise.

Both **columnar** and **stratified nonkeratinized squamous** epithelia cover the cervix.

- The stratified nonkeratinized squamous epithelium covers the ectocervix.
- The columnar epithelium lines the endocervical canal.
- The **squamocolumnar junction** is where the two types of epithelium meet.
- The **transformation zone** is the area of metaplasia where columnar epithelium changes to squamous epithelium. It is the most important cytologic and colposcopic landmark, as this is where over 90% of lower genital tract neoplasias arise.

Blood Supply

Cervical and vaginal branch of the uterine artery, which arises from the internal iliac artery.

Nerve Supply

Hypogastric plexus.

Colposcopy: Magnified view of the cervix, vagina, and vulva.

The uterus is a muscular organ that lies posterior to the bladder and anterior to the rectum in the pelvis of a nonpregnant woman. In pregnancy, the uterus enlarges with the growth of the fetus and progressively becomes an abdominal as well as a pelvic organ.

Total hysterectomy = Uterus and cervix are removed.
Supracervical hysterectomy = Uterus removed, cervix retained (ovarian status unknown).

Components

- **Fundus:** Uppermost region of uterus.
- **Corpus:** Body of the uterus.
- **Cornu:** Part of uterus that connects to the fallopian tubes bilaterally.
- **Cervix:** Inferior part of the uterus that protrudes into the vagina.

Histology

- **Myometrium:** The smooth muscle layer of uterus. It is subdivided into three layers:
  1. Outer longitudinal
  2. Middle oblique
  3. Inner longitudinal
- **Endometrium:** The mucosal layer of the uterus, made up of columnar epithelium.

The ureter travels <u>under</u> the uterine artery. Think "water under the bridge."

Blood Supply

- **Uterine arteries:** Arise from hypogastric artery (internal iliac artery).
- **Ovarian arteries:** Arise from the aorta, and anastamose with uterine vasculature.

Nerve Supply

- **Superior hypogastric plexus**
- **Inferior hypogastric plexus**
- **Common iliac nerves**

The fallopian tubes extend from the superior lateral aspects of the uterus through the superior fold of the broad ligament laterally to the ovaries.

The tubes are occluded at the isthmus for permanent sterilization via laparoscopy.

Anatomic Sections, from Lateral to Medial

- **Infundibulum:** The most distal part the uterine tube. Helps to sweep the egg that is released from the ovary into the tube.
- **Ampulla:** Widest section.
- **Isthmus:** Narrowest part.
- **Intramural part:** Pierces uterine wall and connects to the endometrial cavity.

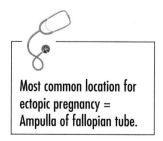

Most common location for ectopic pregnancy = Ampulla of fallopian tube.

HIGH-YIELD FACTS

Reproductive Anatomy

No peritoneum around ovaries leads to fast dissemination of ovarian cancer in the abdomen.

Blood Supply of Ovaries

Aorta → Bilateral ovarian arteries

Left ovarian vein → left renal vein

Right ovarian vein → inferior vena cava

Blood Supply

From uterine and ovarian arteries.

Nerve Supply

Pelvic plexus (autonomic) and ovarian plexus.

OVARIES

The ovaries lie on the posterior aspect of the broad ligament and fallopian tubes. They are attached to the broad ligament by the mesovarium and are not covered by peritoneum. Each ovary functions in ova development and hormone production.

Blood Supply

Both ovarian arteries arise from the aorta at the level of L1. Veins drain into the inferior vena cava on the right side and the renal vein on the left.

Nerve Supply

Derived from the aortic plexus.

Histology

The ovaries are covered by tunica albuginea, a fibrous capsule. The tunica albuginea is covered by germinal epithelium.

LIGAMENTS OF THE PELVIC VISCERA

A 22-year-old G2P1001 at 32 weeks' gestation complains of sharp lower abdominal pain. Pain worsens upon walking and ↓ with rest. Patient denies loss of fluid, vaginal bleeding, fever, trauma, sick contacts, and travel. Her last coitus was 3 weeks ago. Fetal movement is present. Non-stress test (NST) is reassuring and no contractions are recorded. Her cervix is closed on vaginal exam. Urinalysis (UA) is negative. What is this patient's diagnosis?

Answer: Round ligament pain. Round ligament pain is a diagnosis of exclusion. The key is worsening pain with movement and improvement with rest. It can be treated with acetaminophen and rest.

Some ligaments of the pelvis act only as support structures, but others also carry the blood supply for essential organs.

- **Broad ligament:** Peritoneal fold extends from the lateral pelvic wall to the uterus and adnexa. Contains the fallopian (uterine) tube, round ligament, uterine and ovarian blood vessels, lymph, ureterovaginal nerves, and ureter (see Figure 1-2).

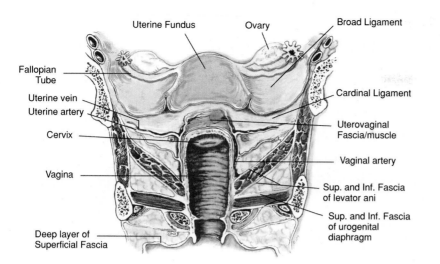

Uterine Fundus — Ovary — Broad Ligament
Fallopian Tube
Uterine vein
Uterine artery
Cervix
Vagina
Deep layer of Superficial Fascia
Cardinal Ligament
Uterovaginal Fascia/muscle
Vaginal artery
Sup. and Inf. Fascia of levator ani
Sup. and Inf. Fascia of urogenital diaphragm

FIGURE 1-2. Supporting structures of the pelvic viscera.

(Reproduced, with permission, from Lindarkis NM, Lott S. *Digging Up the Bones: Obstetrics and Gynecology.* New York: McGraw-Hill, 1998: 2.)

- **Infundibulopelvic (IP) ligament (aka suspensory ligament of the ovary):** Contains the ovarian artery and vein and connects the ovary to the pelvic wall.
- **Round ligament:** The remains of the gubernaculum; extends from the corpus of the uterus down and laterally through the inguinal canal and terminates in the labia majora.
- **Cardinal ligament (Mackenrodt ligament):** Extends from the cervix (near the level of the internal cervical os) and lateral vagina to the pelvic side wall; most **important support** structure of the uterus. It contains the uterine artery and vein.
- **Uterosacral ligaments:** Each ligament extends from an attachment posterolaterally to the supravaginal portion of the cervix and inserts into the fascia over the sacrum. Provides some support to the uterus.

Most hysterectomies start by ligation and transection of the round ligament.

Most common site for ureteral injury during hysterectomy = level of cardinal ligament (ureter passes under the uterine artery).

MUSCLES

Various muscles of the pelvis make up the perineum. Most of the support is provided by the pelvic and urogenital diaphragms.

- **Pelvic diaphragm** forms a broad sling in the pelvis to support the internal organs. It is composed of the levator ani complex (iliococcygeus, puborectalis, pubococcygeus muscles) and the coccygeus muscles.
- **Urogenital diaphragm** is external to the pelvic diaphragm and is composed of the deep transverse perineal muscles, the constrictor of the urethra, and the internal and external fascial coverings. It helps maintain urinary continence.
- **Perineal body** is the central tendon of the perineum, which provides much of the support. The median raphe of the levator ani, between the anus and vagina. Bulbocavernosus, superficial transverse perineal, and external anal sphincter muscles converge at the central tendon.

Pelvic organ prolapse is caused by a defect in the plevic diaphragm.

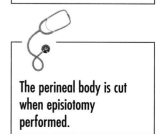

The perineal body is cut when episiotomy performed.

Blood Supply

Internal pudendal artery and its branches, inferior rectal artery, and posterior labial artery.

Nerve Supply

Pudendal nerve, which originates from S2, S3, S4 levels of the spinal cord.

PELVIS

The adult pelvis is composed of four bones: The sacrum, the coccyx, and two innominate bones. The innominate bones are formed from the fusion of the ilium, ischium and pubis (see Figure 1-3).

- **Sacrum:** Consists of five vertebrae fused together to form a single wedge-shaped bone. It articulates laterally with two iliac bones to form the sacroiliac joints. The **sacral promontory** is the first sacral vertebrae, and it can be palpated during a vaginal exam. It is important landmark for clinical pelvimetry.
- **Coccyx:** Composed of four vertebrae fused together to form a small triangular bone that articulates with the base of the sacrum.
- **Ischial spines:** Extend from the middle of the posterior margin of each ischium.

> Pelvimetry assesses the shape and capacity of the pelvis in relation to the ability of a baby to pass through it.

> The ischial spines serve as landmarks in determining the station of the fetus. Leading edge of the fetus head at the ischial spine = 0 station.

Pelvic Shapes

There are four major shapes: **gynecoid, android, platypelloid,** and **anthropoid.** These shapes are differentiated based on the measurements of the pelvis. Gynecoid is the ideal shape for vaginal delivery, having a round to slightly oval pelvic inlet. (See Intrapartum chapter, Table 5-6).

FIGURE 1-3. Bony pelvis.

Diagnosis of Pregnancy

As a physician, it is essential to make the accurate diagnosis of pregnancy and establish the estimated date of delivery. The patient's future prenatal care is dependent on it. This chapter will discuss how to diagnose pregnancy, including symptoms of pregnancy, use of human chorionic gonadotropin (hCG), fetal heart rate (FHR), and ultrasound in its diagnosis.

Naegele's rule assumes two things:
1. A normal gestation is 280 days.
2. All patients have a 28-day menstrual cycle.

When determining the estimated date of delivery (EDD), use the first day of bleeding of the last menstrual period (LMP).

Use Naegele's rule to calculate the estimated due date from the LMP.

EDD = (LMP +1 year + 7 days) – 3 months

Nonpregnant cervix feels like the cartilage of the nose. A pregnant cervix feels like the lips of the mouth. Hegar's sign = softening of the cervix.

NAEGELE'S RULE

A 25-year-old G0P0 presents with complaints of absent menses for 2 months. Prior to this, she reports regular menses every 28 days, lasting for 4 days each month since menarche. She is sexually active but reports using condoms regularly. What is the best test to evaluate her condition?

Answer: Urine pregnancy test (UPT). Pregnancy must be considered in any woman of reproductive age with complaints of amenorrhea or irregular menses and abdominal pain even if she is using contraception. Including or excluding pregnancy will significantly narrow the list of differential diagnoses.

Naegele's rule is used to calculate the estimated date of confinement (EDC; ie, due date) +/– 2 weeks.

- First day of patient's last normal menstrual period (LMP), minus 3 months, plus 7 days, plus 1 year.
- Example: If LMP = July 20, 2006, then EDC = April 27, 2007.

SIGNS AND SYMPTOMS

A woman's body goes through drastic physiological changes from the day she conceives to weeks after the delivery of her baby. It is important to differentiate the physiological changes of pregnancy from other pathological conditions. This section will discuss signs and symptoms that are indicative of pregnancy.

- **Cessation of menses:** Pregnancy is highly likely if 10 or more days have passed from the time of expected menses in a woman who previously had regular cycles.
- **Breast changes:**
  - ↑ breast tenderness.
  - ↑ in breast size.
  - Nipples become larger, more pigmented, and more erectile.
  - Areolae become broader and more pigmented.
  - Colostrum may be expressed from the nipples.
  - Striations on the skin.
- **Skin changes:**
  - Striae gravidarum (aka stretch marks): Reddish, slightly depressed streaks on the abdomen, breast, and thighs.
  - Linea nigra: Midline of the abdominal wall becomes darkly pigmented.
  - Chloasma or melasma gravidarum (aka mask of pregnancy): Irregular brown patches of varying size on the face and neck.
  - Angiomas: Red elevation at a central point with branching vasculature present on the face, neck, chest, and arms due to estrogens.
  - Palmar erythema.

- **Uterine changes:**
  - On bimanual exam, the uterus feels soft and elastic.
  - The uterus ↑ in size throughout the pregnancy (its size correlates to gestational age). By week 12, it is about the size of a grapefruit and the fundus of the uterus becomes palpable above the pubic symphysis (see Table 2-1).
- **Cervical changes:** Cervix becomes softer.
- **Changes in cervical mucus:** Cervical mucus can be dried on a slide and evaluated via microscope.
  - **Fernlike pattern:** Not pregnant—estrogen effect.
  - **Beaded or cellular pattern:** Pregnant—progesterone effect.
- **Vaginal mucosa discoloration:** With pregnancy and ↑ blood flow, the vagina appears dark bluish or purplish-red.
- **Perception of fetal movement:** A primigravida may report fetal movement at approximately 20 weeks gestation, and a multiparous at 18 weeks gestation.
- **Nausea and/or vomiting** (aka morning sickness): Nausea and/or vomiting occurs in approximately 70–85% of pregnancies, most notably at 2–12 weeks gestation. It frequently occurs in the morning, but it can occur through out the day. **Hyperemesis gravidarum** is persistent vomiting that typically occurs early in pregnancy. When severe, it can result in weight loss, dehydration, acidosis (from starvation), alkalosis (from loss of HCl in vomitus), and hypokalemia.
- **Hair growth changes:** Prolonged anagen (the growing hair phase).
- **Fetal heart rate (FHR) detection** (discussed later in this chapter).
- **Urologic changes:** ↑ pressure from the enlarging uterus result in ↑ urinary frequency, nocturia, and bladder irritability.

Estrogen → increased sodium chloride in mucus → crystallization → ferning pattern. Progesterone → decreased sodium chloride in mucus → no crystallization → beading.

Chadwick's sign: Bluish discoloration of the vaginal and cervical mucosa due to vascular congestion in pregnancy.

Quickening: First fetal movements felt by the mother.

TABLE 2-1. Fundal Height During Pregnancy

Weeks Pregnant	Fundal Height
12	Barely palpable above pubic symphysis
15	Midpoint between pubic symphysis and umbilicus
20	At the umbilicus
28	6 cm above the umbilicus
32	6 cm below the xyphoid process
36	2 cm below xyphoid process
40	4 cm below xiphoid process[a]

[a]Due to engagement and descent of the fetal head, the fundal height at 40 weeks is typically less than the fundal height at 36 weeks.

hCG is a glycoprotein hormone composed of α and β subunits.

The hCG α subunit is identical to that in <u>LH</u>, <u>FSH</u>, and <u>TSH</u>.

hCG → supports corpus luteum → produces progesterone → supports early pregnancy

Plasma hCG levels should double every 2 days prior to 10 weeks.

If β-hCG does not rise as expected, consider accidents of pregnancy: spontaneous abortion, missed abortion, ectopic pregnancy.

Do not assay for hCG before a woman has missed a menstrual period because of low test sensitivity before this time.

Serial hCGs are used to follow and make prognosis of first-trimester bleeding.

HUMAN CHORIONIC GONADOTROPIN (hCG)

A 25-year-old female presents with vaginal spotting and right lower quadrant pain. She denies passage of tissue. Her abdomen is tender to mild palpation in the right lower quadrant. There is minimal dark blood in the vaginal vault, and her cervix is closed and thick. Quantitative serum hCG is 4000 mIU/mL. A transvaginal ultrasound (TVUS) shows no evidence of pregnancy inside the uterus. What is the most likely diagnosis?

Answer: Ectopic pregnancy. A gestational sac should be seen inside the uterus on a transvaginal ultrasound with an hCG level of 1500 mIU/mL. If the pregnancy is not in the uterus, then an investigation must be carried out for an ectopic pregnancy.

Detection of hCG in the mother's serum and urine is used to diagnose pregnancy. This section discusses the various aspects of the hormone, as well as how it is used in the diagnosis of abnormal pregnancies.

Overview

- hCG can be detected in maternal serum and urine.
- It is a glycoprotein made by trophoblasts.
- Composed of two subunits—α and β:
    - α subunit is similar in luteinizing hormone (LH), follicle-stimulating hormone (FSH), thyroid-stimulating hormone (TSH).
    - β subunits are unique: Urine and serum tests are based on antibody specificity to β subunit of hCG.
- **Function:** Helps sustain the corpus luteum during the **first 7 weeks.** After the first 7 weeks, the placenta makes its own hormones to sustain the pregnancy.
- Can be detected in the maternal serum or urine 6–12 days after fertilization (3–3.5 weeks after the LMP).
- ↑ by 66–100% every 48 hours prior to 10 weeks. In general, hCG should double every two days.
- Peaks at 10 weeks gestation.
- Nadirs at 14–16 weeks.
- Keep in mind that pregnancy tests not only detect hCG produced by the syncytiotrophoblast cells in the placenta, **but also in:**
    - Hydatidiform mole.
    - Choriocarcinoma.
    - Germ cell tumors.
    - hCG produced by breast cancers and large cell carcinoma of the lung.
- A gestational sac can be visualized with transvaginal ultrasound (TVUS) when hCG levels are >1500. If hCG is >1500 and no evidence of intrauterine pregnancy, think "ectopic pregnancy."

Pregnancy Test Using hCG

hCG can be detected in plasma and urine. Each test has specific uses, which are discussed below.

Urine hCG

- Preferred method to diagnose normal pregnancy.
- Total urine hCG closely parallels plasma concentration.
- First morning specimens are more accurate. hCG concentration is higher in the morning.
- Assays detect 25 mU/mL of hCG, and diagnose pregnancy with 95% sensitivity by 1 week after the first missed menstrual period.
- **False negatives** may occur if:
  - The test is performed too early (ie, before the first missed period).
  - The urine is very dilute.
- **False positives** may occur with:
  - Proteinuria (confirm with plasma hCG).
  - Urinary tract infection (UTI).

Plasma hCG

Used when quantitative information is needed:

- To aid in the diagnosis of ectopic pregnancy.
- Monitoring trophoblastic tumors.
- Screening for fetal abnormalities.
- Serial levels to monitor accidents of pregnancy.
- Do not provide cost-effective additional information in diagnosing routine pregnancy since they are positive < 1 week before urine hCG.

Normal fetal heart rate ranges from 110 to 160 bpm.

FETAL HEART RATE (FHR)

Hearing the fetal heartbeat confirms the presence of a viable pregnancy. **Electronic Doppler device** can detect fetal heart tones as early as 10 weeks gestation.

If fetal heart tones are not auscultated by 10 weeks gestation, an US evaluation should be performed to document a viable intrauterine pregnancy.

Up to 12 weeks, the crown-rump length is predictive of gestational age within 4 days.

ULTRASOUND (US)

US is a noninvasive tool that serves multiple purposes in the setting of a pregnancy:

Indications

- Confirm an intrauterine pregnancy (especially important if an ectopic is suspected).
- Document the viability of embryo. Fetal cardiac motion can be seen when the embryo measures ≥ 5 mm.
- Diagnose multiple gestations.
- Estimate gestational age.
- To screen for fetal structural anomalies.

Early pregnancy US is more precise in establishing the EDD:
US done in T1 can vary by ± 4 days.
US done in T2 can vary by ± 14 days.
US done in T3 can vary by ± 21 days.

Limitations

- Ultrasound dating becomes progressively less accurate after 20 weeks' gestation. It can be used later, keeping in mind its limitations.
- US measures the size of the fetus, not the gestational age.
- Biologic variation in size ↑ as gestation advances.

US dating is used when menstrual data is unreliable or conflicts with clinical findings.

CHAPTER 3

Physiology of Pregnancy

Pregnancy induces changes in the female body from the onset of conception. The body prepares not only for the development and growth of a fetus, but also for delivery. As a result of these alterations, the mother is at risk for developing complications, which can be serious in pregnancy.

Ovulation

Ovulation is necessary for normal fertilization to occur:

- The ovum must leave the ovary and be carried into the fallopian tube.
- The unfertilized ovum is surrounded by its zona pellucida.
- This oocyte has completed its first meiotic division and carries its first polar body.

Fertilization

Fertilization typically occurs within 24 hr after ovulation in the ampulla of the fallopian tube:

- The sperm penetrates the zona pellucida of the ovum. The male and female nuclear material combine to form a single cell called a zygote.
- Fertilization signals the ovum to complete meiosis II and to discharge an additional polar body.

Fertilization occurs in the ampulla of the fallopian tube.

Preimplantation

- The zygote starts to undergo cleavage (divide). At the 16 cells stage, it is called a **morula**.
- The morula divides to form a multicellular **blastomere**.
- The blastomere passes from the fallopian tube into the uterine cavity.
- The embryo develops into a **blastocyst** as it freely floats in endometrial cavity after conception (see Table 3-1).
- Each cell of the preimplantation embryo is **totipotent**; each cell can form all different types of cells in the embryo.

Human chorionic gonadotropin (hCG) is detectable in maternal serum after implantation has taken place, approximately 8–11 days after conception.

Implantation

- On day 5–6 after ovulation, the blastocyst adheres to the endometrium with the help of adhesion molecules on the secretory endometrial surface.
- After attachment, the endometrium proliferates around the blastocyst.

Placentation

- During week 2, cells in the outer cell mass differentiate into **trophoblasts.**
- A trophoblastic shell forms the initial boundary between the embryo and the endometrium.
- The trophoblasts nearest the myometrium form the placental disk; the other trophoblasts form the chorionic membranes.

The decidua produces steroids and proteins that are related to the maintenance and protection of the pregnancy from immunologic rejection.

TABLE 3-1. Embryology

Week	Preembryonic Period
1	Fertilization and start of implantation.
2	Formation of yolk sac and embryonic disk.
3	First missed menstrual period; formation of primitive streak and neural groove.
Embryonic Period	
4	Primitive heartbeat; crown-rump length (CRL) approximately 4.0 mm.
5	Hand and foot plates develop.
6	Hand plates develop digital rays; upper lip, nose, and external ear formed.
7	Umbilical herniation (intestines begin growth outside abdominal cavity).
8	Human appearance; tail has disappeared; CRL approximately 30 mm.
Previable Fetal Period	
9	Eyes closing or closed.
10	Intestines in abdomen; thyroid, pancreas, and gallbladder development.
11	Fetal kidneys begin excreting urine into amniotic fluid; fetal liver begins to function; baby teeth formed in sockets.
12	Sex distinguishable externally; fetal breathing movements begin; colonic rotation; fetus active; first-trimester ends.
14	Head and neck take an erect, straight-line alignment.
16	↑ fetal activity; ultrasound can determine sex; myelination of nerves and ossification of bones begin.
18	Egg cells, ovaries, and uterus develop in females.
20	Head and body (lanugo) visible; testes begin descent in males.
22	Fetus can hear, will reflexively move in response to loud noise.
Viable Fetal Period	
24	Fetal lungs develop alveoli and secrete surfactant, fetus generally capable of breathing air by week 27.
28	Third trimester begins; eyelids unfuse; muscle tone ↑.
30	Cerebral gyri and sulci, which began to form in week 26, are now prominent and begin accelerated formation.

TABLE 3-1. Embryology *(continued)*

WEEK	PREEMBRYONIC PERIOD
32	Fetal immune system functioning and capable of responding to mild infections.
34	Vernix thickens.
36	Fetus capable of sucking; meconium present in fetal intestines.
40	Due date.

Postimplantation

- The endometrium or lining of the uterus during pregnancy is termed *decidua*.
- Maternal RBCs may be seen in the trophoblastic lacunae in the second week postconception.

The Placenta

The placenta continues to adapt over T2 and T3. It is the primary producer of steroid hormones after 7 weeks gestation. The human placenta is **hemochorionic**; transfer of materials between mother and fetus is via maternal blood coming in contact with placental villi. There is no direct mixing of maternal and fetal blood.

First trimester (T1): 1–13 weeks
Second trimester (T2): 14–27 weeks
Third trimester (T3): 28 weeks–term
Term: 37–42 weeks

Most common cause for abnormal maternal serum screen for aneuploidy is incorrect gestational age.

REPRODUCTIVE TRACT

Uterus

- The uterus is a thin-walled, muscular structure that is capable of expanding to hold the fetus, placenta, and amniotic fluid.
- Enlargement of uterus is due to hypertrophy and hyperplasia of the myometrial smooth muscle.
- Early in pregnancy, this process is primarily stimulated with *estrogen*. As pregnancy progresses, ↑ in uterine size is due to mechanical distention.
- Throughout the pregnancy, these muscle cells will spontaneously contract.
  - These contractions, also known as Braxton Hicks contractions, are spontaneous and irregular with an intensity ranging from 5–25 mmHg.
  - They may ↑ in frequency during the last month of pregnancy.
- Perfusion of the placenta depends on uterine blood flow, which comes from uterine and ovarian arteries.
- Blood flow ↑ as a result of vasodilation from the effects of estradiol and progesterone.
- Blood vessels lie between the various layers of uterine muscle. These muscle cells contract after delivery thereby constricting the blood vessels.

The human placenta is hemochorionic—there is NO direct mixing of fetal and maternal blood.

Braxton Hicks contractions do not cause cervical change.

HIGH-YIELD FACTS

Physiology of Pregnancy

Cervix

- The cervix is composed of smooth muscle and connective tissue. ↓ amount of collagen and accumulation of water cause the cervix to soften and become cyanotic.
- Other changes include ↑ vascularity of the entire cervix and hypertrophy and hyperplasia of the glands.
- ↑ in gland activity leads to the formation of a mucous plug.
  - The mucous plug is composed of immunoglobulins and cytokines, which act as a barrier to bacteria.
  - Cervical effacement causes expulsion of the mucous plug as the cervical canal shortens in labor.

Vagina

The vagina also undergoes changes during pregnancy in preparation for labor/delivery.

- The tissue becomes more vascular leading to a purplish tinge—Chadwick's sign.
- The vaginal walls prepare for distention by increasing the thickness of the mucosa, loosening of the connective tissue, and hypertrophy of smooth muscle cells.
- The vaginal secretions become thicker with a white color due to influence of progesterone. Additionally, the secretions are more acidic in nature as a result of ↑ *Lactobacillus acidophilus*. This inhibits growth of most pathogens and favors growth of yeasts.

Skin

The skin undergoes changes in pigmentation and vascularity as a result of pregnancy.

- The ↑ in pigmentation is due to melanocyte-stimulating hormone, estrogen, and progesterone.
  - Linea nigra: Black line/discoloration of the abdomen that runs from umbilicus to pubis.
  - Darkening of the nipple and areola.
  - Facial chloasma/melasma: Light to dark brown hyperpigmentation in exposed areas (face or neck).
- High levels of estrogen cause vascular spiders and palmar erythema.
- Certain dermatologic conditions are unique to pregnancy. See Table 3-2.

Breasts

- Breasts may ↑ in size and become painful.
- After a few months of pregnancy, the breast may express a thick, yellow fluid called colostrum.

METABOLIC CHANGES

- Ideal weight gain:
  T1: 1.5–3 lb gained
  T2 and T3: 0.8 lb/wk

If normal pre-pregnancy weight, patient should gain 25–35 lb during pregnancy. There should be little weight gain in T1, with most of weight gain in T2 and T3.

If pre-pregnancy BMI is <19, weight gain should be 28–40 lb while those with a BMI > 26 should gain no more than 20 lb during the pregnancy.

TABLE 3-2. Pruritic Dermatologic Disorders Unique to Pregnancy

DISEASE	ONSET	PRURITUS	LESIONS	DISTRIBUTION	INCIDENCE	↑ INCIDENCE FETAL MORBIDITY/ MORTALITY	INTERVENTION
Pruritic urticarial papules and plaques of pregnancy (PUPPP) (polymorphic eruption of pregnancy)	T2–T3	Severe	Erythematous urticarial papules and plaques	Abdomen, thighs, buttocks, occasionally arms and legs	Common (1:160–1:300)	No	Topical steroids, antipruritic drugs (hydroxyzine, diphenhydramine, calamine lotion
Intrahepatic cholestasis of pregnancy (bile not properly excreted from the liver)	T3	Severe	Excoriations common	Generalized, palms, soles	Common (1–2%)	Stillbirth	Check serum bile acids, liver function tests, Antipruritics, ursodeoxycholic acid, fetal testing

- As both baby and placenta grow, the mother's body ↑ its energy needs. By the last trimester, requirements ↑ by 300 kcal/day.

Water Metabolism

- Water retention is a normal part of pregnancy. Often, pitting edema of the ankles and legs is seen in pregnant women, especially at the end of the day. This is due to several factors, including:
  - ↑ venous pressure in the lower extremities due to compression of the vena cava and pelvic veins by the gravid uterus.
  - ↓ in interstitial colloid osmotic pressure.
- ↑ hydration of connective tissue leading to laxity and swelling of connective tissue and joints that mainly occur in T3.

Carbohydrate Metabolism

- **First 20 weeks:**
  - Insulin sensitivity ↑ in first half of pregnancy.
  - Lower fasting glucose levels allow for glycogen synthesis and fat deposition.
- **After 20 weeks:**
  - Insulin resistance develops and plasma insulin levels rise.
  - Higher levels of both insulin and glucose stimulate utilization of glucose and lipids for energy.
  - As a result, pregnant women will have mild fasting hypoglycemia, postprandial hyperglycemia, and hyperinsulinemia.

The placental hormone human placental lactogen is thought to cause gestational diabetes because it causes insulin resistance as it ↑ in pregnancy.

The optimal time to screen for glucose intolerance is at 26–28 weeks gestation.

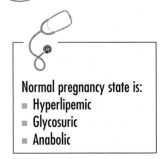

Normal pregnancy state is:
- Hyperlipemic
- Glycosuric
- Anabolic

HIGH-YIELD FACTS

Physiology of Pregnancy

35

A 29-year-old G3P2103 delivers a 7 lb 6 oz baby girl at $38^3/_7$ weeks. The estimated blood loss for the delivery was 950 mL. Vitals remain within normal limits while her hemoglobin ↓ from 12 g/dL to 10 g/dL. What is the explanation for the patient's response to the large blood loss?

Answer: The patient remained hemodynamically stable despite a large blood loss due to the normal ↑ in blood volume that takes place in the second trimester. The ↑ in blood volume buffers the anticipated blood loss at the time of delivery.

Maternal blood volume ↑ more if having twins or higher order gestations as compared to singleton.

If a mother has Beta-thalassemia trait/disease or sickle cell trait/disease, test the father to determine the risk of inheritance for the fetus.

Physiologic anemia of pregnancy develops in T2 due to greater expansion of intravascular volume.

Blood Volume

- Maternal blood volume ↑ during pregnancy to levels that are 50% above that of pre-pregnancy. ↑ blood volume is needed to:
  - Meet the demands of the enlarged uterus.
  - Protect the mother and the fetus against impaired venous return.
  - Protect the mother from blood loss at the time of delivery.
- Expanded volume is composed of plasma and erythrocytes but proportionately more plasma. ↑ erythrocyte production is reflected by ↑ reticulocyte count.
- Both hemoglobin and the hematocrit ↓ slightly.
  - Hemoglobin averages 12.5 g/dL.
  - Levels below 11.0 g/dL, especially late in pregnancy, should be considered abnormal.

Iron

- Iron requirements ↑ in pregnancy to about 1000 mg/day.
- Most of the iron is used for hematopoiesis, especially in the last half of pregnancy.
- The amount of iron from the diet is insufficient to meet the needs of the pregnancy, so patients must take supplemental iron.

Immunology

- During pregnancy, there is suppression of humoral and cell-mediated immunological functions. During T3:
  - ↑ granulocytes, ↑ CD8 T lymphocytes.
  - ↓ in CD4 T lymphocytes, ↓ monocytes.
- The leukocyte count varies during normal pregnancy. Usually, it ranges from 5000 to 12,000/μL. During labor, counts can rise to 25,000/μL; however, it averages 14,000–16,000/μL.
- Markers of inflammatory states such as leukocyte alkaline phosphatase, C-reactive protein, and erythrocyte sedimentation rate (ESR) also rise.

Coagulation

A 36-year-old G3P2002 at 32 weeks gestation presents with a sudden onset of shortness of breath, dyspnea, and palpitations that has been ongoing for 1 hour and is now worsening. She denies sick contacts, cough, fever, or leg swelling. She has no medical conditions and has a negative family history. On exam, she is afebrile, pulse is 120, respirations 25, and BP 120/80. She appears to be in distress. There are absent breath sounds on the right side. Her legs show 1+ pitting edema bilaterally. Fetal heart rate is reassuring. Pulse oximetry is 75% on room air. What is the most likely diagnosis?

Answer: Pulmonary embolus (PE). Estrogen causes an ↑ in clotting factors, resulting in a hypercoagulable state in pregnancy. Pregnant patients are at ↑ risk for pulmonary embolus and deep venous thrombosis (DVT) during the pregnancy and immediately after delivery.

- Pregnancy is a hypercoagulable state (risk factor for stroke, pulmonary emboli, DVT).
    - ↑ concentrations of all clotting factors, except factors XI and XIII.
    - ↑ fibrinogen.
    - ↑ resistance to activated protein C.
    - ↓ protein S.
- The average platelet count is ↓ slightly.

CARDIOVASCULAR SYSTEM

- Changes in cardiac function begin in the first 8 weeks of pregnancy.
- Cardiac output is ↑ as early as the fifth week of pregnancy due to:
    - ↓ systemic vascular resistance.
    - ↑ heart rate.
- As the diaphragm rises, the heart is displaced to the left and upward and rotates slightly.
- Systolic ejection murmurs along left sternal border occur in 96% of pregnant women due to ↑ flow across aortic and pulmonic valves.
- Diastolic murmurs are never normal and should be evaluated by a cardiologist.
- Blood pressure ↓ in midpregnancy and rises during the last trimester. Diastolic pressure ↓ more than systolic.

↑ CO = ↓ SVR + ↑ HR.

Patients with hypertensive heart disease may develop progressive or sudden deterioration in pregnancy.

RESPIRATORY SYSTEM

- As a result of the expanding uterus, diaphragm rises about 4 cm, the subcostal angle widens, and thoracic circumference ↑ about 6 cm.
- Respiratory rate unchanged.
- ↑ tidal volume, minute ventilatory volume, and minute oxygen uptake.
- ↓ functional residual capacity and residual volume due to the elevated diaphragm.
- Normal acid-base status in pregnancy is **respiratory alkalosis** due to more CO_2 being blown off. pH = 7.45

Normal acid-base status in pregnancy = compensated respiratory alkalosis (more CO_2 blown off).

A 31-year-old G1P0 at 24 weeks presents to her obstetrician for her routine prenatal visit. Patient reports no complaints. However, analysis of her urine showed the presence of large nitrites, large leukocytes, and small blood. What is the next step?

Answer: The patient should be empirically treated for a urinary tract infection (UTI). The antibiotics can be modified once the urine culture results are available. Due to the changes caused by progesterone, pregnant women are at ↑ risk for developing asymptomatic bacteriuria, and UTIs can progress to pyelonephritis if left untreated. Pyelonephritis in pregnant women can lead to sepsis and respiratory failure; it is the most common nonobstetric cause for hospitalization in pregnancy, so prevention is key.

In pregnancy, the higher rate of renal clearance leads to reduced effective dose of antibiotics and other medications.

(L)ovarian vein → (L) renal vein
(R)ov → IVC

Kidneys

- ↑ glomerular filtration rate, creatinine clearance, renal plasma flow. ∴
- ↓ serum creatinine, blood urea nitrogen.
- Renal tubules lose some of their resorptive capacity: Amino acids, uric acid, and glucose are not completely absorbed. Sodium is retained in higher levels in the pregnant female.

Ureters

- Dilate due to compression from uterus at the pelvic brim and the effect of progesterone.
- Dilation R > L due to the <u>dextroversion</u> of the uterus.
- Dilated ureters cause ↑ glomerular size and ↑ fluid flow → enlarged kidneys.
- Decreased ureteral peristalsis and increased ureteral compression cause urinary stasis which can lead to asymptomatic bacteriuria and pyelonephritis.

Right hydronephrosis is a normal finding in pregnancy.

Bladder

- ↓ tone, ↑ capacity progressively during pregnancy.
- ↑ urinary frequency is due to bladder compression by an enlarged uterus.
- Stress incontinence develops as a result of relaxation of bladder supports.

Pain from appendicitis may occur much higher in the abdomen because the gravid uterus pushes the appendix up.

- The stomach, appendix, and intestines are displaced upward by the enlarging uterus.
- Effects of progesterone:
    - ↓ lower esophageal sphincter tone → heartburn.
    - ↓ bowel peristalsis → constipation.
- **Hemorrhoids,** common in pregnancy, are caused by constipation and elevated pressure in veins below the level of the uterus.

Liver

- **Alkaline phosphatase** activity in serum almost <u>doubles</u> during pregnancy. Serum aspartate transaminase, alanine transaminase, γ-glutamyl transferase, and bilirubin levels are slightly <u>lower</u>.
- Serum albumin ↓, but total albumin ↑ because of a greater volume of distribution.

Gallbladder

Contractility of the gallbladder is reduced, leading to an increased residual volume and cholestasis.

- Progesterone impairs gallbladder contraction by inhibiting cholecystokinin-mediated smooth muscle stimulation.
- Estrogen inhibits intraductal transport of bile acids, also contributing to cholestasis.

Cholestasis with increased lipids and cholesterol leads to higher incidence of gallstones, cholecystitis, and biliary obstruction.

ENDOCRINE SYSTEM

Pituitary Gland

The pituitary gland ↑ in size and weight during pregnancy

PROLACTIN

- Main function is to ensure milk **production**.
- Levels ↑ throughout pregnancy due to <u>estradiol</u>.

OXYTOCIN

- Responsible for lactation, especially milk **letdown**.
- ↑ throughout the pregnancy.
- Released by nipple stimulation and infant crying.
- Causes uterine contractions.

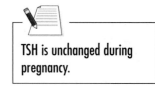

Pitocin is synthetic oxytocin. It is used to start or enhance labor.

Thyroid Gland

- Total thyroxine levels and thyroxine-binding globulin ↑ in response to high estrogen levels. However, *free* thyroxine remains normal and the mother remains euthyroid.
- Thyroxine-stimulating hormone is a sensitive marker for thyroid disease.
- The gland does not ↑ in size; therefore, all goiters need to be investigated.

TSH is unchanged during pregnancy.

Parathyroid Gland

- In the mother, parathyroid hormone ↓ in first trimester but then rises progressively the remainder of the pregnancy. Estrogens block the action of parathyroid hormone on bone resorption, resulting in ↑ hormone levels, which allow the fetus to have adequate calcium supply.
- The fetus has ↑ calcitonin levels allowing for bone deposition.

Mom: ↑PTH

Baby: ↑ calcitonin

Pregnant women have elevated TBG and therefore will have elevated total thyroxine and T_3, normal free T_4, and normal thyroid-stimulating hormone.

CHAPTER 4

Antepartum

42

This chapter focuses on the care provided for the pregnant patient prior to delivery. The prenatal or antepartum course often influences the outcome of the pregnancy. During this time, patients are encouraged to maintain healthy practices and abstain from practices that are harmful for the pregnancy. Regular visits at specific intervals are used to screen patients and fetus for abnormal medical conditions that may develop.

PRENATAL CARE

The goal of prenatal care is as follows:

1. Determine the health status of mother and fetus.
2. Determine gestational age.
3. Initiate plan for obstetrical care (routine vs. high risk).
4. Lower maternal/perinatal morbidity/mortality.
5. Enhance pregnancy, childbirth experience for patient/family.

Definitions

- **Gestational age (GA):** The time of pregnancy counting from the first day of the last menstrual period (LMP).
- **Developmental age:** The time of pregnancy counting from fertilization.
- **First trimester:** 0–13 weeks.
- **Second trimester:** 14–27 weeks.
- **Third trimester:** 28 weeks–birth.
- **Embryo:** Fertilization–8 weeks.
- **Fetus:** 9 weeks–birth
- **Previable:** < 24 weeks.
- **Preterm:** 20–36 weeks.
- **Term:** 37–42 weeks.

Terminology of Reproductive History

The mother's pregnancy history is described in terms of gravidity (G) and parity (P).

- **Gravidity** is the total number of pregnancies, regardless of the outcome.
- **Parity** is the number of pregnancies that have reached a gestational age of ≥ 20 weeks. It can be further subdivided into term births, preterm births, abortions, and living children.
- A woman that is gravida 3, para 1201 (G3P1201) has been pregnant three times, has had one term birth, two preterm births, no abortions, and has one live child.

Frequency of Obstetric Visits

- < 28 weeks: Every month.
- 28–36 weeks: Every 2–3 weeks.
- 36–41 weeks: Once per week.
- 41–42 weeks: Every 2-3 days for fetal testing.
- 42 weeks or more: Plan for delivery.
- See Table 4-1.

Gravidity: The number of times a woman has been pregnant.
Parity: The number of times a woman has had a pregnancy that led to a birth after 20 weeks gestation or an infant > 500 g.

Parity: **TPAL**
Term
Preterm
Abortuses
Living Children

TABLE 4-1. Prenatal Visits

FIRST VISIT	11–13 WEEKS	16–20 WEEKS	26–28 WEEKS

1. History and physical (H&P)
2. Labs:
  ▪ Hct/Hgb
  ▪ Rh factor
  ▪ Blood type
  ▪ Antibody screen
  ▪ Pap smear
  ▪ *Gonorrhea* and *Chlamydia* cultures
  ▪ Urine analysis (protein, glucose, ketones)
  ▪ Urine culture
  ▪ Infection screen: Rubella, syphilis, hepatitis B, human immunodeficiency virus (HIV), tuberculosis (TB)
  ▪ Cystic fibrosis screen
  ▪ Urine drug screen
  ▪ Hemoglobin electrophoresis
	1. H&P
	2. Fetal exam:
	  ▪ Fetal heart tones
	3. Urine dip: Protein, glucose, leukocytes
	4. First-trimester screen
		1. H&P
		2. Fetal exam:
		  ▪ Fetal heart
		  ▪ Fundal height
		3. Urine dip: Protein, glucose, leukocytes
		4. Fetal ultrasound: Anatomy, dating
		5. Quad screen
		6. Genetic amniocentesis (if indicated)
			1. H&P
			2. Fetal exam:
			  ▪ Fetal heart
			  ▪ Fundal height
			3. Labs:
			  ▪ Complete blood count
			  ▪ Ab screen
			  ▪ *Gonorrhea* and *Chlamydia* cultures (optional)
			  ▪ Diabetes screen
			  ▪ Urine dip: Protein, glucose, leukocytes
			  ▪ Syphilis screen (optional)
			4. Give anti D immunoglobulin if indicated (28 weeks)

Week 32	Week 36	Week 38	Week 39	Week 40

1. H&P
2. Fetal exam:
  ▪ Fetal heart
  ▪ Fundal height
3. Urine dip: protein, glucose, leukocytes
	1. H&P
	2. Fetal exam:
	  ▪ Fetal heart
	  ▪ Fundal height
	  ▪ Fetal presentation
	3. Urine dip: Protein, glucose, leukocytes
	4. Group B strep culture
	5. HIV—required in some states
		1. H&P
		2. Fetal exam:
		  ▪ Fetal heart
		  ▪ Fundal height
		  ▪ Fetal presentation
		3. Urine dip: Protein, glucose, leukocytes
		4. Cervical exam (frequency is controversial)
			1. H&P
			2. Fetal exam:
			  ▪ Fetal heart
			  ▪ Fundal height
			  ▪ Fetal presentation
			3. Urine dip: Protein, glucose, leukocytes
				1. H&P
				2. Fetal exam:
				  ▪ Fetal heart
				  ▪ Fundal height
				  ▪ Fetal presentation
				3. Urine dip: Protein, glucose, leukocytes

First Visit

HISTORY

- Biographical: Age, race, occupation, marital status.
- Obstetrical: Gravidity, parity, prior labor/deliveries (vaginal, cesareans), complications, infant status, birth weight.

- Menstrual: Last menstrual period (LMP), menstrual irregularities.
- Contraceptive use: What type and when was it last used?
- Medical: Asthma, diabetes, hypertension, thyroid disease, cardiac disease, seizures, rubella, previous surgeries, sexually transmitted infections, allergies, medications, smoking, alcohol, recreational drugs.
- Family history: Multiple gestations, diabetes, hypertension, bleeding disorders, hereditary disorders, mental retardation, anesthetic problems.

PHYSICAL EXAM

- Vitals: Blood pressure (BP), weight, height, temperature, heart rate.
- Head, neck, heart, lungs, back.
- Pelvic:
  - External genitalia: Bartholin's gland, condyloma, herpes, other lesions.
  - Vagina: Discharge, inflammation.
  - Cervix: Polyps, growths.
  - Uterus: Masses, irregularities, size compared to gestational age.
  - Adnexa: Masses.
  - Clinical pelvimetry: Following are dimensions of a gynecoid pelvis shape:
    - Pelvic inlet: Diagonal conjugate > 12.5 cm. Distance between the inferior border of symphysis pubis to sacral promontory.
    - Midpelvis: Ischial spines blunt, >10 cm.
    - Pelvic outlet: Intertuberous diameter > 8 cm, pubic arch > 90 degrees.

Subsequent Visits

> A 31-year-old G2P1001 at 17 weeks gestation undergoes routine prenatal tests. Her results show that her blood type is A negative, and her antibody screen is positive. She does not report undergoing a blood transfusion in the past or any complications with her last pregnancy. What is the next step in the management of this patient?
>
> **Answer:** The next step is to identify the antibody. There are many types of antibodies, and in a patient that is Rh negative, it should not be assumed that she has Rh antibodies.

HISTORY

Ask each patient the following at each subsequent visit:

- Presence of fetal movement.
- Vaginal bleeding.
- Leakage of fluid.
- Contractions/abdominal pain.
- Preeclampsia symptoms:
  - Headache.
  - Visual disturbances.
  - Right upper quadrant pain.

Remember that alcohol use has the highest correlation with congenital abnormalities.

Patient's history and physical determines whether the patient receives routine or high risk care.

PHYSICAL EXAM

After thorough initial exam, each subsequent exam must record four findings:

- BP
- Urine dip for protein, glucose, leukocytes
- Fundal height
- Fetal heart rate

ROUTINE INITIAL TESTS

- Complete blood count (CBC)
- Blood type
- Rh status
- Antibody screen
- Urinalysis (UA)
- Urine culture
- Urine drug screen (UDS)
- Rapid plasma reagin (RPR)
- Human immunodeficiency virus (HIV)
- Hepatitis B surface antigen (HBsAg)
- Rubella
- Tuberculin skin test
- Wet mount
- Gonorrhea
- Chlamydia
- Pap smear
- Cystic fibrosis screen
- Hemoglobin electrophoresis

ROUTINE TIMED TESTS

Certain prenatal tests should occur at specific times during pregnancy (see Table 4-1):

- 11–13 weeks: First trimester screen; only for Down syndrome.
    - Nuchal translucency (NT) measured via ultrasound.
    - Maternal serum pregnancy-associated plasma protein A (PAPP-A) and free β-human chorionic gonadotropin (β-hCG).
    - In Down syndrome, the NT is ↑, PAPP-A ↓, free β-hCG ↑.
- 16–18 weeks: Quad screen (range 15–21 weeks).
    - Unconjugated estriol
    - α-fetoprotein
    - β-hCG
    - Inhibin A
- 18–20 weeks: Ultrasound for anatomy/dating.
- 26–28 weeks: One hour 50-g glucose tolerance test (GTT) to screen for gestational diabetes.
- 28 weeks: Recheck antibody screen, administer Rhogam if indicated.
- 35–37 weeks:
    - Group B streptococcus (GBS) culture.
    - Third-trimester HIV testing is mandated by law in some states.

Fundal Height

As the fetus grows, the leading edge of the uterus, or the fundus grows superiorly in the abdomen, toward the maternal head. Fundal height (in centimeters) roughly corresponds to gestational age (in weeks).

- Uterus at level of pubic symphysis: 12 weeks
- Uterus between pubic symphysis and umbilicus: 16 weeks
- Uterus at the level of umbilicus: 20 weeks
- Uterine height correlates to weeks gestation: 20–36 weeks

Fundal height (cm) should correlate to gestational age (weeks) ± 3. If not, consider inaccurate dating (most common), multiple gestations, or molar pregnancy. Past approximately 36 weeks gestation, the fundal height may not correspond to the gestational age due to the fetal descent into the pelvis.

Most common cause of size not equal to date—incorrect gestational age. Order an US to establish the correct dates.

FETAL SURVEILLANCE

When the mother is diagnosed with a medical condition that can affect the fetus, or when the fetus is diagnosed with a condition that may result in a poor outcome, several tests can be used to monitor the health of the fetus. They include fetal movement counts, non-stress test (NST), contraction stress test (CST), biophysical profile (BPP), the modified BPP (mBPP), and Doppler ultrasonography. In general, they are performed in T3, but may be done earlier. These tests assess for chronic uteroplacental insufficiency and cannot predict acute events. The choice and frequency of testing depends on indication, gestational age, medical condition, and experience of the practitioner.

Fetal Movement Counts

Fetal movement counts, or kick counts, may be performed at home by the patient in order to monitor the baby's health. The patient should select a time at which the fetus usually is active, usually after a meal. The level of activity differs for each baby, and most have sleep cycles of 20–40 min.

There are several ways to assess fetal movements:

- Ask the patient to record daily how long it takes the fetus to make 10 movements. For most, this is usually achieved in about 2 hr; however, this is variable.
- Alternatively, ask the patient to record the number of fetal movements in 1 hr three times per week. A baseline is established in this way.
- For both of these strategies, a physician should be contacted if there is a change from the normal pattern or number of movements recorded.

Non-stress Test (NST)

- The NST evaluates four components of the fetal heart rate (FHR) tracing:
  - Baseline: Normally 110–160 beats/min.
  - Variability: Beat-to-beat irregularity and waviness of the FHR. Presence of variability reflects an intact and mature brain stem and heart.
  - Periodic changes: Transient accelerations or decelerations:
    - Early deceleration: Vagally mediated, caused by head compression usually at cervical dilation of 4–7 cm.
    - Variable deceleration: Caused by cord compression.

- Late deceleration: Reflects hypoxemia.
  - Acceleration: At least two accelerations of at least 15 beats/min above baseline for 15 sec in a 20-min period. Presence of accelerations = fetal well-being. Reactive NST = two or more accelerations over 20 min.
  - Uterine contractions are also recorded to help interpret the NST.
- Preterm fetuses are frequently nonreactive:
  - 24–28 weeks: Up to 50% nonreactive.
  - 28–32 weeks: 15% nonreactive.
- An NST usually takes 20–40 min to complete. If the NST is nonreactive, the baby may be asleep. If this is suspected, ask the patient to eat or drink to make the baby active if not reactive within 1–2 hours, then additional testing may need to be performed.

Contraction Stress Test (CST)

The contraction stress test (CST) measures how the fetal heart rate (FHR) reacts to uterine contractions. The CST can be performed if the NST is nonreactive. The FHR and the contractions are recorded simultaneously. During a contraction, the blood flow to the placenta briefly ↓. A well-oxygenated fetus can compensate, and there are no decels in the FHR. If the fetus is already compromised with low levels of oxygen, the contraction may cause a late deceleration in FHR, which reflects hypoxemia in the fetus.

- Patient is placed in lateral recumbent position and contractions are stimulated.
  - Administration of oxytocin (pitocin).
  - Nipple stimulation (2 min self-stimulation through clothes every 5 min).
- Adequate contractions:
  - Occur three times in 10 min.
  - Lasting at least 40 sec.
  - Moderate to palpation.
- Interpreted as the presence or absence of late decelerations:
  - **Negative:** No late or significant variable decelerations.
  - **Positive:** Late decelerations following 50% or more of contractions.
  - **Equivocal:** Intermittent late decels or significant variable decelerations.
  - **Unsatisfactory:** Fewer than three contractions in 10 min.
- Contraindications:
  - Preterm labor patients at high risk of delivery.
  - Premature rupture of membranes (PROM).
  - History of extensive uterine surgery or previous cesarean section.
  - Known placenta previa.

A reactive NST has two or more accelerations over 20 min = fetal well-being.

Ultrasound (US)

- Standard US performed for:
  - Fetal number
  - Presentation
  - Fetal viability
  - Gestational age assessment
  - Amniotic fluid volume
  - Fetal biometry
  - Fetal anatomic survey
  - Placental location

- Limited—goal-directed US:
  - Presentation
  - Placental location intrapartum
  - Adjuct to invasive procedures
- Specialized (Level II)—performed when high suspicion of anomaly:
  - Fetal Doppler
  - Biophysical profile

Biophysical Profile (BPP): NST + US

- A biophysical profile (BPP) is the combination of the non-stress test and an ultrasound exam, for a total of five components:
  1. NST: Appropriate variation of fetal heart rate.
  2. Breathing: ≥ 1 episode of rhythmic breathing movements of 30 sec or more within 30 min.
  3. Movement: ≥ 3 discrete body or limb movements within 30 min.
  4. Muscle tone: ≥ 1 episode of extension with return to flexion or opening/closing of a hand.
  5. Determination of amniotic fluid volume: Single vertical pocket of amniotic fluid measuring ≥ 2 cm is considered adequate* (or an amniotic fluid index > 5 cm).
- Each of the category is given a score of 0 or 2 points:
  - 0: Abnormal, absent, or insufficient.
  - 2: Normal and present as previously defined.
  - Total possible score is 10 points.
  - Normal score: 8–10.
  - Equivocal: 6.
  - Abnormal: ≤ 4.

* In the presence of oligohydramnios (largest pocket of amniotic fluid ≤ 2 cm), further investigation is required.

Modified Biophysical Profile (mBPP) NST + AFI

- A modified biophysical profile (mBPP) includes two components: An NST and an amniotic fluid index (AFI).
- Normal amniotic fluid volume varies and ↑ with gestational age. The peak volume is 800–1000 mL at 36–37 weeks gestation. In the late T2 or T3, amniotic fluid volume represents fetal urine output. If there is uteroplacental dysfunction and ↓ oxygenation to the fetus, the fetus preferentially shunts blood to the brain and heart, leaving the fetal kidneys underperfused. This results in ↓ fetal urine output and, as a result, ↓ amniotic fluid. Therefore, the AFI is used as a measure of chronic uteroplacental function.
- The AFI is the sum of amniotic fluid measured in four quadrants of the uterus via the US.
  - AFI > 5 cm: Adequate.
  - AFI ≤ 5 cm: Abnormal (oligohydramnios).
  - AFI ≥ 25 cm: Abnormal (polyhydramnios).
- **Oligohydramnios:**
  - Most common cause: Ruptured membranes.
  - Associated with intrauterine growth restriction 60% of the time.
  - Evaluate for genitourinary malformations.

HIGH-YIELD FACTS

Antepartum

- **Polyhydramnios:**
  - Many causes, including:
    - Fetal malformation (anencephaly, esophageal atresia).
    - Genetic disorders.
    - Maternal diabetes.
    - Multiple gestation.
    - Fetal anemia.
    - Viruses.
  - Associated with uterine overdistention, resulting in:
    - Preterm labor
    - PROM
    - Fetal malposition
    - Uterine atony

Doppler Velocimetry

- Doppler sonography is a noninvasive technique used to assess fetal hemodynamic vascular resistance by imaging specific fetal vessels:
  - Umbilical artery (UA) and umbilical vein.
  - Aorta.
  - Heart.
  - Middle cerebral artery (MCA).
- Commonly measured flow indices are:
  - Peak systolic frequency shift (S).
  - Peak diastolic frequency shift (D).
  - Mean peak frequency shift over the cardiac cycle (A).
  - Systolic to diastolic ratio (S/D).
  - Resistance index (S-D/S).
  - Pulsatility index (S-D/A).
- Flow velocity waveforms differ in normal-sized fetuses as compared to those suffering from growth restriction:
  - Fetuses with normal growth: High-velocity diastolic flow.
  - Fetuses with restricted growth: ↓ velocity diastolic flow, ↑ flow resistance (↑ S/D) in umbilical artery and ↓ resistance (↓ S/D) in MCA.
  - Very severe intrauterine growth restriction: Flow may be absent or even reversed.
- Abnormal flow is usually the result of placental insufficiency and dysfunction, resulting in fetal hypoxia and acidosis. This may induce the phenomenon of brain sparing:
  - ↑ S/D in umbilical artery (↑ resistance).
  - ↓ S/D in MCA (↓ resistance).
  - Adaptive response to fetal hypoxemia.

"Brain sparing" may occur in hypoxic fetuses = ↑ S/D in umbilical artery + ↓ S/D in middle cerebral artery.

SCREENING FOR CONGENITAL ABNORMALITIES

Screening for fetal abnormalities can include testing during the first and second trimesters, and the tests can be noninvasive or invasive. Commonly used techniques are maternal serum screen, ultrasound, amniocentesis, chorionic villus sampling (CVS), and cordocentesis.

First-Trimester Screen (FTS)

- The FTS is an optional noninvasive evaluation performed between weeks 11 and 13. It is a screening test and may require further diagnostic tests if the results are abnormal.
- The FTS combines a maternal blood screening test with a fetal US evaluation to identify risk for Down syndrome (trisomy 21). It can also detect trisomy 13, Turner syndrome, Edwards syndrome (trisomy 18), but not neural tube defects (NTDs).
- The results of maternal hormone levels and fetal US, along with the mother's age, are combined to determine risk factors. The following is assessed in the FTS:
  - Maternal serum: Free or total β-hCG, PAPP-A.
  - US at 11–13 weeks gestation: Nuchal translucency (NT)—measurement of fluid under the baby's skin at the level of the neck (see Figure 4-1).
  - In the case of Down syndrome, β-hCG will be ↑ and PAPP-A will be ↓.
- The FTS is considered the most accurate noninvasive screening method available, with a sensitivity of 85% for Down syndrome.

FTS (11-13)
tri 21
tri 13
tri 18
Turner's

Down (Trisomy 21)
β-hCG ↑
PAPP-A ↓
Nuchal translucency ↑

Quad Screen

A 19-year-old Caucasian female, G1P0, at 16 weeks gestation based on an unsure LMP has an ↑ risk for Down syndrome on her second-trimester quad screen. Her blood pressure is within normal limits, urine protein is negative, and fetal heart tones are 148 bpm. You palpate the fundal height 2 cm above the umbilicus. What is the most likely cause of the abnormal quad screen? What diagnostic tests can confirm the screening test?

Answer: The most common cause for the abnormal quad screen is incorrect dates. This patient's fundal height indicates that her pregnancy is further than what her LMP indicates. The next step is to perform an ultrasound to confirm the gestational age of the fetus and recalculate the quad screen. If the quad screen is abnormal with correct dating, the patient should undergo genetic counseling and be offered a genetic amniocentesis.

A targeted US evaluates the fetus for congenital structural abnormalities that may correlate with abnormal serum screening findings.

The quad screen is a screening test of maternal serum that evaluates the risk a patient has for delivering a baby with Down syndrome (trisomy 21), Edwards syndrome (trisomy 18), or NTDs. The result does not indicate that the fetus does or does not have the indicated condition, only the risk. If the quad screen shows an ↑ risk for any of the screened conditions, further diagnostic tests may be performed to confirm the findings. See Table 4-2 for a summary of quad screen results.

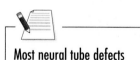

Most neural tube defects are thought to be polygenic or multifactorial.

Quad (16-18)
tri 21
tri 18
NTD

- Ideally performed at 16–18 weeks gestation (range is 15–21 weeks).
- Sensitivity: 81%.
- Evaluates four maternal serum analytes:
  - Maternal serum α feto protein
  - Unconjugated estriol
  - Human chorionic gonadotropin
  - Inhibin A

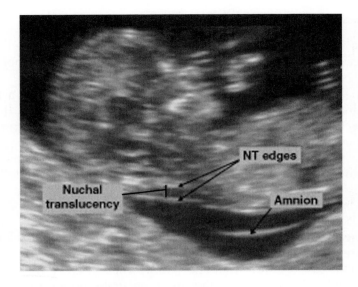

FIGURE 4-1. Nuchal translucency measurement.

(Reproduced, with permission, from Cunningham FG, Leveno KJ, Bloom SL, et al. *Williams Obstetrics*, 23rd ed. New York: McGraw-Hill, 2010: 351.)

> If there is high α-fetoprotein at 16 weeks, a neural tube defect is a likely diagnosis, especially if the woman is older than 35. Low α-fetoprotein is associated with certain chromosomal defects (eg, trisomy 21 or trisomy 18).

- Abnormal quad screen → confirm dates (US) → genetic counseling + targeted US → diagnostic procedure (amniocentesis to obtain fetal cells) → karyotype analysis.
- Most common cause of abnormal quad screen: Incorrect dates.

Maternal Serum α-Fetoprotein (MSAFP)

- MSAFP is first produced in the yolk sac and then by the fetal gastrointestinal tract and liver.
- Normally, it passes by diffusion through the chorion and amnion. It begins to rise at 13 weeks and peaks at 32 weeks.
- In general, MSAFP levels > 2.0–2.5 multiples of the mean (MOM) warrant further investigation, as they are suspicious of NTDs.
- MSAFP screening is most accurate between 16 and 18 weeks.
- High levels are associated with:
  - Underestimation of gestational age.
  - NTDs.
  - Abdominal wall defects (gastroschisis and omphalocele).

TABLE 4-2. Quad Screen Summary

	DOWN (TRISOMY 21)	EDWARDS (TRISOMY 18)	NTD
uE3	↓	↓	Normal
AFP	↓	↓	↑
β-hCG	↑	↓	Normal
Inhibin A	↑	↓	Normal

AFP, α-fetoprotein; β-hCG, β-human chorionic gonadotropin; NTD, neural tube defect; uE3, unconjugated estriol.

- Fetal death.
- Placental abnormalities (eg, abruption).
- Multiple gestations.
- Others: Low maternal weight, fetal skin defects, cystic hygroma, sacrococcygeal teratoma, oligohydramnios.
■ Low levels are associated with:
- Overestimation of gestational age.
- Chromosomal trisomies: Down syndrome (trisomy 21), Edwards' syndrome (trisomy 18).
- Fetal death.
- Molar pregnancy.
- High maternal weight.

Unconjugated Estriol (uE3)

Low levels are associated with:

- **Trisomy 21** (Down syndrome).
- **Trisomy 18** (Edwards syndrome).
- Possibly low in **trisomy 13** (Patau syndrome).

Human Chorionic Gonadotropin (hCG)

- High levels are associated with: Trisomy 21.
- Low levels are associated with: Trisomy 18, anencephaly.

Inhibin A

- This hormone is secreted the placenta and granulosa cells in the female.
- High levels are associated with: Trisomy 21.
- Low levels are associated with: Trisomy 18.

Specialized (Level II) Ultrasound

- Performed by maternal-fetal specialists.
- Evaluates the fetal anatomy for markers of aneuploidy.
- See Figures 4-2 through 4-10 for normal and abnormal US findings.

What can ultrasound determine?
- Diagnosis of early pregnancy
- Determine if fetus is still viable in the setting of vaginal bleeding in early pregnancy
- Determination of gestational age and assessment of fetal size
- Diagnosis of fetal malformation (cleft lip, polydactyly, club foot, fetal sex, NTDs, abdominal wall defects, abdominal renal anomalies)
- Placental localization
- Hydramnios and oligohydramnios

FIGURE 4-2. Normal four-chamber heart.

FIGURE 4-3. **Measurement of biparietal diameter and head circumference**

FIGURE 4-4. Double-bubble sign of duodenal atresia (marker for Down syndrome).

(Reproduced, with permission, from Cunningham FG, Leveno KJ, Bloom SL, et al. *Williams Obstetrics*, 23rd ed. New York: McGraw-Hill, 2010: 359.)

FIGURE 4-5. Anencephaly.

(Reproduced, with permission, from Cunningham FG, Leveno KJ, Bloom SL, et al. *Williams Obstetrics*, 23rd ed. New York: McGraw-Hill, 2010: 354.)

A.

B.

FIGURE 4-6. A. Cleft lip B. Normal lip.

FIGURE 4-7. Measurement of crown-rump length.

FIGURE 4-8. Umbilical cord insertion.

FIGURE 4-9. Omphalocele.

FIGURE 4-10. Gastroschisis.

Amniocentesis

- Amniocentesis is the most frequently employed technique used to obtain fetal cells. A needle is placed through the maternal abdominal wall and uterus with ultrasound guidance (see Figure 4-11). Amniotic fluid is obtained for various purposes. Usually done at 15–20 weeks.
  - **Karyotype:** Fetal cells obtained via amniocentesis are cultured and an evaluation of the chromosomes is performed in the following circumstances:
    - Fetal anomaly suspected on US.
    - Abnormal serum quad screen.
    - Family history of congenital abnormalities.

Ultrasound transducer

Placenta

FIGURE 4-11. Amniocentesis.

(Reproduced, with permission, from Cunningham FG, Leveno KJ, Bloom SL, et al. *Williams Obstetrics*, 23rd ed. New York: McGraw-Hill, 2010: 299.)

- Indicated for patients ≥ 35 years of age because they have a higher risk of aneuploidy.
- **Fetal lung maturity:** Usually done near term in order to deliver the baby.
- **Others:** Rule out infection, check bilirubin.
- **Risks:**
  - Pain/cramping.
  - Vaginal spotting (resolves spontaneously).
  - Amniotic fluid leakage in 1–2% of cases.
  - Symptomatic amnionitis in < 1 in 1000 patients.
  - **Rate of fetal loss is ≤ 0.5% (1 in 200) and is less in experienced hands.**

Chorionic Villus Sampling (CVS)

- CVS is a diagnostic technique in which a small sample of chorionic villi is taken transcervically or transabdominally and analyzed (see Figure 4-12).
- Typically done between 9 and 12 weeks gestation.
- Information on fetal karyotype.
- Biochemical assays or DNA tests can be done earlier than amniocentesis.
- **Complications—0.5–1%:**
  - Preterm delivery.
  - PROM.
  - Fetal injury, especially limb abnormalities if performed before 9 weeks gestation.

DIFFERENCES BETWEEN CVS AND AMNIOCENTESIS

- CVS:
  - Transvaginal or transabdominal aspiration of precursor cells in the intrauterine cavity.
  - Evaluates chromosomal abnormalities but does not evaluate NTDs.
  - Done at 9–12 weeks.

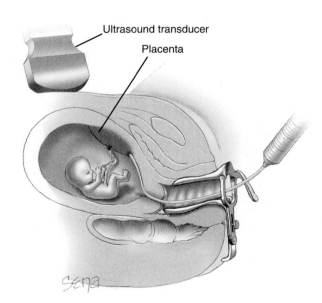

FIGURE 4-12. **Transcervical chorionic villus sampling (CVS).**

(Reproduced, with permission, from Cunningham FG, Leveno KJ, Bloom SL, et al. *Williams Obstetrics*, 23rd ed. New York: McGraw-Hill, 2010: 300.)

- Higher risks (fetal loss has 1% risk, limb defects if done < 9 weeks), diagnosis accuracy is comparable to amniocentesis.
- **Amniocentesis:**
  - Transabdominal aspiration of amniotic fluid using ultrasound-guided needle.
  - Evaluates chromosomal abnormalities.
  - Done at 15–20 weeks.
  - Indicated if > 35-year-old mother at time of delivery.
  - Risks of fetal loss (0.5%).

Cordocentesis

- Cordocentesis is also known as percutaneous umbilical blood sampling (PUBS), fetal blood sampling, and umbilical vein sampling. It is a procedure in which a spinal needle is advanced transabdominally under US guidance into a cord vessel to sample fetal blood (see Figure 4-13). Typically performed after 17 weeks.
- Allows for rapid diagnosis because of the high number of nucleated cells (WBCs) collected which require no culturing.

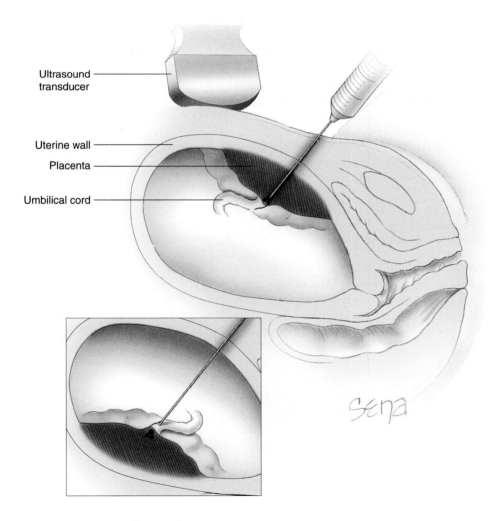

Ultrasound transducer

Uterine wall

Placenta

Umbilical cord

FIGURE 4-13. Cordocentesis.

(Reproduced, with permission, from Cunningham FG, Leveno KJ, Bloom SL, et al. *Williams Obstetrics*, 23rd ed. New York: McGraw-Hill, 2010: 301.)

INDICATIONS

- Fetal karyotyping because of fetal anomalies.
- To determine the fetal hematocrit in isoimmunization or severe fetal anemia.
- To assay fetal platelet counts, acid-base status, antibody levels, blood chemistries, etc.

Genetic Testing

Genetic testing is not required for every pregnancy. There are specific circumstances where it is appropriate to perform. Certain common genetic mutations that are easily screened for can be readily identified using routine scientific techniques.

INDICATIONS

- Advanced maternal age.
- Previous child with abnormal karyotype.
- Known parental chromosome abnormality (balanced translocation or point mutation).
- Fetal structural abnormality on sonogram.
- Unexplained intrauterine growth retardation (IUGR).
- Abnormal quad screen.

TECHNIQUES

- **Fluorescent in situ hybridization (FISH):** A specific DNA probe with a fluorescent label that binds homologous DNA; allows identification of specific sites along a chromosome. **Looks for specific abnormalities. Very sensitive.**
- **Karyotyping:** Allows visualization of chromosome size, banding pattern, and centromere position. **Looks for all chromosomal abnormalities, but not as sensitive.**

NUTRITIONAL NEEDS OF THE PREGNANT WOMAN

Proper nutritional habits are important for every woman; this is especially true for those who are pregnant. ↑ energy needs and specific vitamins are required by the mother to supply the appropriate nutrients essential to the normal development of the fetus. Without proper dietary control, certain common deficiencies and complications in both mother and baby may occur.

Weight Gain

- Weight gain for normal BMI: **25–35 lb.**
- Weight gain of < 15 lb (unless obese) can cause fetal IUGR.
- Weight gain of > 40 lb ↑ morbidity.
- Target weight gain of 1–5 lb in T1; 3–4 lb/month in remaining pregnancy.

Risk factors for IUGR:

- Poor nutrition
- Tobacco smoking
- Drug addiction
- Alcoholism

Advanced maternal age (AMA) is the most common indication for prenatal genetic testing.

Chromosomal abnormalities occur in 0.6% of all live births, account for 5% of stillbirths and 50–60% of spontaneous abortions.

Body Mass Index (BMI)
BMI ≥ 30: Obese
25.0–29.9: Overweight
18.5–24.9: Normal
< 18.5: Underweight

Weight gain in pregnancy:
BMI > 25: 15–25 lbs
BMI normal: 25–35 lbs
BMI < 18: 30–40 lbs

How do you monitor IUGR?
Serial ultrasound

- Severe anemia
- Thrombophilia
- Prolonged pregnancy
- Preeclampsia
- Chromosomal abnormalities
- Placental infarction/hematoma
- Infections
- Multiple gestations

Diet

- The average woman must consume an additional **300 kcal/day** beyond baseline needs and an additional **500 kcal/day when breast-feeding**.
- High protein (70–75 g/day), low simple carbohydrates and fats, high fiber.

Folic Acid

A 32-year-old Hispanic female, G3P2002, at 16 weeks gestation presents for initial obstetric visit. She reports that the last child born 3 years ago has spina bifida. What is the amount of folic acid she should take?

Answer: Women with a previous child with an NTD should take 4 mg/day of folic acid well before conception.

What should be taken to prevent NTDs? Folic acid 400 µg/day or 0.4 mg/day.

- ↑ dietary folate is required to prevent NTDs.
- **400 µg/day** is required. Ideal if started 3 months before pregnancy.
- If previous child with NTD, need folic acid 4 mg/day, starting 4 weeks prior to conception and through T1.

The neural tube is nearly formed by the time of the first missed period. Starting folic acid supplementation when pregnancy is diagnosed is too late.

Minerals

- **30 mg elemental iron per day is recommended in T2 and T3.** Total of 1 g iron is needed for pregnancy (500 mg for ↑ RBC mass, 300 mg for fetus, 200 mg for GI losses).
- The recommended dietary allowance (RDA) for calcium is ↑ in pregnancy to 1200 mg/day and may be met adequately with diet alone.
- The RDA for zinc is ↑ from 15 to 20 mg/day.

Vegetarians

Pregnant women develop iron deficiency anemia due to the ↑ hematopoietic demands of both mother and baby.

- **Lacto-ovovegetarians** in general have no nutritional deficiencies, except possibly iron and zinc.
- **Vegans** must consume sufficient quantities of vegetable proteins to provide all essential amino acids normally found in animal protein. Supplementation of zinc, vitamin B$_{12}$, and iron is necessary.

Pica

Occasionally seen in pregnancy, pica is the compulsive ingestion of nonfood substances with little or no nutritional value, such as ice, clay (geophagia), or starch (amylophagia).

Pica may occur during pregnancy, but all normal dietary and nutritional needs must be met and the substances consumed should be nontoxic (ice). Advise patients against the consumption of nonedible and possibly toxic items, such as dirt.

COMMON QUESTIONS

Pregnancy is a complicated time for most women. Their bodies undergo a transformation which entails many physiologic adaptations. These changes may be alarming to some women, and as a physician, one must be able to discern between normal pregnant physiology and pathophysiologic changes, which may require further investigation or immediate attention in a hospital setting.

Caffeine in Pregnancy

- Contained in coffee, tea, chocolate, cola beverages.
- Ingestion of caffeine (> 300 mg/d) may ↑ risk of early spontaneous abortion among nonsmoking women carrying fetuses of normal karyotype. This risk ↑ according to amount of caffeine ingested.
- Adverse maternal effects include:
  - Insomnia
  - Acid indigestion
  - Reflux
  - Urinary frequency

Exercise

- No data exist to indicate that a pregnant woman must ↓ the intensity of her exercise or lower her target heart rate.
- Women who exercised regularly before pregnancy should continue. Exercise may relieve stress, ↓ anxiety, ↑ self-esteem, and shorten labor.
- The form of exercise should be one with low risk of trauma, particularly abdominal (water exercises are ideal).
- Exercise that requires prolonged time in the supine position should be avoided in T2 and T3.
- Exercise should be stopped if patient experiences oxygen deprivation (manifested by extreme fatigue, dizziness, or shortness of breath).
- Contraindications to exercise include:
  - Evidence of IUGR.
  - Persistent vaginal bleeding.
  - Incompetent cervix.
  - Risk factors for preterm labor.
  - Rupture of membranes.
  - Pregnancy-induced hypertension/preeclampsia/eclampsia.

Hyperemesis gravidarum: Excessive vomiting during pregnancy + dehydration + electrolyte imbalances. A **hypochloremic alkalosis** may occur. What is the treatment? IVF 5% dextrose, antiemetics.

Nausea and Vomiting (N&V)

- Recurrent N&V in T1 occurs in 50% of pregnancies.
- If severe, can result in dehydration, electrolyte imbalance, and malnutrition.
- Management of mild cases includes:
  - Avoidance of fatty or spicy foods.

- Eating small, frequent meals.
- Inhaling peppermint oil vapors.
- Drinking ginger teas.
- Management of severe cases includes:
  - IV fluids (usually with dextrose-containing fluid).
  - Discontinuation of vitamin/mineral supplements until symptoms subside.
  - Antihistamines.
  - Promethazine.
  - Metoclopramide.
  - Intravenous droperidol.

Heartburn

- Occurs in 30% of pregnancies.
- **Etiology:**
  - Normal relaxation of lower esophageal sphincter
  - Mechanical forces
- **Treatment:**
  - Elimination of spicy/acidic foods.
  - Small, frequent meals.
  - Decreasing amount of liquid consumed with each meal.
  - Limiting food and liquid intake a few hours prior to bedtime.
  - Sleeping with head elevated on pillows.
  - Utilizing liquid forms of antacids and H_2-receptor inhibitors.

Constipation

- Common in pregnancy.
- **Management:**
  - Increasing intake of high-fiber foods.
  - Increasing liquids.
  - Use of psyllium-containing products (eg, Metamucil).
  - Avoid enemas, strong cathartics, and laxatives.

Varicosities

- Common in pregnancy, particularly in lower extremities and vulva.
- Can cause chronic pain and superficial thrombophlebitis.
- **Management:**
  - Avoidance of garments that constrict at the knee and upper leg.
  - Use of support stockings.
  - ↑ periods of rest with elevation of the lower extremities.

Hemorrhoids

- Varicosities of the rectal veins are common in pregnancy.
- **Management:**
  - Cool sitz baths.
  - Stool softeners.
  - ↑ fluid and fiber intake to prevent constipation.
  - Hemorrhoidal ointment to ↓ swelling, itching, and discomfort.
  - Topical anesthetic spray or steroid cream for the severe pain of thrombosed hemorrhoids.

Why is dextrose included in the IV fluid for hyperemesis gravidarum? The dextrose helps to ↓ the ketosis, which can cause a vicious cycle of nausea. Dextrose can help break the cycle. "Morning sickness" can occur day or night.

Pregnancy is a hypercoagulable state, and there is an ↑ in clotting factor levels.

Hypercoagulable state and mechanical compression of venous blood flow from the lower extremities cause increased risk of thrombosis.

Most hemorrhoids improve after delivery.

Hemorrhoidectomy can be performed safely during pregnancy if necessary.

Leg Cramps

- Occur in 50% of pregnant women, typically at night and in T3.
- Most commonly occur in the calves.
- Massage and stretching of the affected muscle groups is recommended.

Backache

- Typically progressive in pregnancy (30–50%).
- **Management:**
  - Minimizing time standing.
  - Wearing a support belt over the lower abdomen.
  - Acetaminophen for pain as needed.
  - Exercises to ↑ back strength.
  - Supportive shoes and avoidance of high heels.
  - Gentle back massage.

Round Ligament Pain

- Sharp, bilateral or unilateral groin pain.
- Frequently occurs in T2.
- May ↑ with sudden movement/change in position.
- May be alleviated by patient getting on hands and knees with head on floor and buttocks in air.

Sexual Intercourse

- There are no restrictions during the normal pregnancy.
- Nipple stimulation, vaginal penetration, and orgasm may cause release of oxytocin and prostaglandins, resulting in uterine contractions.
- Contraindications:
  - Ruptured membranes
  - Placenta previa
  - Preterm labor

Employment

- Work activities that ↑ risk of falls/trauma should be avoided.
- Exposure to toxins/chemicals should be avoided.

Travel

- The best time to travel is in T2. Past possible complications of miscarriage in T1 and not yet encountered risk of preterm labor of T3.
- If prolonged sitting is involved, the patient should attempt to stretch her lower extremities and walk for 10 min every 2 hr. This is to avoid DVTs.
- The patient should bring a copy of her medical record.
- Wear seat belt when riding in car.
- Airplane travel in pressurized cabin presents no additional risk to the pregnant woman (if uncomplicated pregnancy). Air travel is not recommended after 35 weeks.
- In underdeveloped areas or when traveling abroad, the usual precautions regarding ingestion of unpurified water and raw foods should be taken. Appropriate vaccines should be given.

Immunizations (Table 4-2)

General principles:

- Delay vaccines until after the first trimester to avoid potential teratogenicity.
- Risk from vaccines is generally small. Always consider whether risk of the disease is worse than the risk of the vaccine.
- Live vaccines are not given in pregnancy.
- Viral vaccines may be safely given to the children of pregnant women.
- Immune globulins are safe in pregnancy and are recommended for women exposed to measles, hepatitis A and B, tetanus, varicella (chickenpox), and rabies.

> Ideally, women should avoid getting pregnant for 4 weeks after receiving live vaccines, such as measles, mumps, rubella (MMR) or varicella.

NOTIFY THE PHYSICIAN

While many physiologic changes in pregnancy are uncomfortable, most are nonemergent. There are, however, some situations when a pregnant woman should contact her obstetrician immediately:

- Vaginal bleeding.
- Leakage of fluid from the vagina.
- Rhythmic abdominal cramping or back pain, > 6/hr that does not improve with hydration and lying supine.
- Progressive and prolonged abdominal pain.
- Fever and chills.
- Dysuria or abnormally cloudy urine (indicative of a urinary tract infection).
- Prolonged vomiting with inability to hold down liquids or solids for > 24 hr.
- Progressive, severe headache; visual changes; or generalized edema (preeclamptic symptoms).
- Seizure (eclampsia).
- Pronounced ↓ in frequency or intensity of fetal movements.

TABLE 4-2. Vaccine Safety in Pregnancy

SAFE	NOT WELL STUDIED IN PREGNANT WOMEN, SO DEFER UNTIL FURTHER RECOMMENDATIONS ISSUED	ADMINISTER ONLY IF RISK OUTWEIGHS BENEFIT	UNSAFE (LIVE)
■ Inactivated polio (IPV)	■ Human papillomavirus (HPV)	■ Yellow fever	■ Oral polio
■ Inactivated typhoid	■ Meningococcus (MPV4)	■ Anthrax	■ Oral typhoid
■ Inactivated influenza	■ Pneumococcus (PPV)	■ Pertussis	■ Intranasal influenza
■ Diphtheria	■ Hepatitis A		■ Measles, mumps, rubella (MMR)
■ Tetanus			■ Varicella
■ Rabies			■ Bacillus Calmette-Guérin (BCG)
■ Meningococcus (MPSV4)			■ Shingles
■ Hepatitis B			

HIGH-YIELD FACTS

Antepartum

CHAPTER 5

Intrapartum

A 25-year-old Hispanic female, G1P0, at 38 weeks gestation presents to triage complaining of contractions that have been increasing in strength and frequency over a 12-hr period. She denies vaginal bleeding, leakage of fluid and preeclampsia symptoms. She reports good fetal movement. Fetal heart rate is reassuring. She is contracting every 2 min on the monitor. Her cervical exam is 6 cm dilated, 50% effaced, 0 station, cephalic by sutures. What stage of labor is she in? If her labor progresses as expected, what should her cervical dilation be at the next vaginal exam in 2 hours?

Answer: She is in the active phase of the first stage of labor. Since she is a primigravida, her cervix should dilate at a minimum of 1.2 cm/hr. So, in 2 hours, she should be 8.4 cm (or 8–9 cm) dilated.

Labor is defined as contractions that result in cervical change. The progression of labor is illustrated in Figure 5-1.

First Stage

- The first stage of labor begins with onset of uterine contractions of sufficient frequency, intensity, and duration to result in effacement and dilation of the cervix, and ends when the cervix is fully/completely dilated to 10 cm.
- The first stage of labor consists of **two phases**:
  1. **Latent phase:** Begins with the onset of labor and ends at approximately 4 cm cervical dilation.

Duration of labor is typically shorter in the multiparous woman than in nulliparous women.

There are three stages of labor, and two phases of stage 1.

Labor is defined as contractions resulting in cervical change.

Remember the three "Ps" that affect the duration of the active phase of labor:
- **Power** (strength and frequency of contractions)
- **Passenger** (size of the baby)
- **Pelvis** (size and shape of mother's pelvis)

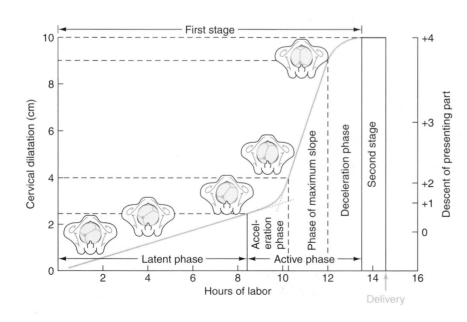

FIGURE 5-1. Progression of labor.

(Reproduced, with permission, from DeCherney AH, Pernoll ML. *Current Obstetrics & Gynecologic Diagnosis & Treatment*. Norwalk, CT: Appleton & Lange, 1994: 211.)

HIGH-YIELD FACTS

Intrapartum

If progress during the active phase is slower than these figures, evaluation for adequacy of uterine contractions, fetal malposition, or cephalopelvic disproportion should be done.

Abnormalities of the second stage may be either protraction or arrest of descent (the fetal head descends < 1 cm/hr in a nullipara and < 2 cm/hr in a multipara).

If 30 min have passed without placental extrusion, manual removal of the placenta may be required.

What are the three signs of placental separation?
1. Gush of blood
2. Umbilical cord lengthening
3. Fundus of uterus rises and firms

- ■ Nulliparous: Prolonged if > 20 hr.
- ■ Multiparous: Prolonged if > 14 hr.
2. **Active phase:** Rapid dilation. Begins at 4 cm dilation and ends at 10 cm.
   - ■ Active phase is further classified according to the rate of cervical dilation: **Acceleration phase, phase of maximum slope,** and **deceleration phase.**
   - ■ Fetal descent begins at 7–8 cm of dilation in nulliparas and becomes most rapid after 8 cm.
   - ■ Average duration of cervical dilation from 4 to 10 cm (minimal normal rate):
     - ■ Nulliparous: < 1.2 cm/hr
     - ■ Multiparous: < 1.5 cm/hr

Second Stage

The second stage of labor is the stage of **fetal expulsion.** It begins when the cervix is fully dilated and ends with the delivery of the fetus.

Average Pattern of Fetal Descent

- ■ Nulliparous: < 2 hr (3 with epidural)
- ■ Multiparous: < 1 hr (2 with epidural)

Third Stage

The main event of the third stage is **placental separation.** It begins immediately after the delivery of the fetus and ends with the delivery of the fetal and placental membranes.

- ■ **Duration:** Usually < 10 minutes; considered prolonged if > 30 minutes.
- ■ The three signs of placental separation are:
  1. Gush of blood from vagina.
  2. Umbilical cord lengthening.
  3. Fundus of the uterus rises up and becomes firm.

TRUE LABOR VERSUS FALSE LABOR

False Labor (Braxton Hicks Contractions)	True Labor
Occur at irregular intervals	Occur at regular intervals that shorten
Intensity remains the same	↑ in intensity
Discomfort in lower abdomen	Discomfort in back and lower abdomen
No cervical change	Cervix dilates
Relieved by medications / sedation	**Not** relieved by medications

History

- Patients without prenatal care require a complete history and physical (H&P), and those with prenatal care require an update and focused physical. Prenatal record should be obtained when possible.
- The following information should always be obtained from a laboring patient:
  - Time of onset and frequency of contractions.
  - Status of fetal membranes. Typical history for ruptured membranes: gush of fluid with continuous leakage. Color may be clear or yellow/green (meconium).
  - Presence/absence of vaginal bleeding. Bloody show is small amount of blood mixed with cervical mucus that is present with cervical dilation and effacement. It should be distinguished from vaginal bleeding.
  - Notation of fetal activity.
  - Symptoms of preeclampsia (headache, visual disturbances, right upper quadrant pain).
  - History of allergies.
  - How long ago patient consumed food or liquids and how much (mostly in case the patient needs to undergo a cesarean delivery).
  - Use of medications.

Vaginal Exam (VE)

- Perform a sterile **speculum** exam first if:
  - Rupture of membranes is suspected.
  - The patient is in preterm labor.
  - Bleeding suspicious for placenta previa is present.
- Otherwise, a sterile **digital** VE may be performed.

Rupture of Membranes

> A 25-year-old G1P0 at 39 weeks presents to labor and delivery triage complaining of a gush of fluid from the vagina followed by constant leakage for 2 hr. The fluid is clear and without odor. What tests can help determine whether the patient has ruptured the membranes and the fluid is amniotic fluid?
>
> **Answer:** Perform a sterile speculum exam, testing for pooling, valsalva, ferning, and nitrazine. If these are positive, the membranes are likely ruptured and the fluid noted on the exam is likely amniotic fluid.

- Perform a sterile speculum exam:
  1. **Pooling:** The presence of fluid collection in the posterior fornix should be noted (positive pooling).
  2. **Valsalva:** Ask the patient to bear down and perform a Valsalva manuever. Note if fluid is seen to come through the cervical os (positive Valsalva).

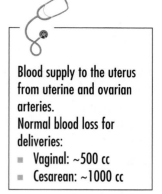

Blood supply to the uterus from uterine and ovarian arteries.
Normal blood loss for deliveries:
- Vaginal: ~500 cc
- Cesarean: ~1000 cc

What can cause a false-positive nitrazine test?
- Vaginal infections with *Trichomonas vaginalis*
- Blood
- Semen

Diagnosis of ROM
The patient's history alone is correct in 90% of patients. Urinary leakage or excess vaginal discharge can be mistaken for ROM.

Spontaneous rupture of membranes (SROM) most often occurs during the course of active labor.

Vernix: The fatty substance consisting of desquamated epithelial cells and sebaceous matter that normally covers the skin of the term fetus.

Meconium: A dark green fecal material that collects in the fetal intestines and is discharged at or near the time of birth.

3. **Ferning:** Place a thin layer of the fluid on a slide. View the dried amniotic fluid under a microscope for a characteristic ferning pattern made by the crystallized sodium chloride in the amniotic fluid (positive ferning). Confirms ROM in 85–98% of cases (see Figure 5-2).

4. **Nitrazine:** Place the vaginal fluid on nitrazine paper to assess the pH. If nitrazine paper turns blue, this indicates basic pH (positive nitrazine). Amniotic fluid has basic pH as compared to vaginal secretions that have acidic pH. Confirms ROM in 90–98% of cases.

■ The presence of pooling, valsalva, ferning, and nitrazine indicates that the membranes are likely ruptured and the fluid noted on the exam is amniotic fluid.

■ Fluid should also be examined for meconium.

■ The presence of meconium in the amniotic fluid may indicate fetal stress.

■ Meconium staining is more common in term and postterm pregnancies than in preterm pregnancies.

■ **Meconium aspiration syndrome (MAS):** Fetal stress, like hypoxia, leads to meconium in the amniotic fluid. With further fetal gasping, the meconium is inhaled into the fetal lungs, causing lung damage. At birth, the infant will present with respiratory distress and can develop pulmonary hypertension. Intubation does not provide adequate oxygenation due to the lung injury and pulmonary hypertension. Infants with MAS may require extracorporeal membranous oxygenation which bypasses the lungs in order to provide oxygen to the baby. Prevent MAS via amnioinfusion intrapartum and fetal nasopharynx suction postpartum.

FIGURE 5-2. Ferning pattern.

Cervical Exam

There are five parameters of the cervix that are examined: dilation, effacement, station, consistency, and position.

DILATION

Describes the size of the **opening** of the cervix at the external os.

- **Ranges:** Ranges from zero to 10 cm dilated (closed to completely dilated). The presenting part of a term-sized infant can usually pass through a cervix that is fully dilated.
- **Determination of dilation:** The index and/or the middle fingers are inserted in the cervical opening and are separated as far as the cervix will allow. The distance (cervical dilation) between the two fingers is estimated.

EFFACEMENT

Describes the **length of the cervix.** With labor, the cervix thins out and softens, and the length is reduced. The normal length is 3–4 cm.

- **Terminology:** When the cervix shortens by 50% (to around 2 cm), it is said to be 50% effaced. When the cervix becomes as thin as the adjacent lower uterine segment, it is 100% effaced.
- **Determination of effacement:** Palpate with finger and estimate the length from the internal to external os.

STATION

Describes the degree of **descent** of the presenting part in relation to ischial spines, which are designated at 0 station.

- **Terminology** (two systems):
  1. The ischial spine is zero station, and the areas above and below are divided into thirds. Above the ischial spines are stations –3, –2, and –1, with –3 being the furthest above the ischial spines and –1 being closest. Positive stations describe fetal descent below the ischial spines. +3 station is at the level of the introitus, and +1 is just past the ischial spines.
  2. Very similar except that the areas above and below the ischial spines are divided by centimeters, up to 5 cm above and 5 cm below. Above are five stations or centimeters: –5, –4, –3, –2, and –1, with –5 being the 5 cm above the ischial spines and –1 being 1 cm above. Positive stations describe fetal descent below the ischial spines. +5 station is at the level of the introitus, and +1 is 1 cm past the ischial spines.
- If the fetus is vertex, the station should be determined by the location of the biparietal diameter (BPD), not the tip top of the head, which may simply be caput and not the head at all. So when the BPD is at the level of the ischial spines, the station is 0.

Know this cervical exam stuff cold for the wards!

CONSISTENCY

Breakdown of collagen bonds in the cervix changes the consistency of the cervix progressively from <u>firm</u> to <u>medium</u> to <u>soft</u>, in preparation for dilation and labor.

POSITION

Describes the location of cervix with respect to the fetal presenting part. It is classified as one of the following:

- **Posterior:** Difficult to palpate because it is behind the presenting part, and usually high in the pelvis.
- **Midposition**.
- **Anterior:** Easy to palpate, low in pelvis.

During labor, the cervical position usually progresses from posterior to anterior.

D E S C P

Bishop Score

A 26-year-old G2P1001 at 41 weeks presents to the hospital for an induction. Her dates are verified, and the infant is noted to be cephalic presentation. Her cervical exam is 3 cm dilation, 70% effaced, −2 station, anterior position, and soft. What is her Bishop score? What is the likelihood of a successful vaginal delivery?

Answer: Her Bishop score is 9 showing that she has a favorable cervix for induction of labor. Her chance of vaginal delivery is similar to those who present in spontaneous labor.

Labor-inducing agents:
- **Vaginal prostaglandins** are inserted for ripening (softening) of cervix.
- **IV pitocin** is used to ↑ strength and frequency of contractions.

This is a scoring system that helps to determine the status of the cervix—favorable or unfavorable—for successful vaginal delivery.

- If induction of labor is indicated, the status of the cervix must be evaluated to help determine the method of labor induction that will be utilized. See Table 5-1 and section on Labor Induction.
- A score of ≥6 indicates that the probability of vaginal delivery with induction of labor is similar to that of spontaneous labor.

TABLE 5-1. Bishop Scoring System

FACTOR	0 POINTS	1 POINT	2 POINTS	3 POINTS
Dilation (cm)	Closed	1–2	3–4	≥ 5
Effacement (%)	0 –30	40 –50	60 –70	≥ 80
Station[a]	−3	−2	−1 to 0	+1 to +3
Consistency	Firm	Medium	Soft	—
Position	Posterior	Midposition	Anterior	—

[a] Station reflects −3 to +3 scale.

Leopold Maneuvers

- Leopold maneuvers are begun in late pregnancy to determine which way the baby is presenting in the uterus. (Figure 5-3). Consist of four parts:
    - **First maneuver** answers the question: "What fetal part occupies the fundus?"
    - **Second maneuver** answers the question: "On what side is the fetal back?"
    - **Third maneuver** answers the question: "What fetal part lies over the pelvic inlet?"
    - **Fourth maneuver** answers the question: "On which side is the cephalic prominence?"
- Four aspects of the fetus are described from the Leopold maneuvers:
    - Lie
    - Presentation
    - Position
    - Attitude

FIGURE 5-3. Leopold maneuvers.

(Reproduced, with permission, from Pernoll ML. *Benson & Pernoll's Handbook of Obstetrics and Gynecology*, 10th ed. New York: McGraw-Hill, 2001: 159.)

LIE

Lie describes the relation of the long axis of the fetus to that of the mother. A **longitudinal** (99% of term or near-term births) lie can be vertex (head first) or breech (buttocks first). The lie may be **transverse** or **oblique**.

PRESENTATION/PRESENTING PART

Describes the portion of the fetus that is foremost within the birth canal. It is normally determined by palpating through the cervix on vaginal examination.

- If the lie is longitudinal, the presentation is either the head (cephalic), buttocks (breech), brow, or face. The most common type of presentation is the **vertex presentation** in which the posterior fontanel is the presenting part.
- If the lie is transverse, the shoulder, back, or abdomen may be the presenting part.

POSITION

Refers to the relation of the presenting part to the right (R) or left (L) side of the birth canal and its direction anteriorly (A), transversely (T), or posteriorly (P).

- The top of the **fetal skull** is composed of five bones: two frontal, two parietal, and one occipital. The anterior fontanel lies where the two frontal and two parietal meet, and the posterior fontanel lies where the two parietal meet the occipital bone.
- For a cephalic presentation, the **occiput** is used as the reference point to determine the position:
  - Occiput anterior (OA)
  - Occiput posterior (OP)
  - Left occiput anterior (LOA)
  - Left occiput posterior (LOP)
  - Left occiput transverse (LOT)
  - Right occiput anterior (ROA)
  - Right occiput posterior (ROP)
  - Right occiput transverse (ROT)
- The **chin** is used as the reference point for face presentation. The **sacrum** is used as the reference point for breech presentation.

ATTITUDE AND POSTURE

In the later months of pregnancy, the fetus assumes a characteristic posture ("attitude/habitus"), which typically describes the position of the arms, legs, spine, neck, and face.

Normal Presentation

VERTEX PRESENTATION (OCCIPUT PRESENTATION)

Vertex presentation is **most common** (96% of term or near-term presentations). The head is flexed so that the chin is in contact with the chest. The **posterior fontanel** is the presenting part. This creates the shortest diameter of the fetal skull that has to pass through the pelvis.

Anterior fontanel: Larger diamond shape

Posterior fontanel: Smaller triangle shape

Interpreting Fetal Positions

Imagine the mother lying in the dorsal lithotomy position (on her back, legs in stirrups) and the baby's occiput in relation to her body. You are at the end of the bed looking between mom's legs. Figure 5-4 represents the mother's birth canal with the fetal head in various positions.

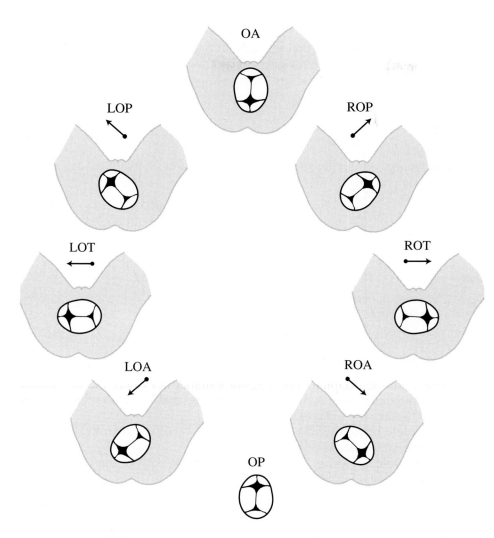

FIGURE 5-4. Vertex positions.

Malpresentations

FACE PRESENTATION

In face presentation (0.3% of presentations at or near term), the fetal neck is sharply extended so the occiput is in contact with the fetal back. The face is the presenting part. Diagnosis is made by palpation of the fetal face on vaginal exam.

SINCIPUT PRESENTATION

The fetal head assumes a position between vertex presentation and face presentation so that the <u>anterior fontanel</u> presents first.

BROW PRESENTATION

The fetal head assumes a position such that the eyebrows present first. This forces a large diameter through the pelvis; usually, vaginal delivery is possible only if the presentation is converted to a face or vertex presentation.

Ninety percent of babies presenting in the occiput **posterior** position spontaneously rotate to occiput **anterior** position.

Vaginal delivery is possible only if the fetus is mentum anterior; mentum posterior cannot deliver vaginally—must be delivered by cesarean section.

A pregnant woman presents at 31 weeks gestation with a breech presentation. What's your next step? Recheck fetal presentation at 36 weeks and then attempt external cephalic version if persistent breech. *Note:* If < 34 weeks, malpresentation not uncommon and not significant.

BREECH PRESENTATIONS

In breech presentations, the presenting fetal part is the **buttocks**. Incidence: 3.5% at or near term but much greater in early pregnancy (14%). Those found in early pregnancy will often spontaneously convert to vertex as term approaches.

RISK FACTORS

- Low birth weight (20–30% of breeches).
- Congenital anomalies such as hydrocephalus or anencephaly.
- Uterine anomalies.
- Multiple gestation.
- Placenta previa.
- Hydramnios, oligohydramnios.
- Multiparity.

DIAGNOSIS

- Leopold maneuvers
- Ultrasound
- Vaginal exam

TYPES OF BREECH (SEE FIGURE 5-5)

- **Frank breech (65%):** The thighs are flexed (bent forward) and knees are extended (straight) over the anterior surfaces of the body (feet are in front of the head or face).
- **Complete breech (25%):** The thighs are flexed (bent) on the abdomen and the knees are flexed (folded) as well.
- **Incomplete (footling) breech (10%):** One or both of the hips are not flexed so that a foot lies below the buttocks.

A   **B**   **C**

FIGURE 5-5. **Types of breech presentations.**

A. Frank breech. B. Complete breech. C. Incomplete breech (single footling). (Reproduced, with permission, from Cunningham FG, Leveno KJ, Bloom SL, et al. *Williams Obstetrics*, 23rd ed. New York: McGraw-Hill, 2010: 528–529.)

- Most frequently, the delivery is via cesarean.
- Frank breech positions with other ideal conditions may deliver vaginally.
- **External cephalic version:** Procedure that maneuvers the infant to a cephalic position by applying pressure through the maternal abdomen. Can be done only if breech is diagnosed before onset of labor and the gestational age is 35–37 weeks. The success rate is 50%, and the risks are placental abruption, fetal heart rate abnormalities, and reversion.

CARDINAL MOVEMENTS OF LABOR

The cardinal movements of labor are movements of the fetal head that allows it to pass through the birth canal. The movements are as follows: engagement, descent, flexion, internal rotation, extension, and external rotation (restitution). Delivery of the shoulders follows (see Figure 5-6).

Engagement

The descent of the biparietal diameter (the largest transverse diameter of the fetal head, 9.5 cm) through the plane of the pelvic inlet. Can occur in late pregnancy or in labor. Clinically if the presenting part is at 0 station, the head is thought to be engagd in the pelvis. *@ ischial spines*

Descent

Occurs when the fetal head passes down into the pelvis. It occurs in a discontinuous fashion. The greatest rate of descent is in the deceleration phase of the first stage of labor and during the second stage of labor.

Flexion

Occurs when the chin is brought close to the fetal thorax. This passive motion facilitates the presentation of the smallest possible diameter of the fetal head to the birth canal.

Internal Rotation

Refers to turning of the head that moves the occiput gradually toward the symphysis pubis or less commonly toward the hollow of the sacrum.

Extension

Extension moves the occiput toward the fetal back:

- Occurs after the fetus has descended to the level of the maternal vulva.
- This action brings the base of the occiput into contact with the inferior margin of the symphysis pubis, where the birth canal curves upward.
- The delivery of the fetal head occurs when it changes from the flexed to the extended position, curving under and past the pubic symphysis.

Complete and incomplete breeches are not delivered vaginally due to risk of umbilical cord prolapse.

Engagement is determined by palpation of the presenting part of the occiput.

The fundal height ↓ at term due to engagement of the fetus.

FIGURE 5-6. Cardinal movements of labor.

(Reproduced, with permission, from Cunningham FG, Leveno KJ, Bloom SL, et al. *Williams Obstetrics*, 22nd ed. New York: McGraw-Hill, 2005: 418.)

External Rotation (Restitution)

Occurs after delivery of the head, when the fetus resumes its normal "face-forward" position with the occiput and spine lying in the same plane. One shoulder is anterior behind the pubic symphysis, and the other is posterior.

Expulsion

After external rotation, further descent brings the anterior shoulder to the level of the pubic symphysis. The shoulder is delivered under the pubic symphysis, and then the rest of the body is quickly delivered.

NORMAL SPONTANEOUS VERTEX VAGINAL DELIVERY

Delivery of the Head

- Place fingers of one hand on the occiput as it is seen passing under the symphysis pubis to control the delivery of the head and avoid lacerations.
- Evaluate the posterior vagina and perineum to assess for the need of an episiotomy. Performing an episiotomy may create more room for the fetus to deliver.
- With maternal effort, the infant's head will deliver and restitute either to the left or the right.
- Bulb suction the infant's mouth first, then the nares. Remember to squeeze the bulb first, place it inside the baby, then release.

Checking for Nuchal Cord

- Occurs when loops of umbilical cord wrap around the fetal neck. To check for this condition, following delivery of the head, a finger should be passed along the fetal neck to ascertain the presence of the cord.
- If nuchal cord is present, a finger should be slipped under the cord and, if loose enough, the cord should be slipped over the infant's head.
- If the cord is wrapped tightly around the infant's neck, it should be cut between two clamps.

Delivery of Shoulders

- Most frequently, the shoulders appear at the vulva just after external rotation and are delivered spontaneously.
- Occasionally, the shoulders must be extracted:
    - The sides of the head are grasped with both hands and *gentle* downward traction is applied until the anterior shoulder descends from under the pubic arch.
    - Next, *gentle* upward traction is applied to deliver the posterior shoulder.

Delivery of the Infant

- The rest of the infant is delivered with maternal pushing.
- Support the infant's head with one hand by grasping the neck, taking care not to grasp the throat.
- Support the infant's buttocks as they are delivered with the other hand.

The anterior shoulder is the one closest to the superior portions of the vagina, while the posterior shoulder is closest to the perineum and anus.

Fundal pressure should never be used to relieve a shoulder dystocia.

Squeeze the bulb between fingers first, then place in fetal mouth/nares.

Know your Apgar scores: Assigns score of 0–2 for the following:
- Color
- Pulse
- Respirations
- Grimace
- Tone

Signs of placental separation typically occur within 5 min of infant delivery.

Placental delivery should *never* be forced before placental separation has occurred; otherwise, uterine inversion may occur.

There are two umbilical arteries and one umbilical vein in the cord.

Proper repair of fourth-degree laceration is essential to prevent future fecal incontinence and rectovaginal fistula.

- Transfer the infant's buttocks in the crook of the elbow of the hand that is holding the head. This frees the other hand to suction the baby and clamp and cut the cord.
- Hand the baby to the nurse or pediatrician.

Delivery of the Placenta

- Obtain arterial pH if indicated, and venous blood for fetal blood typing.
- Monitor for signs of placental separation:
    - There is often a sudden gush of blood.
    - Uterus becomes globular and firmer.
    - The uterus rises in the abdomen after the bulk of the separated placenta passes into the vagina.
    - The umbilical cord lengthens, indicating descent of the placenta.
- Apply pressure with one hand in the suprapubic region and apply gentle traction on the umbilical cord to guide placenta out.
- Once placenta is past the introitus, grasp with hands and gently remove membranes. Inspect the placenta for intact cotyledons and three-vessel cord.
- Perform fundal massage to help the uterus contract down and ↓ the bleeding.

Inspection

Inspect patient for any lacerations or extensions of episiotomy that may need to be repaired. Look at:

- Circumferential cervix
- Vaginal walls
- Labia
- Perineum

Perineal Lacerations

The perineum and anus become stretched and thin, which results in ↑ risk of spontaneous lacerations to the vagina, labia, perineum, and rectum.

- **First degree:** Involve the fourchette, perineal skin, and vaginal mucosa, but not the underlying fascia and muscle (skid mark).
- **Second degree:** First degree plus the fascia and muscle of the perineal body but *not* the anal sphincter.
- **Third degree:** Second degree plus involvement of the anal sphincter.
- **Fourth degree:** Extend through the rectal mucosa to expose the lumen of the rectum.

TABLE 5-2. Midline Versus Mediolateral Episiotomy

CHARACTERISTICS	MIDLINE	MEDIOLATERAL
Surgical repair	Easy	More difficult
Faulty healing	Rare	More common
Postoperative pain	Minimal	Common
Anatomical results	Excellent	Occasionally faulty
Blood loss	Less	More
Dyspareunia	Rare	Occasional
Extensions	Common	Uncommon

(Reproduced, with permission, from Cunningham FG, Leveno KJ, Bloom SL, et al. *Williams Obstetrics*, 22nd ed. New York: McGraw-Hill, 2005: 436.)

Episiotomy

The incision of the perineum and/or labia to aid delivery by creating more room. The classification of episiotomy is the same as perineal lacerations. Table 5-2 compares the two different types of episiotomies:

1. **Midline:** The incision is made in the midline from the posterior fourchette. Most common. ↑ the risk of a fourth-degree laceration.
2. **Mediolateral:** The incision is oblique starting from 5 o'clock or 7 o'clock position of the vagina. Causes more bleeding and pain.

Postdelivery Hemostasis

After the uterus has been emptied and the placenta delivered, hemostasis must be achieved:

- The primary mechanism is myometrial contraction leading to vasoconstriction.
- Fundal massage stimulates uterine contraction.
- Oxytocin (Pitocin) is administered in the third stage of labor. It causes myometrial contractions and reduces maternal blood loss.
- Postpartum hemorrhage: Often defined as > 500 mL of blood loss for vaginal delivery and > 1000 mL for C-section.

Most common cause for postpartum hemorrhage = Uterine atony. Treat with uterotonics like pitocin, methergine, hemabate, misoprostol.

Postpartum hemorrhage causes —
The 4 T's
Tissue: Retained placenta
Trauma: Instrumentation, lacerations, episiotomy
Tone: Uterine atony
Thrombin: Coagulation defects, DIC

MANAGEMENT OF PATIENTS IN LABOR

Vaginal Exams

Vaginal examinations should be kept to the minimum number required for the evaluation of a normal labor pattern, for example, every 4 hr in latent phase and every 2 hr in active phase. Sterile gloves and lubricant should be used.

HIGH-YIELD FACTS

Intrapartum

Inhalation anesthesia may be needed for cesarean delivery or for management of complications in the third stage of labor. Thus, consumption of foods or liquids is discouraged in order to avoid aspiration.

Arrest of labor: Lack of cervical change in active first stage for > 2 hr with > 200 Montevideo units of uterine activity.

The most common cause of maternal mortality in the Western world is postpartum hemorrhage.

Maternal Vital Signs

Maternal blood pressure and pulse should be evaluated and recorded every 10 min.

Other Considerations

Usually, oral intake is limited to small sips of water, ice chips, or hard candies.

MONITORING DURING LABOR

During labor, uterine contractions and fetal heart rate are monitored closely.

Uterine Contractions

Uterine activity is monitored by external or internal uterine monitors.

- **External monitors:**
  - Accurately display the frequency of the contraction.
  - More commonly used unless more detailed information is needed.
- **Intrauterine pressure catheters:**
  - Record frequency, duration, and strength of the contraction.
  - Strength of contraction measured in **Montevideo units.**
    - Calculated by ↑ in uterine pressure above baseline multiplied by contraction frequency over 10 min.
    - If you have time, don't multiply—add every contraction.

Fetal Heart Rate

The **fetal heart rate (FHR)** can be assessed in two ways:

1. **Intermittent** auscultation with a fetal stethoscope or Doppler ultrasonic device.
2. **Continuous** electronic monitoring of the FHR and uterine contractions is most commonly used in United States. The standard fetal monitor tracing records the fetal heart rate on the top portion and the contractions on the bottom.
   - **External (indirect) electronic FHR monitoring:** FHR is detected using a Doppler device placed on the maternal abdomen.
   - **Internal electronic FHR monitoring:** Done with a bipolar spiral electrode attached to fetal scalp, which detects the peak R-wave voltage of the fetal electrocardiogram. This is more invasive and is used if closer fetal monitoring is required.

FETAL HEART RATE PATTERNS

- The normal baseline for the fetal heart rate is 110–160 bpm.
- Baseline rate refers to the most common heart rate lasting ≥ 10 minutes.
- Periodic changes above and below termed **accelerations** (↑ in HR) and **decelerations** (↓ in HR).

- A **reassuring** fetal tracing has two accelerations of at least 15 beats/min above the baseline, lasting for at least 15 sec, in 20 min. It indicates a well oxygenated fetus with an intact neurological and cardiovascular system.

Definitions

- **Hypoxemia:** ↓ oxygen content in blood.
- **Hypoxia:** ↓ level of oxygen in tissue.
- **Acidemia:** ↑ concentration of hydrogen ions in the blood.
- **Acidosis:** ↑ concentration of hydrogen ions in tissue.
- **Asphyxia:** Hypoxia with metabolic acidosis. Goal of fetal monitoring during labor is to avoid metabolic acidosis and asphyxia, which can cause permanent neurological injury.

Decelerations

A 32-year-old G2P1001 at 40 weeks gestation presents to labor and delivery with contractions. She is noted to be 5 cm dilated, 50% effaced, –1 station, cephalic by sutures. The monitor shows contractions every 2 min, and the FHR pattern shows a baseline of 150 beats/min, minimal variability, and gradual decelerations that nadir after the peak of the contractions. No accelerations are noted. What is the most likely cause of the findings on the FHR? What is the next step in management?

Answer: Uteroplacental insufficiency is the most likely cause for this patient's late decelerations. The patient should be turned on her left side to maximize oxygenation to the fetus. Administer oxygen to the mother. Fetal scalp electrode and an intrauterine pressure catheter (internal monitors) will help with the FHR monitoring. A search for the cause of uteroplacental insufficiency should be carried out.

Decelerations during labor have different interpretations depending on when they occur in relation to contractions. (See Table 5-3 and Figure 5-7.)

EARLY DECELERATIONS

- Early decelerations are *normal* and are due to **head compression** during contractions usually between 4 and 7 cm dilation.
- The nadir of the gradual deceleration corresponds to the peak of the contraction.
- The effect is regulated gradual by vagal nerve activation.
- No intervention is necessary.

LATE DECELERATIONS

- Late decelerations are *abnormal* and are due to **uteroplacental insufficiency** (blood without enough oxygen) during contractions.
- They are a gradual decrease below the baseline with onset, nadir, and recovery occurring after uterine contraction onset, peak, and recovery, respectively.
- Can follow epidural (hypotension) or uterine hyperstimulation.

When reading the fetal tracing, **always** note the following:
1. Baseline
2. Variability
3. Presence of accelerations
4. Presence of decelerations
5. Contractions

Reactive: 15 beats/min above the baseline lasting 15 sec; 2 × /20 min.

A fetus < 28 weeks gestation age is neurologically immature and thus is not expected to have a "reactive" FHR.

The left lateral recumbent position is best for maximizing cardiac output and uterine blood flow. (In the supine position, the vena cava and aortoiliac vessels may be compressed by the gravid uterus.)

TABLE 5-3. Types of Decelerations

	EARLY DECELERATION	LATE DECELERATION	VARIABLE DECELERATION
Significance	Benign	Abnormal	Variable
Shape	U shaped	U shaped	Variable (often V or W shaped)
Onset	Gradual	Gradual	Abrupt
Depth	Shallow	Shallow	Variable
When	Nadir of decel = peak of ctx	Start and end after the uterine ctx Nadir of decel after peak of ctx	Variable
Why	Head compression	Uteroplacental insufficiency	Cord compression
Initial treatment	None required	O₂, lateral decubitus position, Pitocin off, close monitoring	Amnioinfusion

Ctx, contraction; decel, deceleration; **gradual**, baseline to nadir > 30 sec; **abrupt**, baseline to nadir < 30 sec.

STOP when you see decelerations:
Sterile vaginal exam
Turn the patient to her left side
Give the patient **O**xygen
Pitocin off

MANAGEMENT

- Change maternal position to the left lateral recumbent position.
- Give oxygen by facemask.
- Stop oxytocin (Pitocin) infusion.
- Provide an IV fluid bolus.
- Consider tocolysis.
- Monitor maternal blood pressure. Treat hypotension with medications.
- Sterile vaginal exam to assess for change in fetal station or position.
- If repetitive (> 50% of the contractions have late decelerations) and no other reassuring finding present, consider immediate delivery.

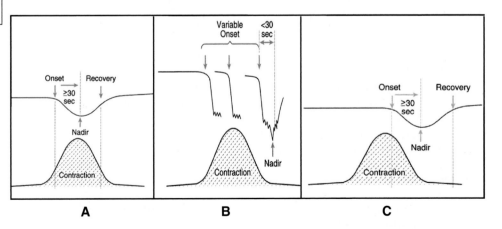

FIGURE 5-7. Features of early (A), variable (B), and late (C) decelerations on fetal heart monitoring.

(Reproduced, with permission, from Cunningham FG, Leveno KJ, Bloom SL, et al. *Williams Obstetrics*, 22nd ed. New York: McGraw-Hill, 2005: 452–454.)

84

TABLE 5-4. Classification of Variable Decelerations

Mild	Lasts < 30 sec and depth > 70–80 beats/min
Moderate	Lasts 30–60 sec and depth < 70–80 beats/min **OR** Lasts > 60 sec and depth = 70–80 beats/min
Severe	Lasts > 60 sec and depth < 70 beats/min

VARIABLE DECELERATIONS

- Variable decelerations are *abnormal* and can be mild, moderate, or severe (Table 5-4).
- They are due to **cord compression** and can be seen with oligohydramnios or a nuchal cord.
- Abrupt deceleration that looks like a "v".
- They can occur at any time.

MANAGEMENT

- **Amnioinfusion:** Infuse normal saline into the uterus through the intrauterine pressure catheter to alleviate cord compression. Most commonly used for severe variable decelerations.
- Change maternal position to side/Trendelenburg position.
- Plan delivery of fetus soon if worsening or nonreassuring.

PROLONGED DECELERATIONS

Isolated decelerations that last 2–10 min. Causes include:

- Cervical examinations.
- Uterine hyperactivity.
- Maternal hypotension leading to transient fetal hypoxia.
- Umbilical cord compression.

MANAGEMENT

- Stop oxytocin and prostaglandins.
- Change maternal position.
- Administer IV fluids.
- If mother is hypotensive, administer vasopressors.
- Administer maternal O_2.
- Sterile vaginal exam to exclude cord prolapse, sudden cervical dilation, or fetal descent.

Fetal Tachycardia

- Baseline HR > 160 beats/min for ≥ 10 min.
- Causes:
  - Fetal hypoxia
  - Intrauterine infection
  - Maternal fever
  - Drugs

If an FHR of 160 beats/min lasts for ≥ 10 min, then tachycardia is present.

Scalp stimulation is done between decelerations to elicit a reactive acceleration and rule out metabolic acidosis.

Internal FHR monitoring is the best way to determine BTBV.

Short-term variability is thought to be the most important predictor of fetal outcome.

No BTBV = *fetal acidosis,* and the fetus must be delivered immediately.

Beat-to-Beat Variability (BTBV)

- **The single most important characteristic of the baseline FHR.**
- Variation of successive beats in the FHR BTBV is controlled primarily by the autonomic nervous system. ↑ in FHR is due to activation of the sympathetic nervous system. The ↓ in the FHR is due to the activation of the parasympathetic nervous system. The constant push and pull of the sympathetic and parasympathetic systems creates the BTBV, which indicates intact fetal CNS.
- At < 28 weeks gestational age, the fetus is neurologically immature; thus, ↓ variability is expected.

DECREASES IN BTBV

Beat-to-beat variability ↓ with:

- Fetal acidemia.
- Fetal asphyxia.
- Maternal acidemia.
- Drugs (narcotics, magnesium sulfate [$MgSO_4$], barbiturates, etc.).
- Acquired or congenital neurologic abnormality.

INCREASES IN BTBV

Beat-to-beat variability ↑ with mild fetal hypoxemia.

Short-Term Variability (STV)

- Reflects instantaneous beat-to-beat (R wave to R wave) changes in FHR.
- The *roughness* (STV present) or *smoothness* (STV absent) of the FHR tracing.
- May be ↓/absent due to alterations in the CNS or inadequate fetal oxygenation.

Long-Term Variability (LTV)

- Describes the oscillatory changes that occur in 1 min.
- Results in waviness of baseline.
- Normal: 3–6 cycles/min.

ABNORMAL LABOR PATTERNS

Dystocia

A 32-year-old G3P2002 at 38 weeks is admitted to labor and delivery for active labor. Two hours ago her cervical exam was 5 cm/80% effaced/−2 station. Her exam now is 6 cm/80% effaced/−2 station. What is her labor pattern? What is the next step in management?

Answer: She has a protracted active phase. Since she is a multipara, she should dilate 1.5 cm/hr at a minimum and should have been 8 cm over a span of 2 hr. The next step in management is to determine if there are adequate contractions, if the fetal size and position are amenable for a vaginal delivery, and whether the pelvis is adequate for a normal vaginal delivery.

TABLE 5-5. Abnormal Labor Patterns

LABOR PATTERN	NULLIPARAS	MULTIPARAS
Prolongation disorder (prolonged latent phase)	> 20 hr	> 14 hr
Protraction disorder		
1. Protracted active phase dilatation	< 1.2 cm/hr	< 1.5 cm/hr
2. Protracted descent	< 1 cm/hr	< 2 cm/hr
Arrest disorders		
1. Dilatation	> 2 hrs	> 2 hrs
2. Descent	> 1 hr	> 1 hr
3. Failure of descent (no descent in deceleration phase or second stage of labor)	> 1 hr	> 1 hr

Dystocia literally means difficult labor and is characterized by abnormally slow or no progress of labor.

- **Prolonged latent phase** (see Table 5-5).
- **Active phase abnormalities:** May be due to cephalopelvic disproportion (CPD), excessive sedation, conduction analgesia, and fetal malposition (ie, persistent OP).
- **Protraction disorders:** A slow rate of cervical dilation or descent.
- **Arrest disorders:** Complete cessation of dilation or descent (see Table 5-5).
- With the diagnosis of protraction or arrest disorder of labor, assess the following:
  - Contraction strength: Start or ↑ pitocin to obtain stronger contractions.
  - Fetal size and position: Baby too big to pass through pelvis? Position abnormal?
  - Pelvis: Does pelvimetry indicate adequate pelvis?

CAUSES

1. Abnormalities of the expulsive forces:
   - Uterine dysfunction can lead to uterine forces insufficiently strong or inappropriately coordinated to efface and dilate cervix.
   - Inadequate voluntary muscle effort during second stage of labor.
2. Abnormalities of presentation, position, or fetal development.
3. Abnormalities of the maternal bony pelvis.
4. Abnormalities of the birth canal.

PELVIC SHAPES

See Table 5-6.

Dystocia is the most common indication for primary cesarean delivery.

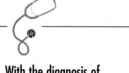

With the diagnosis of abnormal labor pattern, assess the three Ps:
- Power (contractions)
- Passenger (fetus)
- Pelvis

HIGH-YIELD FACTS

Intrapartum

TABLE 5-6. Pelvis Shapes

	GYNECOID	ANDROID	ANTHROPOID	PLATYPELLOID
	⬭	♡	⬭	⬭
Frequency	In 50% of all females	One third of white women; one sixth of nonwhite women	One fourth of white women; one half of nonwhite women	Rarest, < 3% of women
Inlet shape	Round	Heart shaped	Vertically oriented oval	Horizontally oriented oval
Sidewalls	Straight	Convergent	Convergent	Divergent, then convergent
Ischial spines	Not prominent (diameter ≥ 10 cm)	Prominent (diameter < 10 cm)	Prominent (diameter < 10 cm)	Not prominent (diameter > 10 cm)
Sacrum	Inclined neither anteriorly nor posteriorly	Forward and straight with little curvature	Straight = pelvis deeper than other three types	Well curved and rotated backward; short = shallow pelvis
Significance	Good prognosis for vaginal delivery	Limited posterior space for fetal head → poor prognosis for vaginal delivery	Good prognosis for vaginal delivery; commonly seen with OP position	Poor prognosis for vaginal delivery

INDUCTION OF LABOR

In some cases, an immature fetus may be delivered due to maternal illness.

Indications

Medically indicated induction of labor is performed when the benefits of delivery to either the maternal or fetal status outweigh the risks of continuing the pregnancy.

- **Maternal:**
  - Fetal demise.
  - Prolonged pregnancy.
  - Chorioamnionitis.
  - Severe preeclampsia/eclampsia.
  - Maternal conditions: Diabetes, renal disease, chronic pulmonary disease, chronic hypertension, antiphospholipid syndrome.
- **Fetal:**
  - Intrauterine growth retardation (IUGR).
  - Abnormal fetal testing.
  - Infection.

- Isoimmunization.
- Oligohydramnios.
- Postterm.
- Premature ROM.

Contraindications

- **Maternal:**
  - Placenta or vasa previa.
  - Prior uterine surgery/malpresentation.
  - Classical cesarean delivery.
  - Active genital herpes infection.
  - Previous myomectomy.
- **Fetal:**
  - Acute distress.
  - Transverse fetal lie.
  - Cord prolapse.

Confirmation of Fetal Maturity

Elective induction and/or cesarean should have fetal maturity documented by accurate dating criteria or amniocentesis. Elective indicates that there is no medical reason for delivery of fetus; it is more for convenience.

DATING CRITERIA

1. Documented fetal heart tones for:
   - 20 weeks by nonelectronic fetoscope.
   - 30 weeks by Doppler.
2. 36 weeks since a positive urine or serum pregnancy test.
3. Ultrasound of crown-rump length at 6–11 weeks dates the pregnancy and supports a gestational age of 39 weeks or more (gestational age is determined by the ultrasound).
4. Ultrasound at 12–20 weeks confirms a gestational age of 39 weeks or more determined by clinical history (LMP) and physical exam (ultrasound gestational age is consistent with LMP).

Induction Methods

OXYTOCIN

- A synthetic polypeptide hormone that stimulates uterine contraction.
- Acts promptly when given intravenously. Half-life about 5 min.

COMPLICATIONS

- Potent antidiuretic effects of oxytocin in high doses can cause water intoxication (ie, hyponatremia), which can lead to convulsions, coma, and death. Oxytocin is related structurally and functionally to vasopressin or antidiuretic hormone.
- Risk of hyperstimulation: Frequent, strong contractions that cause an abnormality in the FHR.

The term *cephalopelvic disproportion* (CPD) has been used to describe a disparity between the size of the maternal pelvis and the fetal head that precludes vaginal delivery. This condition can rarely be diagnosed with certainty and is often due to malposition of the fetal head (ie, asynclitism).

Cephalopelvic disproportion (CPD) leads to failure to progress and cesarean delivery.

The most common reason for cesarean delivery (CD) = previous CD

The skin incision that you see on the maternal abdomen does not tell you the type of uterine incision that the patient received. For example, a woman may have a midline skin incision but a low-transverse uterine incision.

PROSTAGLANDINS

- Misoprostol, a synthetic PGE$_1$ analog:
  - Can be administered intravaginally or orally.
  - Used for cervical ripening and induction.
- PGE$_2$ gel and vaginal insert:
  - Both contain dinoprostone.
  - Used for cervical ripening in women at or near term.

MECHANICAL

- Foley balloon: Passed through the internal cervical os into the extra-amniotic space, inflated and rested with traction on the internal os to cause dilation.
- Laminaria: Organic/synthetic material that slowly hygroscopically expands when placed in the cervix.

CESAREAN DELIVERY (CD)

The birth of a fetus through incisions in the abdominal wall (laparotomy) and the uterine wall (hysterotomy).

Types (See Figure 5-8)

1. Low-transverse cesarean section (LTCS):
   - Horizontal incision made in lower uterine segment.
   - Most common type performed.
2. Classical:
   - Vertical incision made in the contractile portion of uterine corpus.
   - Performed when:
     - Lower uterine segment is not developed (ie, prematurity).
     - Fetus is transverse lie with back down.
     - Placenta previa.

Indications

- Prior cesarean (elective repeat, previous classical).
- Dystocia or failure to progress in labor.
- Breech presentation.

FIGURE 5-8. Types of uterine incisions.

A. Low Transverse. B. Classical. (Reproduced, with permission, from Gabbe S, Niebyl J, Simpson J. *Obstetrics: Normal and Problem Pregnancies*, 5th ed. Philadelphia: Churchill Livingstone, 2007, Fig 19-3. Copyright © Elsevier.)

- Transverse lie.
- Concern for fetal well-being (ie, nonreassuring fetal heart tones).
- Uterine malformations/scars.

TRIAL OF LABOR AFTER CESAREAN (TOLAC)

TOLAC is associated with a small but significant **risk of uterine rupture** with poor outcome for mother and infant:

- Classical uterine incision: 10% risk.
- Low-transverse incision: 1% risk.
- Maternal and infant complications are ↑ with a failed trial of labor followed by cesarean delivery.

Remember, if a young woman has an 18- or 20-week-size uterus but a negative pregnancy test, the most likely diagnosis is a fibroid uterus.

Candidates for TOLAC

- One LTCS.
- Clinically adequate pelvis.
- No other uterine scars or previous rupture.
- Physician immediately available throughout active labor capable of monitoring labor and performing an emergency CD.
- Availability of anesthesia and personnel for emergency CD.

Contraindications to TOLAC

- Prior classical or T-shaped incision or other transmyometrial uterine surgery.
- Contracted pelvis.
- Medical/obstetric complication that precludes vaginal delivery.
- Inability to perform emergency CD because of unavailable surgeon, anesthesia, sufficient staff, or facility.

OPERATIVE VAGINAL DELIVERY

Forceps Delivery

Forceps are an important tool to allow for a vaginal delivery. The cervix must be fully dilated.

INDICATIONS

- Lack of progress in the second stage of labor.
- Fetal distress.
- Maternal factors: Exhaustion, heart disease, pulmonary edema, aneurysm, etc.
- After coming head for a breech delivery.

CONTRAINDICATIONS

- Presenting part is not engaged.
- Position of head is not precisely known.
- Membranes are not ruptured.
- Cervix is not fully dilated.
- Presence of cephalopelvic disproportion.

Cephalohematoma:
Collection of blood under periosteum of the skull; therefore, it does not cross the sutures on the fetal head. Due to rupture of vessels; resolves spontaneously over several weeks.
Vs.

Caput succedaneum:
Temporary swelling of fetal head from prolonged engagement of the head; does cross suture lines. Resolves in 1–2 days.

The peripheral branches of the pudendal nerve provide sensory innervation to the perineum, anus, and the medial and inferior parts of the vulva and clitoris.

Vacuum Delivery

- Same indications and contraindications as forceps.
- A safe, effective alternative to forceps delivery.
- A vertex fetus is required.
- Delivery should not be one that will require rotation or excessive traction.
- Prior scalp sampling is a contraindication.

ADVANTAGES

- Simpler to apply with fewer mistakes in application.
- Less force applied to fetal head.
- Less anesthesia is necessary (local anesthetic may suffice).
- No increase in diameter of presenting head.
- Less maternal soft-tissue injury.
- Less parental concern.

DISADVANTAGES

- Traction is applied only during contractions.
- Proper traction is necessary to avoid losing vacuum.
- Possible longer delivery than with forceps.
- Small ↑ in incidence of cephalohematomas.

PAIN CONTROL DURING LABOR AND DELIVERY

Three essentials of obstetric pain relief are simplicity, safety, and preservation of fetal homeostasis.

Lower Genital Tract Innervation

During the second stage of labor, much of the pain arises from the lower genital tract:

- Painful stimuli from the lower genital tract are primarily transmitted by the **pudendal nerve,** which passes beneath the posterior surface of the sacrospinous ligament (just as the ligament attaches to the ischial spine).
- The sensory nerve fibers of the pudendal nerve are derived from the ventral branches of the second, third, and fourth sacral nerves.

Nonpharmacological Methods of Pain Control

Women who are free from fear and who have confidence in their obstetrical staff require smaller amounts of pain medication:

- An understanding of pregnancy and the birth process.
- Appropriate antepartum training in breathing.
- Appropriate psychological support (eg, by a friend or family member).
- Considerate obstetricians and labor assistants who instill confidence.

Intravenous Analgesia and Sedation

Pain relief with an opiate or opioid plus an antiemetic is typically sufficient, with no significant risk to the mother or infant:

- Discomfort is still felt during uterine contractions but is more tolerable.
- Slight ↑ in uterine activity.
- Does *not* prolong labor.

Local Anesthesia

Administered before an episiotomy or after a delivery to repair a laceration.

Regional Anesthesia

Nerve blocks that provide pain relief for women in labor and delivery without loss of consciousness.

Pudendal Block

- Local infiltration of the pudendal nerve with a local anesthetic agent (eg, lidocaine) by obstetrician.
- Allows pinching of the lower vagina and posterior vulva bilaterally without pain.
- Effective, safe, and reliable method of providing analgesia for spontaneous delivery.
- Can be used along with epidural analgesia.
- **Complications:** Inadvertent intravascular injection will cause systemic toxicity, hematoma, infection.

Paracervical Block

- Agent is injected at the 3 o'clock and 9 o'clock positions around the cervix.
- Provides good relief of pain of uterine contractions during first stage of labor.
- Requires additional analgesia for delivery because the pudendal nerves are not blocked.
- **Complication:** Fetal bradycardia (usually transient).

Spinal (Subarachnoid) Block

- Introduction of local anesthetic into the subarachnoid space.
- Used for uncomplicated cesarean delivery and vaginal delivery.
- Provides excellent relief of pain from uterine contractions.
- Preceded by infusion of 1 L of crystalloid solution to prevent hypotension.
- Complications:
    - Maternal hypotension (common).
    - Total spinal blockade.
    - Spinal (postpuncture) headache—worse with sitting or standing.
    - Seizures.
    - Bladder dysfunction.
- Contraindications:
    - Severe preeclampsia: Hypotension from anesthesia can cause ischemic stroke.
    - Coagulation/hemostasis disorders.
    - Neurologic disorders.
    - Infection at the puncture site.
    - Surgical emergency.

Uterine contractions and cervical dilation cause discomfort.

Always pull back on the syringe prior to injection of anesthetic to look for blood flow into the syringe; if present, you are in a vessel and must reposition your needle.

When vaginal delivery is anticipated in 10 to 15 min, a rapidly acting agent is given through the epidural catheter to effect perineal analgesia.

EPIDURAL ANALGESIA

- Injection of local anesthetic into the epidural or peridural space:
  - **Lumbar epidural analgesia:** Injection into a lumbar intervertebral space.
  - **Caudal epidural analgesia:** Injection through the sacral hiatus and sacral canal.
- Relieves pain of uterine contractions, abdominal delivery (block begins at the eighth thoracic level and extends to first sacral dermatome) or vaginal delivery (block begins from the tenth thoracic to the fifth sacral dermatome).
- Complications:
  - Inadvertent spinal blockade (puncture of dura with subarachnoid injection).
  - Ineffective analgesia.
  - Hypotension.
  - Seizures.
- Effects on Labor:
  - Longer duration of labor.
  - ↑ incidence of:
    - Chorioamnionitis
    - Low-forceps procedures
    - Cesarean deliveries
    - Maternal pyrexia
- Contraindications
  - Same as spinal contraindications above.

General Anesthesia

General anesthesia should not be induced until all steps preparatory to actual delivery have been completed, so as to minimize transfer of the agent to the fetus, thereby avoiding newborn respiratory depression.

CONCERNS

- **Fetal:** All anesthetic agents that depress the maternal CNS cross the placenta and depress the fetal CNS.
- **Maternal:** Induction of general anesthesia can cause aspiration of gastric contents, resulting in airway obstruction, pneumonitis, pulmonary edema, and/or death.

Prophylactic measures to avoid aspiration:
- Fasting for 6 hrs.
- Administer antacids.
- Cricoid pressure before induction of anesthesia.

CHAPTER 6

Postpartum

The **puerperium** is the period of confinement between birth and 6 weeks after delivery. During this time, the reproductive tract returns anatomically to a normal nonpregnant state.

Uterus

INVOLUTION OF THE UTERINE CORPUS

Immediately after delivery, the fundus of the contracted uterus is slightly below the umbilicus. After the first 2 days postpartum, the uterus begins to shrink in size. Within 2 weeks, the uterus has descended into the cavity of the true pelvis. The contraction of the uterus immediately after delivery is critical for the achievement of hemostasis. "Afterpains" due to uterine contraction are common and may require analgesia. They typically ↓ in intensity by the third postpartum day.

ENDOMETRIAL CHANGES

 A 27-year-old woman undergoes a normal spontaneous vaginal delivery and spontaneous placental delivery without any lacerations. An hour later she has persistent vaginal bleeding. What is the likely diagnosis? What is the next step?

Answer: Most likely cause is retained placental tissue. An ultrasound may help with the diagnosis. Palpate the endometrium to remove any retained placenta. The patient may need to undergo a curettage of the uterus to remove any retained products. Tissue, Trauma, Tone, Thrombin

Within 2–3 days postpartum, the remaining decidua becomes differentiated into two layers:

1. Superficial layer becomes necrotic, sloughs off as vaginal discharge = *lochia*.
2. Basal layer (adjacent to the myometrium) becomes new endometrium.

PLACENTAL SITE INVOLUTION

Within hours after delivery, the placental site consists of many thrombosed vessels. Immediately postpartum, the placental site is the size of the palm of the hand and rapidly ↓ in size.

Sidebar notes (High-Yield Facts / Postpartum)

Late postpartum hemorrhage due to atony occurs when uterine involution is defective. Presents with vaginal bleeding and boggy uterus. Treat with oxytocin.

Uterine size:
- In pregnancy: > 36 weeks fundal height
- Postdelivery: Just below umbilicus (20 weeks)
- Returns to normal in 6 weeks

Lochia (lóke-ah) is decidual tissue that contains erythrocytes, epithelial cells, and bacteria. See Table 6-1.

TABLE 6-1. Lochia

TYPE	DESCRIPTION	WHEN OBSERVED
Lochia rubra	Red due to blood in the lochia	Days 1–3
Lochia serosa	More pale in color	Days 4–10
Lochia alba	White to yellow-white due to leukocytes and reduced fluid content	Day 11 →

CHANGES IN UTERINE VESSELS

Large blood vessels are obliterated by hyaline changes and replaced by new, smaller vessels.

Cervix

- The external os of the cervix contracts slowly and has narrowed by the end of the first week. The multiparous cervix takes on a characteristic fish mouth appearance.
- As a result of childbirth, the cervical epithelium undergoes much remodeling. Approximately 50% of women with high-grade cervical dysplasia will show regression after a vaginal delivery due to the remodeling of the cervix.

Vagina

Gradually diminishes in size, but rarely returns to nulliparous dimensions:

- Rugae reappear by the third week.
- The rugae become obliterated after repeated childbirth and menopause.

Peritoneum and Abdominal Wall

- The broad ligaments and round ligaments slowly relax to the nonpregnant state.
- The abdominal wall is soft and flabby due to the prolonged distention and rupture of the skin's elastic fibers; it resumes pre-pregnancy appearance in several weeks. However, the silver striae persist.

Urinary Tract

- The puerperal bladder has an ↑ capacity and is relatively insensitive to intravesical fluid pressure. Hence, overdistention, incomplete bladder emptying, and excessive residual urine are common and can result in a urinary tract infection (UTI).
- Between days 2 and 5 postpartum, "puerperal diuresis" typically occurs to reverse the ↑ in extracellular water associated with normal pregnancy.
- Dilated ureters and renal pelves return to their pre-pregnant state 2–8 weeks postpartum.

Hematology/Circulation

- **Leukocytosis** occurs during and after labor (up to 30,000/µL).
- During the first few postpartum days, the **hemoglobin** and **hematocrit** fluctuate moderately from levels just prior to labor.
- **Plasma fibrinogen** and the **erythrocyte sedimentation rate** may remain elevated for ≥ 1 week postpartum.
- The **cardiac output** is higher than during pregnancy for ≥ 48 hours postpartum due to ↓ blood flow to the uterus (much smaller) and ↑ systemic intravascular volume.
- By 1 week postpartum, the **blood volume** has returned to the patient's nonpregnant range.

The thinned-out lower uterine segment (that contained most of the fetal head) contracts and retracts over a few weeks and forms the uterine isthmus. The uterine isthmus is located between the uterine corpus above and the internal cervical os below.

At the completion of involution, the cervix does not resume its pregravid appearance:
- Before childbirth, the os is a small, regular, oval opening.
- After childbirth, the os is a horizontal slit.

Instrument-assisted delivery, regional and general anesthesia are risk factors for postpartum urinary retention.

All postpartum women who cannot void should be promptly catheterized.

The likelihood of cardiac overload is most likely in the immediate postpartum period, due to the autotransfusion of blood.

Hemostasis is obtained primarily by mechanical clamping of vessels by contracted myometrium.

Inadequate postpartum uterine contraction (= atony) is a major cause of early postpartum bleeding.

Blood can accumulate within the uterus without visible vaginal bleeding: *Watch for:* Palpable uterine **enlargement** during the initial few hours postpartum.

Sitz baths: Soaking the perineum in plain warm water or water with Epsom salts.

Body Weight

Most women approach their pre-pregnancy weight 6 months after delivery, but still retain approximately 1.4 kg of excess weight.

- Five to six kilograms are lost due to uterine evacuation and normal blood loss.
- Two to three kilograms are lost due to diuresis.

ROUTINE POSTPARTUM CARE

Immediately After Labor

FIRST HOUR

- Take blood pressure (BP) and heart rate (HR) at least every 15 min.
- Monitor the amount of vaginal bleeding.
- Palpate the fundus to ensure adequate contraction. If the uterus is relaxed, it should be massaged through the abdominal wall until it remains contracted. Massaging the uterus leads to ↑ release of oxytocin, which helps promote uterine contraction.

First Several Hours

EARLY AMBULATION

Women are out of bed (OOB) within a few hours after delivery. Advantages include:

- **Reduced** frequency of puerperal venous thrombosis and pulmonary embolism.
- ↓ bladder complications.
- Less frequent constipation.

CARE OF THE VULVA

The patient should be taught to cleanse and wipe the vulva from front to back (toward the anus).

IF EPISIOTOMY/LACERATION REPAIR

- An ice pack should be applied for the first several hours to reduce edema and pain.
- At 24 hr postpartum, moist heat (eg, via warm sitz baths) can ↓ local discomfort.
- The episiotomy incision is typically well healed and asymptomatic by week 3 of the puerperium.

BLADDER FUNCTION

Ensure that the postpartum woman has voided within 4-6 hr of delivery. If not:

- This indicates further voiding trouble to follow.
- An indwelling catheter may be necessary.
- Bladder sensation and capability to empty may be diminished due to anesthesia.
- Consider a hematoma of the genital tract as a possible etiology.

The First Few Days

BOWEL FUNCTION

Lack of a bowel movement may be due to a cleansing enema administered prior to delivery. Encourage early ambulation and feeding to ↓ the possibility of constipation. Ask the patient about flatus.

IF FOURTH-DEGREE LACERATION

Fecal incontinence may result, even with correct surgical repair, due to injury to the innervation of the pelvic floor musculature. Keep the patient on a stool softener and a low residue diet to avoid straining and ↓ risk of fistula formation. Avoid enemas or suppositories which can disrupt the repair.

DISCOMFORT/PAIN MANAGEMENT

During the first few days of the puerperium, pain may result from:

- Afterpains: Contractions of the uterus as it involutes. Treat with non-steroidal anti-inflammatory drugs (NSAIDs).
- Episiotomy/laceration pain: May require a narcotic medication, but NSAIDs or plain acetaminophen can help.
- Breast engorgement: Well-fitted with brassiere. NSAIDs.
- Postspinal puncture headache: Positional headache that is worse when upright, improved when lying down. Caffeine may help. Occasionally, patient may need a blood patch (performed by an anesthesiologist).
- Constipation: Treat with stool softeners over 2–3 weeks. May discontinue iron supplementation because it may cause constipation.
- Urinary retention: May need intermittent bladder catheterizations. Evaluate the patient for causes and treat accordingly

ABDOMINAL WALL RELAXATION

Exercise may be initiated any time after vaginal delivery and after abdominal discomfort has diminished after cesarean delivery.

DIET

- There are *no* dietary restrictions/requirements for women who have delivered vaginally. Two hours postpartum, the mother should be permitted to eat and drink. Those with an uncomplicated CD can be given clear liquids and regular diet as tolerated.
- Continue iron supplementation for a minimum of 3 months postpartum.

IMMUNIZATIONS

- The non-isoimmunized D-negative mother whose baby is D-positive is given 300 µg of anti-D immune globulin within 72 hours of delivery.
- Mothers not previously immunized against/immune to rubella should be vaccinated prior to discharge. Rubella vaccine is not given during the pregnancy because it is a live attenuated virus.
- Unless contraindicated, mothers may receive a diphtheria–tetanus toxoid booster prior to discharge.

Kleihauer-Betke test detects fetal-maternal hemorrhage in Rh-negative mothers; 300 µg of anti-D immune globulin neutralizes 30 mL of fetal whole blood or 15 mL of Rh-positive RBCs.

The uterine cavity is sterile before rupture of the amniotic sac.

Endometritis is relatively uncommon following vaginal delivery, but 5–10 times more frequent after C-section.

Following delivery, the bladder and lower urinary tract remain somewhat hypotonic, resulting in residual urine and reflux, which predisposes to urinary tract infection.

GBS colonization leads to 80% greater likelihood of postpartum endometritis.

> A 30-year-old G1P1001 is postpartum day 1 from a vaginal delivery over an intact perineum. On rounds, she reports pain in the lower abdomen. She denies cough, back pain, leg pain, dysuria, or breast pain. She has a temperature of 100.1°F (37.8°C) 4 hr ago, and now has a temperature of 101.0°F (38.3°C). Her lungs are clear to auscultation, breasts are soft, costovertebral angle tenderness (CVAT) is not present and has no tenderness in her legs. She has fundal tenderness and foul-smelling lochia. She has no suprapubic tenderness. She was admitted with ruptured membranes at 2 cm dilation and delivered after 20 hr in labor. Fetal heart tones were concerning for late decelerations, so she had internal monitors. She pushed for 3 hr before the infant was delivered. What is the most likely diagnosis? What risk factors did this patient have?
>
> **Answer:** Endometritis. Fever, fundal tenderness, and foul-smelling lochia in the absence of other findings is consistent with endometritis. This patient's risk factors include prolonged rupture of membranes and internal monitors, and she likely had multiple vaginal exams during her long labor course.

Pelvic infections are **ascending infections**. The bacteria responsible for pelvic infections are those that normally reside in the bowel and colonize the perineum, vagina, and cervix.

CAUSES

- **Gram-positive cocci:** Group A, B, and D streptococci.
- **Gram-positive bacilli:** *Clostridium* species, *Listeria monocytogenes.*
- **Aerobic gram-negative bacilli:** *Escherichia coli, Klebsiella, Proteus* species.
- **Anaerobic gram-negative bacilli:** *Bacteroides bivius, B fragilis, B disiens.*
- **Other:** *Mycoplasma hominis, Chlamydia trachomatis.*

RISK FACTORS

- Prolonged rupture of membranes > 18 hr.
- Prolonged second stage.
- Cesarean delivery/uterine manipulation.
- Colonization of the lower genital tract with certain microorganisms (ie, group B streptococci [GBS], *C trachomatis, M hominis,* and *Gardnerella vaginalis*).
- Premature labor.
- Frequent vaginal exams.
- Foreign body.
- Diabetes.

DIAGNOSIS

- Fever > 100.4°F (38°C).
- Soft, tender uterus.
- Lochia has a foul odor.

- Leukocytosis (WBC > 10,000/µL) (remember physiologic leukocytosis; look for trends).
- Identify source of infection (urinalysis, culture of lochia).

MANAGEMENT

Broad-spectrum antibiotics.

Types of Postpartum Infections

ENDOMETRITIS (METRITIS, ENDOMYOMETRITIS)

- A postpartum uterine infection involving the decidua, myometrium, and parametrial tissue.
- More common after cesarean delivery than vaginal delivery. Hypoxic tissue and foreign body (suture) with cesarean delivery are ideal for infections.
- Typically develops postpartum day 2–3.
- Treat with IV antibiotics until patient is afebrile for 24–48 hr.
- GBS colonization ↑ risk of endometritis.

URINARY TRACT INFECTION

- Caused by catheterization, birth trauma, conduction anesthesia, and frequent pelvic examinations.
- Presents with dysuria, frequency, urgency, and low-grade fever.
- Rule out pyelonephritis (costovertebral angle tenderness, pyuria, hematuria).
- Obtain a urinalysis and urinary culture (*E coli* is isolated in 75% of postpartum women).
- Treat with appropriate antibiotics.

CESAREAN DELIVERY: SURGICAL SITE INFECTION (SSI)

> A 30-year-old G2P2002 is 2 weeks postoperative from a repeat cesarean delivery and presents to the office for an incision check. She reports induration around the incision site and ↑ tenderness. Her pain medications do not help. She reports a small amount of white malodorous drainage from the incision. She is tolerating her diet well and voiding spontaneously. On physical exam, she is afebrile. Her surgical site is indurated 2 cm around the incision and erythematous 3 cm around the incision. Purulent drainage is noted from a 1-cm opening at the right margin. What is the next step in management?
>
> **Answer:** Next step is to differentiate whether this is a superficial or deep surgical site infection. The wound should be opened further and should be probed to evaluate whether the fascia is intact. Cultures should be obtained and the patient should receive antibiotics.

- Classification:
  - **Superficial SSI:** Involves skin and subcutaneous tissue.
  - **Deep SSI:** Involves fascia and muscle.

Postdelivery causes of fever:

The 5 W's + B

- Wind: Atelectasis, 1–2 days postop
- Water: Urinary tract infections, 2–3 days postpartum
- Wound: Surgical site infection—cellulitis, purulence, fluctuance, tenderness; 5–7 days postpartum
  - Cesarean: Abdominal incision
  - Vaginal: Episiotomy
- Walking: Deep vein thrombosis (DVT) and subsequent pulmonary embolus, 4–10 days postpartum
- Wonder drugs: Drug fever, 7–10 days postpartum
- Breast: Engorgement, mastitis, abscess, 3 days–4 weeks postpartum

Wound infection occurs in 4–12% of patients following C-section.

Antibiotic prophylaxis with IV cefazolin is commonly employed during cesarean deliveries.

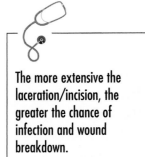

DIAGNOSIS

- Fever, wound erythema and persistent tenderness, purulent drainage.
- Management: Obtain Gram stain and cultures from wound material.
- Wound should be drained, irrigated, and debrided.
- Antibiotics should be given along with:
  - Superficial SSI: Wet-to-dry packing placed. Consider closure of incision when wound healthy.
  - Deep SSI: May need debridement in the operating room under anesthesia. Consider necrotizing fasciitis.

EPISIOTOMY INFECTION

- Look for pain at the episiotomy site, disruption of the wound, and a necrotic membrane over the wound.
- Rule out the presence of a rectovaginal fistula with a careful rectovaginal exam.
- Open, clean, and debride the wound to promote granulation tissue formation.
- Sitz baths are recommended.
- Reassess for possible closure after granulation tissue has appeared.

DISCHARGE FROM HOSPITAL

Vaginal Delivery

One to two days postdelivery, if no complications. Return to the office at 4–6 weeks for postpartum exam.

Cesarean Delivery

Two to three days postdelivery, if no complications. Return to the office in 2 weeks to check the incision and 4–6 weeks for postpartum exam.

Discharge Instructions

The patient should call the doctor or go to hospital if she develops:

- Fever > 100.4°F (37°C).
- Excessive vaginal bleeding—soaking a pad an hour. Suspicious for retained placenta.
- Lower extremity pain and/or swelling: Suspicious for DVT.
- Shortness of breath: Suspicious for pulmonary embolus (PE).
- Chest pain—can occur with PE.

COITUS IN POSTPARTUM

- After 6 weeks, coitus may be resumed based on patient's desire and comfort. A vaginal lubricant prior to coitus may improve comfort.
- Dangers of premature intercourse:
  - Pain due to continued uterine involution and healing of lacerations/episiotomy scars.
- ↑ likelihood of hemorrhage and infection.

Contraception

A 25-year-old G1P1001 is postpartum day 2 from a vaginal delivery. She is overall healthy and is breast-feeding. She wants contraception that is easy to use. She reports that she had used a combination oral contraceptive pill prior to conceiving this baby and had no bad side effects. She is afraid of needles. What is the best contraceptive option for this patient?

Answer: Progestin-only pill. Progestin does not have an effect on breast milk, and it is easy to use.

- Do not wait until first menses to begin contraception; ovulation may come before first menses.
- Contraception is essential after the first menses unless a subsequent pregnancy is desired.
- See contraception chapter.

LACTATIONAL AMENORRHEA METHOD OF CONTRACEPTION

Lactational amenorrhea involves exclusive breast-feeding to prevent ovulation. It can be used as a contraceptive method. It is 98% effective for up to 6 months if:

- The mother is not menstruating.
- The mother is nursing > 2–3 times per night, and more than every 4 hr during the day without other supplementation.
- The baby is < 6 months old.

ORAL CONTRACEPTIVE PILLS IN POSTPARTUM

- **Combined oral contraceptive pills** reduce the amount of breast milk, and very small quantities of the hormones are excreted in the milk.
- **Progestin-only oral contraceptive pills** are 95% effective with typical use without substantially reducing the amount of breast milk. Need to take it the same time every day.

DEPO-MEDROXYPROGESTERONE

A progesterone-containing injection, given every 3 months, does not have any effect on breast milk production; 99% effective.

INTRAUTERINE DEVICE

Not used while the uterus in undergoing involution due to risk of expulsion and uterine perforation.

IMPLANON

A progestin-releasing implant that is placed in the arm; lasts for 3 yr.

Nursing mothers rarely ovulate within the first 10 weeks after delivery. Non-nursing mothers typically ovulate 6–8 weeks after delivery.

Prior to discharge:

- Follow-up care arrangements should be made.
- All laboratory results should be normal, including:
  - Coombs' test.
  - Bilirubin.
  - Hemoglobin and hematocrit.
  - Blood glucose.
  - Maternal serologic tests for syphilis and HbsAg should be nonreactive.
- Initial HBV vaccine should be administered.
- All screening tests required by law should be done (eg, testing for phenylketonuria [PKU] and hypothyroidism).
- Patient education regarding infant immunizations and well-baby care.

Development of Milk-Secreting Machinery

Progesterone, estrogen, placental lactogen, prolactin, cortisol, and insulin act together to stimulate the growth and development of the milk-secreting machinery of the mammary gland:

- Midpregnancy: Lobules of alveoli form lobes separated by stromal tissue, with secretion in some alveolar cells.
- T3: Alveolar lobules are almost fully developed, with cells full of proteinaceous secretory material.
- Postpartum: Rapid ↑ in cell size and in the number of secretory organelles. Alveoli distend with milk.

Milk Development

- At delivery, the abrupt, large ↓ in progesterone and estrogen levels allow for milk production. All vitamins, except vitamin K, are found in human milk, necessitating neonatal administration of vitamin K to prevent hemorrhagic disease of the newborn.
- **Colostrum** can be expressed from the nipple by the second postpartum day and is secreted by the breasts for 5 days postpartum. It has more minerals and protein than breast milk. It has less sugar and fat when compared to breast milk. Antibodies in colostrum protect the infant against enteric organisms.

Mature Milk and Lactation

- Colostrum is composed of protein, fat, carbohydrates (lactose), secretory IgA, and minerals.
- Milk comes in within the first week postpartum and is composed of protein, fat, carbohydrates (lactose), and water.
  - Protein: Colostrum > milk.
  - Fat: Milk > colostrum.
  - Carbs: Milk > colostrum.

Colostrum is a yellow—colored liquid secreted by the breasts that contains minerals, protein, fat, antibodies, complement, macrophages, lymphocytes, lysozymes, lactoferrin, and lactoperoxidase.

Milk letdown may be provoked by the cry of the infant and suckling and inhibited by stress or fright.

- Colostrum is gradually converted to mature milk by 4 weeks postpartum. Subsequent lactation is primarily controlled by the repetitive stimulus of nursing and the presence of prolactin.
- Breast engorgement with milk is common on days 2–4 postpartum:
  - Often painful.
  - Often accompanied by transient temperature elevation.
  - Often present in non-breast-feeding women.
- Suckling stimulates the neurohypophysis to secrete oxytocin in a pulsatile fashion, causing contraction of myoepithelial cells and small milk ducts, which leads to milk expression.

Oxytocin stimulates milk letdown/ejection. **Prolactin** stimulates milk production. **Progesterone** has an inhibitory effect on production of milk.

Lactation Suppression

> A 26-year-old female, 1 month postpartum, presents to the office with complaints of fever of 100.9°F (37.3°C) and breast tenderness for 1 day. She has been breast-feeding without problems and reports no other symptoms. On physical exam, her temperature is 100.8°F (38.2°C). Her left breast has a 4-cm area of induration and erythema at the 3 o'clock position that is tender to palpation. Milk expressed from that breast is white. What is the most likely diagnosis? What is the treatment?
>
> **Answer:** Mastitis. Focal area of breast infection and fever approximately 1 month postpartum is consistent with mastitis. Milk should be cultured, and the patient should be started on dicloxacillin empirically until culture and sensitivities are available.

What is Sheehan syndrome? Postpartum pituitary dysfunction, possibly due to intrapartum ischemia. These patients cannot breast-feed due to the absence of prolactin.

Women who do not want to breast-feed should wear a well-fitting brassiere, breast binder, or "sports bra." Pharmacologic therapy with bromocriptine is not recommended due to its associations with strokes, myocardial infarction, seizures, and psychiatric disturbances.

Bromocriptine no longer FDA approved for suppression of lactation.

Breast Fever

Breast engorgement is a result of milk collecting in the breast.

- Occurs within 2–4 days of delivery. Seldom persists for > 24 hrs.
- Presents with **bilateral** painful, firm, globally swollen breasts.
- Rule out other causes of postpartum fever.
- Treat with supportive bra, 24 hr demand feedings, ice packs.
- **Mastitis** is an infection of the breast. It affects 1–2% of postpartum women. Approximately 10% of women with mastitis develop breast abscess.
  - Caused by:
    - *Staphylococcus aureus* from the infant's nasopharynx (40%). More likely to cause an abscess.
    - *Staphylococcus* coagulase negative, *Streptococcus viridans* (60%).
  - Presents approximately 4 weeks postpartum with fever, chills.
  - **Focal** area of erythema and induration. No fluctuance.
  - Culture milk to identify the organism.
  - Treat with dicloxacillin for 7–10 days. Continue breast-feeding. Resolves within 48 hr.

- **Breast abscess** may follow mastitis:
  - Suspected when fever does not defervesce within 48–72 hr with antibiotics.
  - Palpable mass may be present.
  - Ultrasound can visualize the fluid collection.
  - Treat with broad-spectrum antibiotics and incision and drainage or ultrasound-guided needle aspiration.

Breast-Feeding

Human milk is the ideal food for neonates for the first 6 months of life. Breast-fed infants are less prone to enteric infections than are bottle-fed babies.

RECOMMENDED DIETARY ALLOWANCES

Lactating women need an extra 500 nutritious calories per day. Food choices should be guided by the Food Guide Pyramid, as recommended by the U.S. Department of Health and Human Services/U.S. Department of Agriculture.

BENEFITS

- Uterine involution: Nursing accelerates uterine involution (increases oxytocin).
- Immunity:
  - Colostrum and breast milk contain secretory IgA antibodies against *Escherichia coli* and other potential infections.
  - Milk contains memory T cells, which allows the fetus to benefit from maternal immunologic experience.
  - Colostrum contains interleukin-6, which stimulates an ↑ in breast milk mononuclear cells.
- Nutrients: All proteins are absorbed by babies, and all essential and nonessential amino acids available.
- Gastrointestinal (GI) maturation: Milk contains epidermal growth factor, which may promote growth and maturation of the intestinal mucosa.

CONTRAINDICATIONS TO BREAST-FEEDING

Mothers with the following infections:

- HIV infection.
- Breast lesions from active herpes simplex virus.
- Tuberculosis (active, untreated).
- Breast-feeding not contraindicated:
  - Cytomegalovirus (CMV): Both the virus and antibodies are present in breast milk.
  - Hepatitis B virus (HBV): If the infant receives hepatitis B immune globulin.
  - Hepatitis C: 4% risk of transmission same for breast- and bottle-fed infants.
- **Medications:** Mothers ingesting the following contraindicated medications (not an exhaustive list):
  - Bromocriptine.
  - Cyclophosphamide.
  - Cyclosporine.
  - Doxorubicin.
  - Ergotamine.

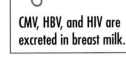

CMV, HBV, and HIV are excreted in breast milk.

A common misperception: Mothers who have a common cold should not breast-feed (false).

- *Lithium.*
- Methotrexate.
- Estrogen-containing oral contraceptives (OCPs).
- **Drug abuse:** Mothers who abuse the following drugs should not breast-feed:
    - Amphetamines
    - Cocaine
    - Heroin
    - Marijuana
    - Nicotine
    - Phencyclidine
    - Ethanol
- **Radiotherapy:** Mothers undergoing radiotherapy with the following should not breast-feed:
    - Gallium
    - Indium
    - Iodine
    - Radioactive sodium
    - Technetium

What type of oral contraceptives are okay with breast-feeding? Progesterone-only OCPs

Most drugs given to the mother are secreted in breast milk. However, the amount of drug ingested by the infant is typically small.

POSTPARTUM PSYCHIATRIC DISORDERS

Maternity/Postpartum Blues

A 25-year-old G1P1001 presents 1 week postpartum to the office with complaints of tearfulness, inability to sleep, fatigue, and decreased appetite. She has enough support at home and is still very involved in taking care of her infant. What is the most likely diagnosis? What therapy should be offered?

Answer: Postpartum blues. She should be given supportive therapy with monitoring for more severe signs of depression.

A self-limited, mild mood disturbance due to biochemical factors and psychological stress:

- Affects 50% of women.
- Begins within 3–6 days after parturition.
- May persist for up to 10 days.
- May be related to progesterone withdrawal.

Thirty percent of adolescent women develop postpartum depression.

SYMPTOMS

Similar to depression, but milder (see below).

TREATMENT

- Supportive—acknowledgment of the mother's feelings and reassurance.
- Monitor for the development of more severe symptoms (ie, postpartum depression or psychosis).

Postpartum Depression

Similar to minor and major depression that can occur at any time:

- Classified as "postpartum depression" if it begins within 3–6 months after childbirth.
- Eight to fifteen percent of postpartum women develop postpartum depression within 2–3 months.
- Up to 70% recurrence.

SYMPTOMS

Symptoms are the same as major depression.

NATURAL COURSE

- Gradual improvement over the 6-month postpartum period.
- The mother may remain symptomatic for months to years.

TREATMENT

- Pharmacologic intervention is typically required:
  - Antidepressants
  - Anxiolytic agents
  - Electroconvulsive therapy
- Mother should be comanaged with a psychiatrist (ie, for psychotherapy to focus on any maternal fears or concerns).

Postpartum Psychosis

- Mothers cannot discern real vs. unreal (can have periods of lucidity). Hearing voices, seeing things.
- Occurs in 1–4 in 1000 births.
- Peak onset: 10–14 days postpartum, but may occur months later.

RISK FACTORS

- History of psychiatric illness.
- Family history of psychiatric disorders.
- Younger age.
- Primiparity.

COURSE

Variable and depends on the type of underlying illness; often 6 months.

TREATMENT

- Psychiatric care.
- Pharmacologic therapy.
- Hospitalization (in most cases).

Postpartum thyroiditis is a transient lymphocytic thyroiditis in 5–10% of women during the first year after childbirth. The **two clinical phases** of postpartum thyroiditis are **thyrotoxicosis** and **hypothyroidism** (see Table 6-2).

TABLE 6-2. Thyrotoxicosis vs. Hypothyroidism

	THYROTOXICOSIS	HYPOTHYROIDISM
Onset	1–4 months postpartum	4–8 months postpartum
Mechanism	Destruction-induced hormone release	Thyroid insufficiency
Symptoms	Small, painless goiter Palpitations, fatigue	Goiter, fatigue, inability to concentrate
Treatment	β-blocker	Thyroxine for 6–12 months
Sequela	Two-thirds euthyroid One-third hypothyroid	One-third permanent hypothyroidism

HIGH-YIELD FACTS

Postpartum

Medical Conditions in Pregnancy

- Diabetes that existed before pregnancy:
  - Type 1 diabetes: Absolute insulin deficiency.
  - Type 2 diabetes: Defective insulin secretion or insulin resistance.
- Classes B through H in the White Classification (see Table 7-1).

DIAGNOSIS

- Classic symptoms:
  - Polyuria
  - Polydipsia
  - Unexplained weight loss
- Fasting > 126 mg/dL; random > 200 mg/dL.

MATERNAL COMPLICATIONS

- Gestational hypertension
- Preeclampsia
- Preterm delivery
- Cesarean section
- Polyhydramnios
- Infections
- Impaired wound healing

FETAL COMPLICATIONS

- Preterm birth.
- Macrosomia.
- Fetal-growth restriction.

Most common medical complication of pregnancy = diabetes (gestational + pregestational).

Women with pregestational diabetes have significant maternal and fetal complications when compared to those with gestational diabetes.

TABLE 7-1. Classification of Diabetes Complicating Pregnancy

		PLASMA GLUCOSE LEVEL		
CLASS	**ONSET**	**FASTING**	**2-HR POSTPRANDIAL**	**THERAPY**
A₁	Gestational	< 105 mg/dL	< 120 mg/dL	Diet controlled
A₂	Gestational	> 105 mg/dL	> 120 mg/dL	Insulin
CLASS	**AGE OF ONSET**	**DURATION (YR)**	**VASCULAR DISEASE**	**THERAPY**
B	Over 20	< 10	None	Insulin
C	10 to 19	10–19	None	Insulin
D	Before 10	> 20	Benign retinopathy	Insulin
F	Any	Any	Nephropathy	Insulin
R	Any	Any	Proliferative retinopathy	Insulin
H	Any	Any	Heart	Insulin

(Reproduced, with permission, from Cunningham FG, Leveno KJ, Bloom SL, et al. *Williams Obstetrics*, 22nd ed. New York: McGraw-Hill, 2005: 1171.)

HIGH-YIELD FACTS

Medical Conditions in Pregnancy

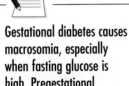

Diabetic ketoacidosis may be induced in type 1 diabetics by:
- Corticosteroids (for lung maturity).
- β mimetics (for tocolysis).
- Hyperemesis gravidarum.
- Infections.

Gestational diabetes causes macrosomia, especially when fasting glucose is high. Pregestational diabetes causes growth restriction especially due to concurrent maternal vascular disease.

Insulin requirements ↑ during the second trimester due to the antagonistic effect of pregnancy hormones. Immediately following delivery, insulin requirements dramatically ↓.

- Congenital anomalies:
  - Caudal regression—absence of the sacrum with variable defects of the lower spine.
  - Cardiac anomalies.
  - Neural tube defects (NTDs).
  - ↑ risk of fetal anomalies in diabetics is due to poor glycemic control prior to conception and in early pregnancy.
- Stillbirths—unexplained.
- Perinatal deaths.
- Neonatal hypoglycemia—chronic maternal hyperglycemia → hyperplasia of fetal β-islet cells → increased fetal insulin → rapid decline in fetal plasma glucose after delivery.
- Respiratory distress syndrome—likely due to earlier gestational age at delivery.
- Neonatal hypocalcemia.
- Neonatal hyperbilirubinemia.
- Polycythemia.

MANAGEMENT

Preconception
- Optimize glycemic control:
  - Preprandial: 70–100 mg/dL.
  - Postprandial: < 140 mg/dL and < 120 mg/dL at 1 and 2 hr, respectively.
  - Goal HbA_{1C} is < 6 mg/dL.
- HbA_{1C} levels > 10% significantly increase the risk of congenital malformations.
- Folic acid 0.4 mg/day during preconception and early pregnancy to ↓ risk of NTDs.
- Baseline 24-hr urine for total protein and creatinine clearance.
- Ophthalmology exam.
- Electrocardiogram (ECG).
- Thyroid-stimulating hormone (TSH).

First Trimester
- Start individualized insulin regimen.
- Check fasting and 2-hr postprandial glucose.

Second Trimester
- 16–20 weeks: Offer quad screen.
- 18–20 weeks: Get targeted ultrasound (US), then US every 4 weeks for growth.
- 22 weeks: Fetal echocardiogram looking for cardiac anomalies.

Third Trimester
- Antenatal testing at 32–34 weeks or when poor glycemic control.
- Consider amniocentesis for fetal lung maturity and delivery at 37 weeks if poor glycemic control.
- Consider delivery at 38 weeks without fetal lung maturity without amniocentesis if good glycemic control.
- Consider cesarean delivery if estimated fetal weight is > 4500 g.
- Start insulin drip in labor for glycemic control.

Thyroid hormone is essential for the normal development of the fetal brain and mental function. The incidence of hyperthyroidism, hypothyroidism, and thyroiditis is each about 1%.

- TSH:
  - Essential for diagnosis of thyroid dysfunction in pregnancy.
  - Unchanged in pregnancy.
  - Does not cross the placenta.
- Free thyroxine (T_4): Unchanged in pregnancy.
- Thyroid-binding globulin ↑ in pregnancy.

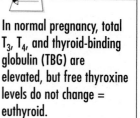

Free T_4 and TSH do not change in pregnancy and are the most sensitive markers to detect thyroid disease.

Hyperthyroidism

A 32-year-old G2P1001 at 16 weeks gestation presents with complaints of palpitations, nervousness, insomnia, and fatigue. On physical exam a fine tremor is noted in her hand, and her heart rate is 120 beats/min. What is the most likely diagnosis? What is the best treatment?

Answer: She has symptoms most consistent with hyperthyroidism. Although this patient has many symptoms that are normal for pregnancy, she should be screened for thyroid disorder with TSH and free T_4. Hyperthyroidism should be treated with PTU in pregnancy.

In normal pregnancy, total T_3, T_4, and thyroid-binding globulin (TBG) are elevated, but free thyroxine levels do not change = euthyroid.

- Twenty-five percent mortality rate.
- Thyrotoxicosis complicates 1 in 2000 pregnancies.
- Graves' disease is the most common cause of thyrotoxicosis in pregnancy.
- Precipitating factors are infection, labor, and C-section.

TREATMENT

- Ablation with radioactive iodine **contraindicated.**
- Propylthiouracil (PTU):
  - Drug of choice for treatment during pregnancy.
  - Inhibits conversion of T_4 to T_3.
  - Small amount transfer across the placenta.
- Methimazole:
  - Readily crosses placenta.
  - Associated with aplasia cutis in fetus.
- Thyroidectomy:
  - Seldom done in pregnancy.
  - For women who fail medical management.

COMPLICATIONS

- Women who remain hyperthyroid despite treatment have higher incidence of preeclampsia, heart failure, and adverse perinatal outcomes (stillbirth, preterm labor).
- Neonatal thyrotoxicosis: 1% risk due to placental transfer of thyroid-stimulating antibodies.
- Fetal goiter/hypothyroid—from propylthiouracil (PTU).

- Preterm delivery.
- Stillbirth.
- Preeclampsia.
- **Thyroid storm:** An acute, life-threatening, hypermetabolic state in patients with thyrotoxicosis. Often associated with heart failure. Treatment in intensive care unit (ICU) setting:
  - PTU orally or nasogastric tube.
  - β blocker to control tachycardia.
  - Sodium iodide inhibits release of T_3 and T_4 (lithium if iodine allergic).
  - Dexamethasone blocks peripheral conversion of T_4 to T_3.

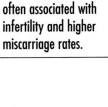

Hyperthyroidism ($\uparrow$ free T_4, $\downarrow$ TSH) are noted in hyperemesis gravidarum and gestational trophoblastic disease.

Hypothyroidism: $\uparrow$ TSH, $\downarrow$ Free T4

Subclinical Hypothyroidism: $\uparrow$ TSH, normal free T4

Overt hypothyroidism is often associated with infertility and higher miscarriage rates.

Hypothyroidism

- Hashimoto's thyroiditis is the most common cause of hypothyroidism during pregnancy.
- Subclinical hypothyroidism is more common than overt hypothyroidism.
  - Overt hypothyroidism is diagnosed by $\uparrow$ TSH and $\downarrow$ free T_4.
  - Subclinical hypothyroidism is an $\uparrow$ TSH with normal free T_4.
- Diagnosis may be difficult, as many of the symptoms of hypothyroidism (weight gain, fatigue, constipation, etc.) are also symptoms of pregnancy.
- The American College of Obstetricians and Gynecologists recommends **against** routine prenatal screening for subclinical hypothyroidism.

TREATMENT

Levothyroxine replacement:

- TSH is monitored every 8 weeks after the initiation of treatment or a change in dosage.
- TSH is monitored every trimester if no change in medication is needed due to increased thyroxine requirements in advancing pregnancy.

COMPLICATIONS

- Preeclampsia
- Placental abruption
- Cardiac dysfunction
- Low birth weight
- Still births

A 37-year-old G3P2002 at 37 weeks by an unsure last menstrual period (LMP) comes to triage complaining of a severe headache for 1 day that is unrelieved with acetaminophen. Her prenatal course has been complicated by chronic hypertension that has been well controlled with Aldomet (methyldopa). Her blood pressures are normally 140/90. She had no proteinuria during her prenatal visits. She denies any visual changes, right upper quadrant pain, contractions, vaginal bleeding, leakage of fluid. She reports good fetal movement. Her blood pressure is 180/110 and 175/100. She has 3+ proteinuria. Fetal heart rate is reassuring. What is the most likely diagnosis?

Answer: Chronic hypertension with superimposed preeclampsia. Women with chronic hypertension are at high risk for developing preeclampsia; worsening blood pressure and proteinuria can indicate the development of superimposed preeclampsia.

- Hypertension prior to 20th week of gestation.
- Prevalence is markedly ↑ in obese and diabetic patients.

PRECONCEPTION

Evaluate for renal and cardiac function:

- Echocardiography: Women with left ventricular hypertrophy or cardiac dysrhythmias indicate long-standing or poorly controlled hypertension leading to ↑ risk for congestive heart failure (CHF) in pregnancy.
- Serum creatinine and proteinuria: Abnormal results indicate risk for adverse pregnancy outcome.

COMPLICATIONS

- Superimposed preeclampsia: Development of preeclampsia in the setting of chronic hypertension. Infant should be delivered for maternal interest, even if markedly premature.
- Abruptio placenta: ↑ risk with severe hypertension. Smoking compounds the risk.
- Fetal growth restriction: Directly related to the severity of hypertension.
- Preterm delivery.

MANAGEMENT

- Fetus should undergo testing to assess for adequate perfusion.
- Fetus should receive ultrasounds to monitor growth.
- Unless other complications develop, patients with chronic hypertension should deliver at term.
- Vaginal delivery is preferred to cesarean.

Poorer control of hypertension and presence of end organ damage = ↑ adverse outcomes in pregnancy.

Blood pressure is dynamic during pregnancy. It normally ↓ in T_2. If a patient with chronic hypertension is seen for the first time in T_2, she may appear normotensive.

Development of complications may require the delivery of a very premature infant.

HIGH-YIELD FACTS

Medical Conditions in Pregnancy

MEDICATIONS

- Labetalol: α- and β-adrenergic blocker.
- α-Methyldopa: Generally not used outside obstetrics.
- Hydralazine: Vasodilator.
- Nifedipine: Calcium channel blocker. Also used for tocolysis in preterm labor.
- Angiotensin-converting enzyme (ACE) inhibitors/angiotensin receptor blockers (ARBs): Not given due to teratogenic potential (hypocalvaria and renal defects).

α-Methyldopa (centrally acting agent): One of the most common antihypertensives used in pregnancy.

CARDIOVASCULAR DISEASE

- Pregnancy-induced hemodynamic changes have profound effects on underlying heart disease. Cardiac output ↑ by 50% in midpregnancy.
- Need to monitor for CHF.
- Some congenital heart lesions are inherited. There is a 4% risk of congenital heart disease in the infant of a woman with a particular defect.
- Pain control:
  - Essential during labor and delivery to decrease the cardiac workload.
  - Continuous epidural anesthesia is recommended.
  - General anesthesia can cause hypotension.
- Vaginal delivery (spontaneous, forceps, vacuum) desired over cesarean delivery.

Pain control of choice during labor and delivery: Epidural anesthesia.

Mitral Stenosis (MS)

- ↑ preload due to normal ↑ in blood volume results in left atrial overload. ↑ pressure in the left atrium is transmitted into the lungs, resulting in **pulmonary hypertension (HTN).**
- Tachycardia associated with labor and delivery exacerbates the pulmonary HTN because of decreased filling time. May lead to pulmonary edema.
- Twenty-five percent of women with mitral stenosis have cardiac failure for the first time during pregnancy.
- Fetus is at risk for growth restriction.
- **Peripartum period is the most hazardous time.**
- Consider intrapartum endocarditis prophylaxis.

Mitral Valve Prolapse

- Normally asymptomatic.
- Have a systolic click on physical exam.
- Generally safe pregnancy.
- Consider intrapartum endocarditis prophylaxis.

Think: PPSS
Prolapse—okay to be **P**regnant
Stenosis—**S**ick in pregnancy

Aortic Stenosis

- Similar problems with mitral stenosis.
- Avoid tachycardia and fluid overload.
- Give antibiotic prophylaxis.

Eisenmenger Syndrome and Conditions with Pulmonary Hypertension

- Extremely dangerous to the mother.
- This condition may justify the termination of pregnancy on medical grounds.
- Maternal mortality can be as high as **50%**, with death usually occurring postpartum.

PULMONARY DISEASE

The adaptations to the respiratory system during pregnancy must be able to satisfy the $\uparrow O_2$ demands of the hyperdynamic circulation and the fetus. Advanced pregnancy may worsen the pathophysiological effects of many acute and chronic lung diseases.

Asthma

- Asthmatics have a small but significant $\uparrow$ in pregnancy complications.
- Fetal growth restriction $\uparrow$ with the severity of asthma.
- Arterial blood gases analysis provides objective information as to severity of asthma.

EPIDEMIOLOGY

- One to four percent of pregnancies are complicated by asthma.
- Twenty-five percent of asthmatics worsen in pregnancy.
- Twenty-five percent improve.
- Fifty percent have no change.

TREATMENT

- Generally, asthma is exacerbated by respiratory tract infections, so killed influenza vaccine should be given.
- Pregnant asthmatics can be treated with β agonists, epinephrine, and inhaled steroids (same medications used outside of pregnancy).

F-series prostaglandins exacerbate asthma, so avoid in pregnancy.

Pneumonia

COMPLICATIONS

- Premature rupture of membranes.
- Preterm delivery due to acidemia.

Severe pneumonia is a common cause of acute respiratory distress syndrome (ARDS).

MANAGEMENT

- **Any pregnant woman suspected of having pneumonia should undergo chest radiography (CXR) with an abdominal shield.**
- Abnormalities seen on CXR may take up to 6 weeks to resolve.
- Pneumococcal vaccine is not recommended for healthy pregnant patients. Use in patients who are immunocompromised or have severe cardiac/renal/pulmonary disease.
- Influenza vaccine is recommended for prevention in all trimesters.
- For bacterial pneumonia empirical therapy with erythromycin IV then PO is reportedly effective in 99% of uncomplicated pneumonia cases.

- Severe disease may require β-lactams + macrolide (amoxicillin-clavulanate), or third-generation cephalosporins (ceftriaxone).
- Vancomycin is added for community-acquired methicillin-resistant *Staphylococcus aureus* (MRSA).

RENAL AND URINARY TRACT DISORDERS

Pregnancy causes hydronephrosis (dilatation of renal pelvis, calyces, and ureters; <u>R</u> > L):

- Pregnant uterus compresses the lower ureter.
- Hormonal milieu ↓ ureteral tone.
- May cause urinary stasis and ↑ vesicoureteral reflux leading to symptomatic upper urinary tract infections (UTIs).

Asymptomatic Bacteriuria

- Five percent incidence.
- If untreated, 25% will develop pyelonephritis.
- Routine screening at the first prenatal visit recommended.

Pyelonephritis

A 23-year-old G3P2002 at 25 weeks gestation presents to triage with fever, nausea, and vomiting for 1 day. She complains of back pain and lower abdominal pain. She has a fever of 101.2°F (38.9°C), clear lungs, and right costovertebral tenderness. Fetal heart rate is reassuring. The monitor shows contractions every 2 min. Cervix is closed/thick/high. Urine dip shows many bacteria, leukocytes, nitrites, and ketones. What is the most likely diagnosis? What is the next step in management?

Answer: The clinical presentation is most consistent with pyelonephritis. She should be admitted to the hospital and given IV hydration and IV antibiotics.

- Acute pyelonephritis is the most common serious medical complication of pregnancy.
- Unilateral, right-sided > 50% of the time.
- *Escherichia coli* cultured 80% of the time.
- Bacteremia in 15–20% of women with acute pyelonephritis.

COMPLICATIONS

- Renal dysfunction: ↑ creatinine.
- Pulmonary edema: Endotoxin-induced alveolar injury.
- ARDS.
- Hemolysis.
- Preterm labor.

DIFFERENTIAL DIAGNOSIS

- Preterm labor
- Chorioamnionitis

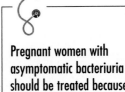

Pregnant women with asymptomatic bacteriuria should be treated because of their ↑ risk of developing pyelonephritis.

Hydronephrosis: Usually R > L

Highest incidence of asymptomatic bacteriuria: African-Americans with sickle-cell trait.

Most common cause of septic shock in pregnancy: Urosepsis.

- Appendicitis
- Placental abruption
- Infracted myoma

MANAGEMENT

- Hospitalization.
- IV antibiotics usually cephalosporins.
- IV hydration for adequate urinary output.
- Consider long-term antibiotic suppression for remainder of pregnancy for recurrent pyelonephritis.

Most common cause of persistent pyelonephritis despite adequate therapy: Nephrolithiasis.

GASTROINTESTINAL DISORDERS

During advanced pregnancy, gastrointestinal (GI) symptoms become difficult to assess, and physical findings are often obscured by the enlarged uterus.

Differential Diagnosis of Acute Abdomen

- Pyelonephritis
- Appendicitis
- Pancreatitis
- Cholecystitis
- Ovarian torsion
- Ectopic pregnancy (early pregnancy)
- Labor

Increased estrogen in pregnancy → increased cholesterol saturation in bile → increased biliary stasis and gallstones.

Appendicitis

- Appendicitis is the most common surgical condition in pregnancy (occurs in 1 in 2000 births).
- Incidence is same throughout pregnancy, but rupture is more frequent in third trimester (40%) than first (10%).
- Symptoms of appendicitis, such as nausea, vomiting, and anorexia, may also be a part of normal pregnancy complaints, making diagnosis difficult.
- Uterus displaces the appendix superiorly and laterally. Pain may not be located at McBurney's point (RLQ).
- Physical exam may be obscured from the enlarging uterus.

Most common indications for surgery in pregnancy:
- Appendicitis
- Adnexal masses
- Cholecystitis

COMPLICATIONS

- Abortion.
- Preterm labor.
- Maternal-fetal sepsis → neonatal neurologic injury.

TREATMENT

- Immediate appendectomy.
- Laparoscopy (early pregnancy when uterus is small).
- Laparotomy in later pregnancy.

Cholelithiasis and Cholecystitis

- Incidence of cholecystitis is 1 in 1000 pregnancies (more common than nonpregnant).
- Same clinical picture as nonpregnant.
- Medical management unless common bile duct obstruction or pancreatitis develops, in which case a cholecystectomy should be performed.
- High risk of preterm labor.

COMPLICATIONS

- Women with epilepsy taking anticonvulsants during pregnancy have double the general population risk of fetal malformations and preeclampsia.
- Women with a seizure disorder have an ↑ risk of birth defects even when they do not take anticonvulsant medications.
- Pregnant epileptics are more prone to seizures due to the associated stress and fatigue of pregnancy.
- The fetus is at risk for megaloblastic anemia.

TREATMENT

- Management of the epileptic female should begin with pre-pregnancy counseling.
- Anticonvulsant therapy should be reduced to the minimum dose of the minimum number of anticonvulsant medications.
- Folic acid supplementation should be taken by those women taking anticonvulsants.
- Once pregnant, the fetus should be screened for NTDs and congenital malformations.
- Blood levels of anticonvulsant medications should be checked at the beginning of pregnancy to determine the drug level that controls epileptic episodes successfully.

A 27-year-old G1 at 26 weeks presents to the office with swelling of the left leg and thigh since the previous night. She denies any trauma. She denies any dyspnea or chest pain. She is afebrile and in no apparent distress. Her left calf measures 4 cm more than the right. The fetal status is reassuring. What is the most likely diagnosis?

Answer: Deep vein thrombosis.

Deep Vein Thrombosis (DVT)

SIGNS AND SYMPTOMS

- Calf/leg swelling.
- Calf pain.
- Palpate cords in leg.

> Remember that maternal seizure disorder ↑ the risk of congenital anomalies.

> Contrast venography is the gold standard for diagnosis of lower-extremity DVT.

HIGH-YIELD FACTS

Medical Conditions in Pregnancy

DIAGNOSIS (FIGURE 7-1)

- Venography: Gold standard. Many complications, time consuming, cumbersome.
- Impedance plethysmography: Better for larger veins.
- Compression ultrasonography: Test most often used currently.

COMPLICATIONS

Pulmonary embolism develops in about 25% of patients with untreated DVT.

TREATMENT

- Anticoagulation with unfractionated or low-molecular-weight heparin (LMWH) during pregnancy.
- Heparin should be suspended during labor and delivery and restarted after 12–48 hr, depending on the degree of trauma to the genital tract.
- Convert to warfarin postpartum (do **not** use warfarin when pregnant).
- Anticoagulation ↓ the risk of pulmonary embolism to less than 5%.

Warfarin is a terotogen, so not used in pregnancy. Can breast-feed with it postpartum.

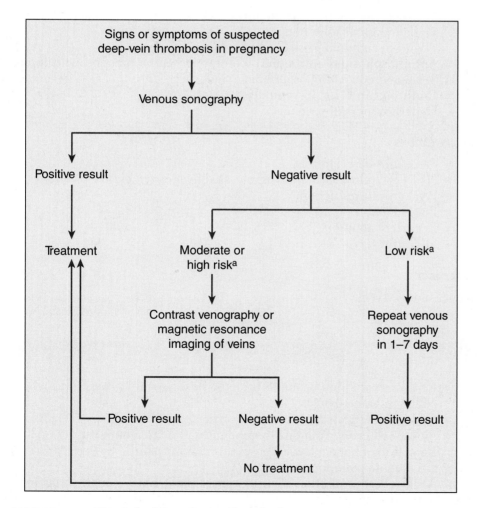

FIGURE 7-1. Diagnosis of Deep Venous Thrombosis

(Reproduced, with permission, from Lockwood C: *Clinical Updates in Women's Health Care: Thrombosis, Thrombophilia, and Thromboembolism*, Vol. VI, No. 4. American College of Obstetricians and Gynecologists, October 2007.)

HIGH-YIELD FACTS

Medical Conditions in Pregnancy

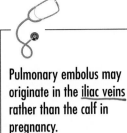

Pulmonary embolus may originate in the iliac veins rather than the calf in pregnancy.

Antithrombin deficiency: Most thrombogenic of the heritable coagulopathies.

Most common thrombophilia: Factor V Leiden mutation, often diagnosed when an asymptomatic woman starts combination oral contraceptive pills.

How do you treat a pregnant woman with a deep vein thrombosis (DVT)? Heparin or low-molecular-weight heparin. **Do not use** coumadin.

Pulmonary Embolism (PE)

- **Symptoms:** Dyspnea, chest pain, cough, syncope, hemoptysis.
- **Signs:** Tachypnea, tachycardia, apprehension, rales, hypoxemia.
- **Diagnosis:** Spiral CT.
- **Complications** include maternal death.
- **Treatment:** Anticoagulation with heparin/LMWH.
- Half of women presenting with a DVT will have a "silent" PE.

Thrombophilias

- ↑ risk of thrombus formation and associated complications.
- **Antithrombin III deficiency:** The most thrombogenic of the heritable coagulopathies.
- **Protein C deficiency:** 6- to 12-fold ↑ risk of first venous thromboembolism (VTE) in pregnancy.
- **Protein S deficiency:** 2- to 6-fold ↑ risk of first VTE in pregnancy.
- **Factor V Leiden mutation:**
  - Most common heritable thrombophilia; 5–8% of the general population.
  - Heterozygous inheritance.
  - Four to eightfold ↑ risk of first VTE in pregnancy.
- **Antiphospholipid antibodies:** Commonly seen in patients with lupus. See section on Antiphospholipid Syndrome.
- **Prothrombin G20210A mutation.**
- **Hyperhomocysteinemia.**

COMPLICATIONS

- Preeclampsia/eclampsia.
- HELLP syndrome (hemolysis, elevated liver enzymes, low platelets).
- Fetal growth restriction.
- Placental abruption.
- Recurrent abortion.
- Stillbirth.

TREATMENT

Heparin or LMWH.

SICKLE CELL DISEASE

- Red cells with hemoglobin S undergo sickling with ↓ oxygen leading to cell membrane damage.
- One in 12 African-Americans are carriers.
- **Sickle-cell crisis:** Pain due to ischemia and infarction in various organs. Infarction of bone marrow causes severe bone pain.
- Crisis more common in pregnancy.
- Acute chest syndrome: Pleuritic chest pain, fever, cough, lung infiltrates, hypoxia.

PREGNANCY COMPLICATIONS

- Thromboses (cerebral vein thrombosis, DVT, PE).
- Pneumonia.
- Pyelonephritis.

- Sepsis syndrome.
- Gestational HTN.
- Preeclampsia.
- Eclampsia.

DELIVERY COMPLICATIONS

- Placental abruption
- Preterm delivery
- Fetal growth restriction
- Stillbirth

MANAGEMENT

- Supplementation with 4 mg/day of folic acid to accommodate for rapid cell turnover.
- IV hydration and pain control for crises.
- Oxygen given via nasal cannula administered in an attempt to ↓ sickling.
- Prophylactic blood transfusions throughout pregnancy are **controversial.**

ANEMIA

- Physiologic anemia is normal anemia in pregnancy due to hemodilution from volume expansion.
- Anemia for a pregnant woman is a drop in hemoglobin below 10 g/dL or hematocrit < 30%.

INCIDENCE

Twenty to sixty percent of pregnant women; 80% is iron deficiency type.

COMPLICATIONS

- Preterm delivery.
- Intrauterine growth restriction (IUGR).
- Low birth weight.

TREATMENT

Two hundred milligrams of elemental iron daily from either ferrous sulfate, fumarate, or gluconate.

The two most common causes of anemia during pregnancy and the puerperium are iron deficiency and acute blood loss.

ANTIPHOSPHOLIPID SYNDROME

DIAGNOSIS

Clinical Criteria
- Arterial and venous thrombosis.
- Pregnancy morbidity:
  - At least one otherwise unexplained fetal death at or beyond 10 weeks.
  - At least one preterm birth before 34 weeks.
  - At least three consecutive spontaneous abortions before 10 weeks.

- Puerperium:
  - Fe deficiency.
  - Acute blood loss.

Laboratory Criteria
- Lupus anticoagulant.
- Medium to high titers of anticardiolipin antibody.
- Anti-β_2 glycoprotein.
- Each of these findings must be present in plasma, on at least two occasions > 12 weeks apart.

MANAGEMENT

Ranges from no treatment to daily low-dose aspirin to heparin, depending on the patient's past history of thrombosis and pregnancy morbidity.

SYSTEMIC LUPUS ERYTHEMATOSUS

COMPLICATIONS

Significant ↑ in maternal morbidity/mortality and other complications:

- Preeclampsia.
- Preterm labor.
- Fetal growth restriction.
- Anemia.
- Thrombophilia.
- Neonates may have symptoms of lupus for several months after birth.
- **Congenital heart block** may be seen in the offspring of women with anti-Ro (SS-A) and anti-La (SS-B).

Presence of anti-Ro (SS-A) and anti-La (SS-B) are associated with fetal congenital heart block.

MANAGEMENT

- Patients should be counseled to get pregnant while their disease is in remission.
- Monitor for disease flares and hypertensive episodes.
- Unless there is evidence of fetal compromise, the pregnancy should progress to term.
- High-dose methylprednisolone can be given for a lupus flare.
- Azathioprine is an immunosuppressant that can be used safely in pregnancy.
- Cyclophosphamide, methotrexate, and mycophenolate mofetil should be avoided, or at least not started until after 12 weeks gestation.

Rule of thumb for pregnant patients with lupus: one-third get better, one-third get worse, and one-third remain the same.

PRURITIC URTICARIAL PAPULES AND PLAQUES OF PREGNANCY (PUPPP)

INCIDENCE

- The most common pruritic dermatosis in pregnancy.
- One in 200 singleton pregnancies, ↑ to 8 in 200 with multiples.
- Seldom occurs in subsequent pregnancies.

- Intensely pruritic cutaneous eruption that usually appears late in pregnancy.
- Erythema, vesicles, and eczematous target lesions may be seen.
- Begins on the abdomen and spread to arms and legs. Rarely may involve face, palms, and soles.

TREATMENT

- Oral antihistamines and topical steroids are the mainstays of treatment.
- May require systemic corticosteroids for severe pruritus.
- Rash usually disappears shortly before or a few days after delivery.

CANCER THERAPY DURING PREGNANCY

Surgery

As long as the reproductive organs are not involved, surgery is generally well tolerated by both the mother and fetus during pregnancy and should not be delayed.

Radiation

- Therapeutic radiation can cause significant complications in the fetus, such as carcinogenesis, cell death, and brain damage.
- The most susceptible period is during organogenesis.
- The site of the tumor is important as well; radiation to head and neck cancers can be done relatively safely but if directed toward abdominal tumors, it may cause fetal death.

Chemotherapy

- Risks to the fetus include malformations, growth restriction, mental retardation, and the risk of future malignancies.
- Risk is highest during organogenesis, and few adverse outcomes are seen if chemotherapeutic agents are used after the first trimester.

HIGH-YIELD FACTS

Medical Conditions in Pregnancy

CHAPTER 8

Obstetric Complications

What is the treatment of choice for seizure prophylaxis in pregnant female with pregnancy-induced HTN? Magnesium sulfate (MgSO$_4$)
What is its antidote in the case of toxicity? Calcium gluconate

Hypertensive Diseases of Pregnancy

A 28-year-old G2P1001 at 37 weeks gestation complains of severe headaches and black spots in her visual field. Her blood pressures are 165/95 and 163/96 and she has 4+ protein on urine dipstick. Her cervical exam is closed, thick, and high. The fetal heart tones are reassuring and she has no contractions. The ultrasound (US) shows a fetus that is appropriate for 37 weeks, with normal amniotic fluid index (AFI), and in cephalic position. What is the next best step?

Answer: This patient has signs and symptoms of severe preeclampsia and should be delivered immediately, especially when term. Vaginal delivery is usually attempted. Patients with preeclampsia can have a seizure at any point before, during, or after labor, so seizure prophylaxis with magnesium sulfate is indicated.

Hypertensive disorders of pregnancy include gestational hypertension (HTN), mild and severe preeclampsia, HELLP (hemolysis, elevated liver enzymes, low platelets), and eclampsia. These may all be a spectrum of the same disease process that manifest at different levels of severity at different gestational ages.

Hypertension-related deaths in pregnancy account for 15% of maternal deaths (second after pulmonary embolism).

There are four categories of HTN in pregnancy:

1. **Preexisting or chronic HTN during pregnancy:**
   - Preexisting HTN begins prior to pregnancy or before the 20th week of gestation.
   - Defined as a sustained systolic BP ≥ 140 mm Hg and/or diastolic BP ≥ 90 mm Hg documented on more than one occasion *prior* to the 20th week of gestation, HTN that existed before pregnancy, or HTN that persists > 12 weeks after delivery.
   - Usually not associated with significant proteinuria or end-organ damage if well controlled.

2. **Gestational hypertension** (most benign):
   - Also called transient HTN and pregnancy-induced HTN.
   - A sustained or transient systolic blood pressure (BP) ≥ 140 mm Hg and/or diastolic BP ≥ 90 mm Hg occurs after the 20th week of gestation.
   - No proteinuria or end-organ damage.

3. **Preeclampsia:**
   - Defined as hypertension with proteinuria after the 20th week of gestation.
   - **Mild preeclampsia** is defined by:
     - A systolic BP ≥ 140 mm Hg or a diastolic BP ≥ 90 mm Hg twice > 6 hr apart at bed rest.
     - Proteinuria: 1+ on dipstick or ≥ 300 mg/24 hr.
     - Usually no other subjective symptoms.
   - **Severe preeclampsia** is defined by:
     - A systolic BP ≥ 160 mm Hg or a diastolic BP ≥ 110 mm Hg twice 6 hr apart at bed rest with or without the following end organ findings.

Chronic HTN:
- ↑ BP outside of pregnancy.
- ↑ BP prior to 20 weeks gestation.
- ↑ BP persisting after 12 weeks postpartum.

Superimposed preeclampsia:
Preeclampsia in the presence of preexisting chronic hypertension. Diagnosed with worsening blood pressures and proteinuria. Patients with chronic hypertension are at ↑ risk of developing superimposed preeclampsia.

- Neurologic: Frontal headaches, scotomata, eclampsia (seizure due to preeclampsia).
- Renal: Proteinuria ($\geq$ 5.0 g/24 hr), oliguria (< 500 cc/24 hr).
- Gastrointestinal (GI): Epigastric or right upper quadrant (RUQ) pain (hepatocellular ischemia and edema that stretches Glisson's capsule). ↑ aspartate transaminase (AST), alanine transaminase (ALT).
- Pulmonary: Edema, cyanosis.
- Hematologic: Thrombocytopenia (< 100,000), microangiopathic coagulopathy, hemolysis (↑ LDH).
- Fetal: IUGR or oligohydramnios.

4. **Superimposed preeclampsia:**
   - Preeclampsia (mild or severe) in patients with chronic HTN in pregnancy.
   - Twenty-five percent of patients with chronic HTN in pregnancy develop preeclampsia.
   - Patients can have seemingly benign HTN (no proteinuria or evidence of end-organ damage) in early pregnancy and then develop preeclampsia.
   - Increasing proteinuria in the setting of HTN after the 20th week of gestation is preeclampsia, regardless of the timing of the onset of the HTN.
   - Often occurs earlier in pregnancy, has more severe fetal growth restriction than preeclampsia without chronic HTN, and is also associated with ↑ risk of placental abruption.

Symptoms of severe preeclampsia include:
- **Headache**
- **Visual disturbances**
- **Epigastric/RUQ pain**

PATHOPHYSIOLOGY

Vasospasm in various organs (brain, kidneys, lungs, uterus) causes most of the signs and symptoms of preeclampsia; however, the cause of the vasospasm is unknown.

Preeclampsia is usually asymptomatic; it is critical to pick it up during routine prenatal visits.

COMPLICATIONS

- Abruption.
- Eclampsia with intracranial hemorrhage, blindness.
- Coagulopathy.
- Renal failure.
- Hepatic subcapsular hematoma.
- Uteroplacental insufficiency.

The only definitive treatment for preeclampsia is delivery.

TREATMENT

See Figure 8-1 for a management algorithm.

- The only cure for preeclampsia and its variants is **delivery** of the fetus.
- Preexisting HTN/transient HTN/chronic HTN in pregnancy: Antihypertensive medications vs. close observation.
- Antihypertensive medications have not been found to be helpful, and in some cases adversely affect fetal growth.
- **Magnesium sulfate (MgSO$_4$)** is started for **seizure prophylaxis** when decision is made to deliver fetus. It is **not** a treatment for HTN.

Magnesium toxicity (7–10 mEq/L) is associated with loss of patellar reflexes, respiratory depression, and cardiac arrest. Treat with calcium gluconate 10% solution 1 g IV.

FIGURE 8-1. **Management of hypertension in pregnancy.**

(Reproduced, with permission, from Lindarkis NM, Lott S. *Digging Up the Bones: Obstetrics and Gynecology.* New York: McGraw-Hill, 1998: 60.)

Magnesium sulfate prevents seizures in preeclampsia; does not treat HTN.

When patients are put on MgSO₄ for seizure prophylaxis, they must be closely monitored for magnesium toxicity by obtaining magnesium levels and watching for hyporeflexia.

HTN may be absent in 20% of women with HELLP syndrome and severe in 50%.

- **Mild preeclampsia:**
  - Preterm: Close monitoring for worsening disease.
    - Fetal testing (non-stress tests [NSTs] and biophysical profiles [BPPs]) to ensure fetal well-being.

- Bed rest is not necessary, although ↓ physical activity is recommended.
- Term: delivery.
  - Vaginal delivery is usually attempted; cesarean delivery for other obstetrical reasons.
  - Start MgSO$_4$ for seizure prophylaxis.
- **Severe preeclampsia:**
  - Very preterm (< 28 weeks): Close monitoring in hospital in select cases only.
  - Preterm or term: Delivery.
    - Delivery may not be in the best interest of the premature baby, but it is indicated to prevent worsening maternal disease.
    - Vaginal delivery is usually attempted; cesarean delivery for other obstetrical reasons.
    - Start MgSO$_4$ for seizure prophylaxis.

HELLP Syndrome

- HELLP syndrome is a manifestation of severe preeclampsia with:
  - **H**emolysis,
  - Elevated **L**iver enzymes
  - **L**ow **P**latelets.
- It is associated with high morbidity, and immediate delivery is indicated. It may occur with or without HTN.

Eclampsia

Defined as seizure or coma without another cause in a patient with preeclampsia. Eclampsia → hemorrhagic stroke → death.

TREATMENT

- Airway, breathing, and circulation (ABCs).
- Rule out other causes: Head trauma is a possible confounder; others include cerebral tumors, cerebral venous thrombosis, drug overdoses, epilepsy, and cerebrovascular accidents.
- Control seizures with magnesium sulfate (the only anticonvulsant used).
- Delivery is the only definitive treatment.
  - If diagnosis of eclampsia made, no expectant management regardless of gestational age.
  - Vaginal delivery is recommended.
  - Women often go into spontaneous labor after onset of seizures, and/or have a shorter duration of labor.
- Control BP with hydralazine or labetalol.

RISK FACTORS FOR HYPERTENSIVE DISEASES IN PREGNANCY

- Nulliparity.
- Age > 40 yr.
- African-American race.
- Family history of preeclampsia.
- Chronic HTN.

Objectives in management of severe preeclampsia:
1. Prevent eclampsia which can cause intracranial hemorrhage and damage to other vital organs
2. Deliver a healthy infant

Diuretics are not used in pregnancy because they ↓ plasma volume and this may be detrimental to fetal growth. Salt restriction also ↓ plasma volume and is not recommended.

Angiotensin-converting enzyme (ACE) inhibitors are contraindicated because they are teratogenic. Use other classes of antihypertensives to control HTN in pregnancy.

- Chronic renal disease.
- Antiphospholipid syndrome.
- Diabetes mellitus.
- Multiple gestation.
- Angiotensinogen gene T235 (homozygous > heterozygous).

Antihypertensive Agents Used in Pregnancy

SHORT-TERM CONTROL

- **Hydralazine:** IV or PO, direct vasodilator. Side effects: systemic lupus erythematosus (SLE)-like syndrome, headache, palpitations.
- **Labetalol:** IV or PO, nonselective β_1 and α_1 blocker. Side effects: headache and tremor.

LONG-TERM CONTROL

- **Methyldopa:** PO, false neurotransmitter. Side effects: postural hypotension, drowsiness, fluid retention.
- **Nifedipine:** PO, calcium channel blocker. Side effects: edema, dizziness.

Eclampsia:
- 25% of seizures are before labor.
- 50% of seizures are during labor.
- 25% of seizures are postdelivery (may be encountered up to 10 days postpartum).

GESTATIONAL DIABETES MELLITUS

A 33-year-old G4P3003 at 26 weeks gestation undergoes the 50-g glucose challenge test. The result is 160 mg/dL. What is the next step in management?

Answer: She should undergo the 3-hr glucose tolerance test since her 1-hr result was > 140 mg/dL.

What is a major fetal complication of gestational diabetes mellitus?
Macrosomia

- **Pregestational diabetes (DM):** Patient diagnosed with DM prior to pregnancy.
- **Gestational diabetes (GDM):** Patient develops diabetes only during pregnancy.
  - White Classification A1: Controlled with diet.
  - White Classification A2: Requires insulin.

SCREENING

When obtaining a patient's history, look for signs of overt diabetes that has not yet been diagnosed. If these signs are present, the patient should not receive the routine screening during pregnancy.

- **Signs of overt diabetes:**
  - Polydipsia.
  - Polyuria.
  - History of insulin or oral hypoglycemic agents between pregnancies.
  - History of "touch of sugar" between pregnancies.
  - Overt glycosuria.
  - Frequent infections (vaginal candidiasis, cellulitis).
- If overt diabetes is suspected, perform a fingerstick (FS) glucose level without a glucose load.

- If fasting FS is > 110 mg/dL or random > 150 mg/dL, diagnosis of diabetes.
- If fasting is > 140 mg/dL or random > 200 mg/dL, consider hospitalization for glycemic control.
- See Chapter 7 regarding Pregestational Diabetes.
- **Risk factors:** Early screen at 16 weeks when:
  - Age > 30.
  - Prior pregnancy with gestational diabetes.
  - Family history of diabetes.
  - Obesity (> 20% ideal body weight).
  - Previous infant > 4000 g (8¾ lb).
  - History of stillbirth or child with cardiac defects (poor obstetrical outcome).
  - Race: Black, Hispanic, Native American.
- **Glucose challenge test** at 24–28 weeks:
  - Give 50-g glucose load (nonfasting state).
  - Draw glucose blood level 1 hr later.
  - If ≥ 140, a 3-hr glucose tolerance test (GTT) is then required to diagnose GDM.
  - If > 200, patient is diagnosed with GDM type A1 and a diabetic diet is initiated.
- **3-hr GTT**—if glucose challenge test is ≥ 140 and < 200:
  - Unrestricted diet for 3 days, carbohydrate load prior to test.
  - Fasting for 8–14 hr.
  - Draw fasting glucose level.
  - Give 100-g glucose load.
  - Draw glucose levels at 1 hr, at 2 hr, and at 3 hr.
  - Diagnosis of gestational diabetes made if two or more values are equal to or greater than those listed (see Table 8-1). Either criteria can be used to make the diagnosis.

MATERNAL EFFECTS

- Four times ↑ risk of preeclampsia.
- ↑ risk of bacterial infections.
- Higher rate of C-section.
- ↑ risk of polyhydramnios.
- ↑ risk of birth injury.

Diabetes is the most common medical complication of pregnancy.

Gestational diabetes probably results from **human placental lactogen** secreted during pregnancy, which has large glucagon-like effects.

If a pregnant woman has an abnormal one hour glucose challenge test, then check a 3-hr GTT.

Thirty percent of women with gestational diabetes develop diabetes mellitus in later life.

TABLE 8-1. Diagnosis of Gestational Diabetes

	NATIONAL DIABETES PLASMA DATA GROUP CRITERIA (mg/dL)	CARPENTAR/COUSTAN CRITERIA (mg/dL)
Fasting	105	95
1 hr	190	180
2 hr	165	155
3 hr	145	140

FETAL EFFECTS

- ↑ risk of perinatal death (A2 > A1).
- Fetal anomalies not ↑ in gestational diabetes (as opposed to pregestational diabetes).
- Two to three times ↑ risk of preterm delivery.
- Hyperinsulinemia → fetal macrosomia → birth injury (shoulder dystocia).
  - Hyperglycemia affects most fetal organs except brain.
  - Excessive fat on shoulders and trunk.
- Metabolic derangements at birth (hypoglycemia, hypocalcemia).

MANAGEMENT

The key factors involved in successful management of these high-risk pregnancies include:

- A glucose control log should be checked at each prenatal visit.
- Maintain fasting glucose < 95 and 2-hr postprandial (breakfast, lunch, dinner) glucose < 120.
- If A1 with continued ↑ in glucose, start insulin. Oral hypoglycemic agents (glyburide, metformin) have been studied.
- If A2 with continued ↑ in glucose, ↑ insulin dose.
- Fasting glucose most important for fetal and maternal effects.
- **At 32–34 weeks for A2 gestational diabetics:**
  - Fetal testing (BPP).
  - US for growth every 4 weeks.
- **Delivery:**
  - A1 gestational diabetics: Await labor. Fetal testing between 41 and 42 weeks. Consider delivery between 41 and 42 weeks.
  - A2 gestational diabetics: Consider delivery at 39–42 weeks if good dating. If poor glycemic control, consider amniocentesis for fetal lung maturity and delivery at term.
  - Maintain euglycemia during labor (insulin drip for A2).
  - May offer cesarean delivery if fetal weight ≥ 4500 g.

The CNS anomaly most specific to DM is **caudal regression.**

SHOULDER DYSTOCIA

A 25-year-old G1P0 is delivering her first child. Her labor course was protracted and she pushed for 3 hr. The head is seen to deliver and then retracts, forming the turtle sign. The infant's shoulder does not deliver with gentle symmetric traction. What is the diagnosis? What is the next step in management?

Answer: Shoulder dystocia. Calling for help is essential to perform the additional maneuvers.

Shoulder dystocia = obstetric emergency

Shoulder dystocia is diagnosed when the fetal shoulder is lodged behind the pubic symphysis after the fetal head has been delivered, and the delivery cannot be completed. This is an obstetric emergency. If infant is not delivered quickly, it may suffer neurologic injury or death from hypoxia.

RISK FACTORS

- Maternal factors leading to ↑ fetal birth weight:
  - Obesity
  - Multiparity
  - Gestational diabetes
- Fetal: Post-term pregnancy (> 42 weeks).
- Intrapartum: Prolonged first and/or second stage of labor.

COMPLICATIONS

- Brachial plexus nerve injuries.
- Fetal humeral/clavicular fracture.
- Hypoxia/death.

TREATMENT

Several maneuvers can be done to dislodge the shoulder:

- **McRoberts maneuver:** Maternal thighs are sharply flexed against maternal abdomen. This flattens the sacrum and the symphysis pubis and may allow the delivery of the fetal shoulder.
- **Suprapubic pressure** slightly superior to the symphysis pubis and in the direction of the desired shoulder rotation.
- **Woods corkscrew maneuver:** Pressure is applied against scapula of posterior shoulder to rotate the posterior shoulder and "unscrew" the anterior shoulder.
- **Posterior shoulder delivery:** Hand is inserted into vagina and posterior arm is pulled across chest, delivering posterior arm and shoulder. This creates a shorter distance between the anterior shoulder and posterior axilla, allowing the anterior shoulder to be delivered.
- **Break clavicle:** Apply pressure with the fingers to the fetal clavicle.
- **Zavanelli maneuver:** If the above measures do not work, the fetal head can be returned to the uterus by reversing the cardinal movements of labor. At this point, a C-section can be performed.
- Maneuvers that do not require direct contact with the fetus should be done first because they have lower morbidity for the fetus. Manipulation of the fetus to accomplish a delivery in a shoulder dystocia has ↑ morbidity.

Shoulder dystocia management — HELPERRR

Help — Call for **Help**
Episiotomy
Legs up (McRobert's position)
Pressure suprapubically
Enter vagina for shoulder rotation (Woods corkscrew)
Reach for posterior arm
Rupture clavicle or pubic symphysis
Return head into vagina for C-section (Zananelli).

Do not apply fundal pressure in shoulder dystocia. It causes further impaction of the shoulder behind the symphysis pubis.

HYPEREMESIS GRAVIDARUM

- Severe vomiting that results in:
  - Weight loss.
  - Dehydration.
  - Metabolic derangements.
- Due to high levels of human chorionic gonadotropin (hCG), estrogens, or both.
- Psychiatric component present.
- **Management:**
  - Rule out other causes (molar pregnancy, thyrotoxicosis, GI etiology).
  - First line: Vitamin B$_6$ with doxylamine (antihistamine/emetic)
  - IV hydration, thiamine replacement, antiemetics.
  - Parenteral nutrition.

First step in management of isoimmunized pregnant patient: Check paternal erythrocyte antigen status.

Kell **K**ills, **D**uffy **D**ies, **L**ewis **L**ives.

 A 29-year-old G2P1001 at 16 weeks gestation presents for prenatal care. Her blood type is A negative with a positive antibody screen. What is the next step in management?

Answer: Identify the antibody. Some can be dangerous for the fetus and some are benign.

- In each pregnancy, a woman should have her blood type, Rh status, and antibody screen evaluated at the initial prenatal visit. If the antibody screen is positive, the next step is to identify the antibody. Some antibodies pose no harm to the fetus (ie, anti-Lewis), while others can cause hemolytic disease of the newborn (HDN) and be fatal (ie, anti-D, anti-Kell, anti-Duffy).
- Along with antibodies to antigens on fetal red blood cells (RBCs), antibodies may be directed against fetal platelets. If the antibodies are not harmful to the fetus, no further workup needs to be done. If antibodies are known to cause harm to the fetus, next step is to determine the titer of the antibodies. A **critical titer**, usually 1:16 at most institutions, is the titer associated with a significant risk for HDN. Fetal surveillance with possible therapeutic interventions may be needed (see Figure 8-2).

Anti-D Isoimmunization

An understanding of D (or Rho) RBC antigen compatibility is a crucial part of prenatal care. If a mother and developing child are incompatible, very serious complications can cause fetal death. This section will review the appropriate screening and therapy for anti-D isoimmunization.

WHAT IS RH OR D?

- The surface of the human RBC may or may not have a Rho (Rh) antigen. If a patient with blood type A has a Rho antigen, the blood type is A+. If that person has no Rho antigen, the blood type is A–. In the following discussion, the Rh antigen will be referred to as D.
- Half of all antigens on fetal RBCs come from the father, and half come from the mother. That means that the fetus may have antigens to which the mother's immune system is unfamiliar.

THE PROBLEM WITH D SENSITIZATION

- If the mother is D negative and the father is D positive, there may be a chance that the baby may be D positive.
- If the mother is D negative and her fetus is D positive, she may become sensitized to the D antigen and develop antibodies against the baby's RBCs.
- These antibodies cross the placenta and attack the fetal RBCs, resulting in fetal RBC hemolysis. The hemolysis results in significant fetal anemia, resulting in fetal heart failure and death. This disease process is known as hemolytic disease of the newborn (HDN).

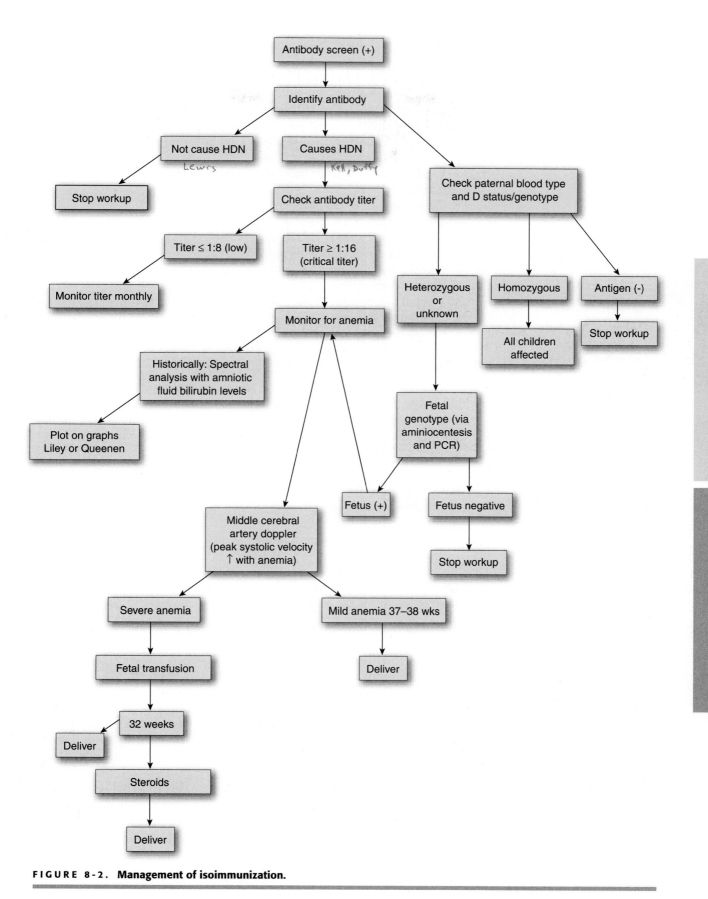

FIGURE 8-2. Management of isoimmunization.

- Sensitization is the development of maternal antibodies against D antigens on the fetus RBC. Sensitization may occur whenever fetal blood enters the maternal circulation. The fetus of the pregnancy when sensitization occurred usually suffers no harm because the maternal antibody titers are low. The subsequent pregnancies with a D-positive fetus are at significantly higher risk of HDN because the mother has already developed memory cells that quickly produce anti-D antibodies against the fetus RBCs.
- The following conditions can cause fetal-maternal bleeding, and lead to sensitization:
  - Chorionic villus sampling.
  - Amniocentesis.
  - Spontaneous/induced abortion.
  - Threatened/incomplete abortion.
  - Ectopic pregnancies.
  - Placental abruption/bleeding placenta previa.
  - Vaginal or cesarean delivery.
  - Abdominal trauma.
  - External cephalic version.

ANTI-D IMMUNE GLOBULINS (IgG) (BRAND NAME: RHOGAM)

Anti-D immune globulins are collected from donated human plasma. When a mother is given a dose of anti-D IgG, the antibodies bind to the fetal RBCs that have the D antigen on them and clear them from the maternal circulation. The goal is to prevent the mother's immune system from recognizing the presence of the D antigen and forming antibodies against it.

- Give to D-negative mothers, who have not formed antibodies against D antigen.
- **Not** indicated for patients who already have anti-D antibodies and are sensitized.
- Indicated for patients who might be sensitized to other blood group antigens.

MANAGEMENT OF THE UNSENSITIZED D-NEGATIVE PATIENT (THE D-NEGATIVE PATIENT WITH A NEGATIVE ANTIBODY SCREEN)

1. Antibody screen should be done at the initial prenatal visit and at 28 weeks.
2. If antibody screen negative, the fetus is presumed to be D positive, and one dose of anti-D IgG immune globulin is given to the mother at 28 weeks to prevent development of maternal antibodies. Anti-D immune globulins last for ~12 weeks, and the highest risk of sensitization is in T3.
3. At birth, the infant's D status is noted. If the infant is D negative, no anti-D IgG is given to the mother. If the infant is D positive, anti-D IgG is given to the mother within 72 hr of delivery. The dose of anti-D IgG is determined by KB test.
4. Administration of anti-D IgG at 28 weeks gestation and within 72 hr of birth, reduces sensitization to 0.2%.

Kleihauer-Betke test determines the number of fetal RBCs in the maternal circulation (see section on RhoGAM).

The standard dose of RhoGAM is 300 µg. It is sufficient for 15 mL of D-positive fetal RBCs (30 mL of whole fetal blood). Kleihauer-Betke (KB) test estimates the number of fetal RBCs that are present in the maternal circulation. The dose of anti-D IgG is based on the results of the KB test.

Management of the Sensitized D-Negative Patient (Antibody Screen Positive for Anti-D Antibody)

> 👤 A 35-year-old G4P2012 at 26 weeks gestation is diagnosed with anti-Kell antibodies with the titer of 1:32. Amniocentesis shows that the fetus is positive for the Kell antigen. In addition to fetal testing with a biophysical profile, what other testing is critical for this fetus?
>
> **Answer:** The fetus should be monitored with middle cerebral artery Dopplers, which indicate the severity of anemia.

1. If antibody screen at initial prenatal visit is positive, and is identified as anti-D,
2. Check the antibody titer. Critical titer is 1:16.
   - If titer remains stable at < 1:16, the likelihood of hemolytic disease of the newborn is low. Follow the antibody titer every 4 weeks.
   - If the titer is ≥ 1:16 and/or rising, the likelihood of hemolytic disease of the newborn is high. Amniocentesis is done.
3. Amniocentesis:
   - Fetal cells are analyzed for D status.
   - Historically, amniotic fluid was analyzed by spectral analysis, which measured the light absorbance by bilirubin. Absorbance measurements were plotted on a graph to predict the severity of disease. The preferred method now is to perform middle cerebral artery (MCA) Dopplers to assess for anemia.
4. Serial US monitoring for:
   - Anatomy scan for hydrops fetalis.
   - MCA Doppler for presence or severity of anemia (see Figure 8-3). Consider blood transfusion to fetus if very premature.
5. Delivery:
   - Mild anemia: Induction of labor at 37–38 weeks.
   - Severe anemia: Deliver at 32–34 weeks.
     - Most babies > 32 weeks do well in the neonatal intensive care unit (NICU).

Hemolytic Disease of the Newborn

Hemolytic disease of the newborn (HDN)/fetal hydrops occurs when the mother lacks an antigen present on the fetal RBC → fetal RBCs in maternal circulation trigger an immune response → maternal antibodies lyse fetal RBCs → fetal anemia → fetal hyperbilirubinemia + kernicterus + heart failure, edema, ascites, pericardial effusion → death.

Fetal hydrops = collection of fluid in two or more body cavities:
- Scalp edema
- Pleural effusion
- Pericardial effusion
- Ascites

FIGURE 8-3. Middle cerebral artery.

A. Doppler B. Waveform. (Reproduced, with permission, from Cunningham FG, Leveno KJ, Bloom SL, et al. *Williams Obstetrics*, 23rd ed. New York: McGraw-Hill, 2010: 365.)

- Weigh risks for continued cord blood sampling and transfusions with neonatal risks of preterm delivery.
- Administer steroids to mother to enhance fetal lung maturity.

Kell Isoimmunization

With the use of anti-D immune globulin, there is an $\uparrow$ of isoimmunization caused by minor antigens acquired by incompatible blood transfusion. Some minor antigens cause HDN, and some do not. Those that do cause HDN are managed the same way as anti-D isoimmunized mothers. Kell isoimmunization is an exception because:

- It is less predictable and results in more severe anemia than alloimmunization due to other erythrocyte antigens.
- Maternal Kell antibody titers and amniotic fluid delta OD_{450} are not predictive of the severity of fetal anemia as with anti-D sensitization.
- MCA Dopplers are accurate in predicting severe anemia with Kell isoimmunization.

PRETERM LABOR

CRITERIA

Gestational age (GA) < 37 weeks with regular uterine contractions and:
- Progressive cervical change

or

- A cervix that is 2 cm dilated

or

- A cervix 80% effaced

or

- Ruptured membranes.

Braxton Hicks contractions (irregular, nonrhythmic, usually painless contractions that begin at early gestation and $\uparrow$ as term approaches) may make it difficult to distinguish between true and false labor.

RISK FACTORS

- Previous history of preterm delivery.
- Hydramnios.
- Multiple gestations.
- Cocaine.
- Urinary tract infection (UTI).
- Vaginal infections.
- Abruption.

ASSESSMENT

- Evaluate for causes such as infection (gonococcus, bacterial vaginosis), abruption.
- Confirm GA of fetus (ie, by US).
- Predictors of preterm labor:
  - Transvaginal cervical length measurement:
    - > 35 mm: Low risk of preterm delivery.
    - < 25 mm (especially with funneling): High risk of preterm delivery.

- Fetal fibronectin assay:
  - Vaginal swab of posterior fornix prior to digital exam.
  - If negative, 99% predictability for no preterm delivery within 1 week.

Management of Preterm Labor

HYDRATION

Not proven to reduce preterm labor, but hydration may decrease uterine irritability. Dehydration causes antidiuretic hormone (ADH) secretion, and ADH mimics oxytocin, which causes uterine contractions.

TOCOLYTIC THERAPY

Tocolysis is the pharmacologic inhibition of uterine contractions. Tocolytic drugs have not been shown to decrease neonatal morbidity or mortality, but may prolong gestation for 2–7 days to allow time for administration of steroids and transfer to a facility with a neonatal ICU. It is used when fetus is < 34 weeks gestation.

TOCOLYTIC AGENTS

- **Magnesium sulfate:** Suppresses uterine contractions. *& suppresses seizures*
  - Unknown mechanism of action: Competes with calcium, inhibits myosin light chain.
  - Maternal side effects: Flushing, lethargy, headache, muscle weakness, diplopia, dry mouth, pulmonary edema, cardiac arrest. Toxicity is treated with calcium gluconate.
  - Fetal side effects: Lethargy, hypotonia, respiratory depression.
  - Contraindications: Myasthenia gravis.
- **Nifedipine:** Oral calcium channel blocker.
  - Maternal side effects: Flushing, headache, dizziness, nausea, transient hypotension.
  - Fetal side effects: None yet noted.
  - Contraindications: Maternal hypotension, cardiac disease; use with caution with renal disease. Avoid concomitant use with magnesium sulfate.
- **Ritodrine, terbutaline, β agonist:** β_2 receptor stimulation on myometrial cells → ↑ cyclic adenosine monophosphate (cAMP) → ↓ intracellular Ca → ↓ contractions:
  - Maternal side effects: Pulmonary edema, tachycardia, headaches.
  - Fetal side effect: Tachycardia.
  - Contraindications: Cardiovascular disease, hyperthyroidism, uncontrolled diabetes mellitus.
- **Indomethacin,** prostaglandin inhibitors: For < 32 weeks.
  - Maternal side effects: Nausea, heartburn.
  - Fetal side effects: Premature constriction of ductus arteriosus, pulmonary HTN, reversible ↓ in amniotic fluid.
  - Contraindications: Renal or hepatic impairment, peptic ulcer disease.

Most infants born after 34 weeks GA will survive (the survival rate is within 1% of the survival rate beyond 37 weeks).

Tocolytics have not been proven to prolong pregnancy.

Contraindications to tocolysis—
BAD CHU
- Severe **B**leeding from any cause
- Severe **A**bruptio placentae
- Fetal **D**eath/life-incompatible anomaly
- **C**horioamnionitis
- Severe pregnancy-induced **H**ypertension
- **U**nstable maternal hemodynamics

CORTICOSTEROIDS

- Given to patients in preterm labor from 24 to 34 weeks unless they have an infection.
- Actions: Accelerate fetal lung maturity (↓ RDS), and reduce intraventricular hemorrhage.

ASSESSING FETAL LUNG MATURITY

An amniocentesis may be performed to assess fetal lungs for risk of RDS. Fetal lungs are mature if:

- Phosphatidylglycerol is present in amniotic fluid.
- Surfactant-albumin in amniotic fluid at a ratio > 55.
- Lecithin-sphingomyelin in amniotic fluid at a ratio > 2.

PREVENTION OF PRETERM LABOR

17α-hydroxyprogesterone is often given as weekly IM injections starting at 16–20 weeks to women with risk factors or history of preterm labor.

- Relaxes the myometrium.
- Prevents rejection of the fetus by suppressing lymphocyte production of cytokines.

PREMATURE RUPTURE OF MEMBRANES

> A 24-year-old G3P1102 at 38 weeks presents to triage with a complaint of leakage of clear fluid from the vagina for the past 24 hr. She reports good fetal movement, no vaginal bleeding, no contractions. She is afebrile. On sterile speculum exam, pooling, ferning, and positive nitrazine is noted. Sterile vaginal exam is 1 cm, long cervix, −3 station, cephalic. Fetal heart rate (FHR) is reassuring, and no contractions are noted. What is the diagnosis?
>
> **Answer:** Premature rupture of membranes is diagnosed when the membranes rupture prior to the onset of labor. Rupture of membranes is confirmed by the sterile speculum exam. Based on the vaginal exam and the absence of contractions, the patient is not in labor. Considering that the fetus is term, the next step should be induction of labor in order to prevent chorioamnionitis.

Premature rupture denotes spontaneous rupture of fetal membranes before the onset of labor. This can occur at term (PROM) or preterm (PPROM).

- **ROM:** Rupture of membranes.
- **PROM:** Premature rupture of membranes (ROM before the onset of labor).
- **PPROM:** Preterm (< 37 weeks) premature rupture of membranes.
- **Prolonged rupture of membranes:** Rupture of membranes present for > 18 hr.

Maternal corticosteroid administration with:
- **Preterm labor 24–34 weeks**
- **Preterm premature rupture of membranes (PPROM) 24–32 weeks**

Fetal benefits:
- ↓ respiratory distress syndrome (RDS).
- ↓ intraventricular hemorrhage.

PPROM: Most common diagnosis associated with preterm delivery.

ETIOLOGY

- Unknown but hypothesized:
  - Vaginal and cervical infections.
  - Incompetent cervix.
  - Nutritional deficiencies.

COMPLICATIONS

- Prematurity: If PROM occurs at < 37 weeks, the fetus is at risk of being born prematurely with its associated complications.
- Pulmonary hypoplasia: If PROM occurs at < 24 weeks → oligohydramnios → **pulmonary hypoplasia.** *Survival at this age is low.*
- Chorioamnionitis.
- Placental abruption.
- Neonatal infection.
- Umbilical cord prolapse.
- Preterm labor.

MANAGEMENT OF ALL PROM PATIENTS

- Avoid vaginal exams if possible to ↓ risk of chorioamnionitis.
- Evaluate patient for chorioamnionitis (common etiology of PROM): Fever > 100.4°F (38°C), leukocytosis, maternal/fetal tachycardia, uterine tenderness, malodorous vaginal discharge.
- If chorioamnionitis present, delivery is performed despite GA, and broad-spectrum antibiotics (ampicillin, gentamicin) are initiated.

SPECIFIC MANAGEMENT FOR PROM AT TERM

Ninety percent of term patients go into spontaneous labor within 24 hr after rupture:

- Patients in active labor should be allowed to progress.
- If labor is not spontaneous, it should be induced. Cesarean delivery should be performed for other indications.

SPECIFIC MANAGEMENT OF PPROM

> An 18-year-old G1P0 at 30 weeks gestation presents to triage with complaints of clear fluid leaking from her vagina. Testing is positive for pooling, ferning, and nitrazine. The cervix is visually closed. FHR is reassuring. No contractions are noted on the monitor. The US shows a singleton, viable fetus, in the breech position. What is the next step in management?
>
> **Answer**: The patient has preterm premature rupture of membranes. She should be admitted to the hospital. Steroids should be administered to ↓ the risk of RDS in the fetus, and antibiotics should be given to ↑ the latency period.

- Fifty percent of preterm patients go into labor within 24 hr after rupture.
- Generally, one needs to balance the risks of premature birth against the risk of infection (which ↑ with the time that membranes are ruptured before birth).
- Amniotic fluid assessment for fetal lung maturity from vaginal pooling. Consider delivery if mature.
- US to assess GA, anomalies, presentation of baby, and AFI.

Prolonged rupture of membranes may be due to premature rupture (PROM) *or* an abnormally long labor (not PROM).

Nitrazine test may be falsely positive if contaminated with blood, semen.

- Monitor in hospital for infection, abruption, fetal distress and preterm labor.
- If < 32 weeks gestation, give steroids to ↓ the incidence of RDS.
- Antibiotic coverage to prolong latency period (time between ROM and onset of labor) to give a premature fetus time to mature in utero.
- Fetal testing to ensure fetal well-being.
- Delivery:
  - If infection, abruption, fetal distress noted.
  - At 34 weeks gestation. At this GA, most babies with little risk of RDS; avoid the risk of other complications.

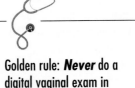

Golden rule: **Never** do a digital vaginal exam in third-trimester bleeding until placenta previa is ruled out.

THIRD-TRIMESTER BLEEDING

INCIDENCE

Occurs in 2–5% of pregnancies.

WORKUP

Apt, Kleihauer-Betke, and Wright's stain tests determine if blood is fetal, maternal, or both.

- History, including trauma.
- Vitals: Signs of hypovolemia include hypotension and tachycardia.
- Labs: Complete blood count (CBC), coagulation profile, type and crossmatch, urinalysis, drug screen.
- US to look for placenta previa, as well as monitoring for fetal well-being.
- See Figure 8-4 for management of third-trimester bleeding.
- Determine whether blood is maternal, fetal, or both:
  - **Apt test:** Put blood from vagina in tube with KOH: Turns brown for maternal; turns pink for fetus.
  - **Kleihauer-Betke test:** Take blood from mother's arm and determine percentage of fetal RBCs in maternal circulation: > 1% = fetal bleeding. Maternal cells are washed out (ghost cells); fetal cells are bright red (due to fetal hemoglobin).
  - **Wright's stain:** Vaginal blood; nucleated RBCs indicate fetal bleed.

Whose blood is lost with a ruptured vasa previa? Fetal-placental circulation more than maternal

DIFFERENTIAL

- **Obstetric causes:**
  - Placental abruption.
  - Placenta previa.
  - Vasa previa/velamentous insertion.
  - Uterine rupture.
  - Circumvillate placenta.
  - Extrusion of cervical mucus ("bloody show").
- **Nonobstetric causes:**
  - Cervicitis
  - Polyp
  - Neoplasm

2 most common causes of third-trimester bleeding = Placenta previa and abruption

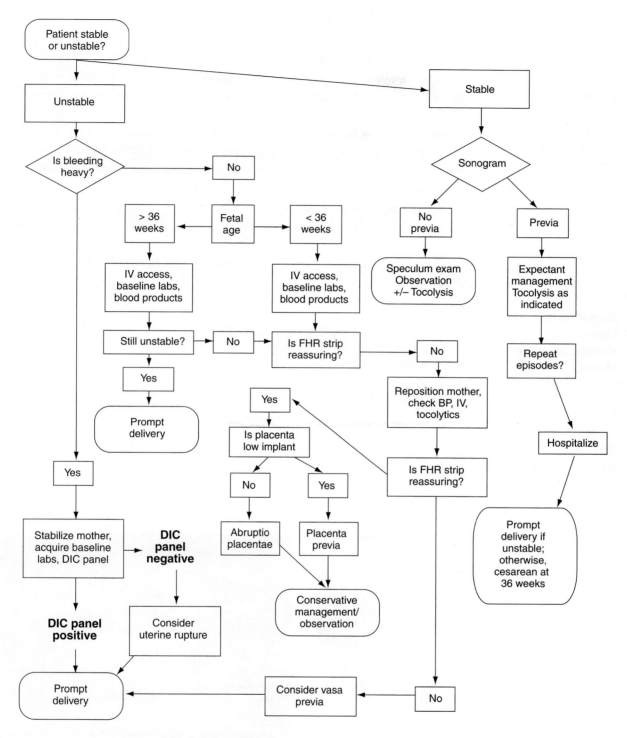

FIGURE 8-4. Management of third-trimester bleeding.

Placental Abruption (Abruptio Placentae)

Most nonobstetric causes result in relatively little blood loss and minimal threat to the mother and fetus.

> A 32-year-old G2P1001 at 34 weeks gestation is brought to triage after a motor vehicle crash. She was a restrained driver who was rear-ended while going 65 miles per hour on the freeway. The airbags were deployed. She has dark red vaginal bleeding and severe abdominal pain. Her vitals are stable. Abdomen is firm all throughout and tender to palpation. FHR shows a baseline of 130, ↓ variability, no accelerations, and late decelerations are present. Contractions are not well recorded. US shows a fundal grade 2 placenta. What is the most likely diagnosis?
>
> **Answer:** Placental abruption.

Pregnant woman + vaginal bleeding + pain = abruption until proven otherwise.

Premature separation of placenta from uterine wall before the delivery of baby (see Figure 8-5).

INCIDENCE

0.5–1.3%; severe abruption can lead to death (0.12%).

RISK FACTORS

- Trauma (usually shearing, such as a car accident).
- Previous history of abruption.
- Preeclampsia (and chronic HTN).
- Smoking.
- Cocaine abuse.
- High parity.

FIGURE 8-5. Placental abruption.

(Courtesy of SUNY at Buffalo School of Medicine, Residency Program in Emergency Medicine.)

A 28-year-old woman at 35 weeks gestation is brought in by ambulance following a car accident. She is complaining of severe abdominal pain, and on exam she is found to have vaginal bleeding. An US shows a fundal placenta and a fetus in the cephalic presentation. What is most likely the cause?

Answer: Placental abruption. Microangiopathic hemolytic anemia seen on maternal blood smear. What is occurring? Disseminated intravascular coagulation (DIC). What is the next step? Transfuse blood products (PRBCs, platelets, FFP) and expedite a vaginal delivery. Want to avoid major surgery in the setting of DIC.

- Vaginal bleeding (maternal and fetal blood present).
- Constant and severe abdominal pain.
- Irritable, tender, and typically hypertonic uterus.
- Evidence of fetal distress (if severe).
- Maternal shock.
- Disseminated intravascular coagulation.

DIAGNOSIS

- US shows retroplacental hematoma or placental thickening only part of the time.
- Clinical findings most important.

MANAGEMENT

- Correct shock (IV fluids, packed RBCs, fresh frozen plasma, cryoprecipitate, platelets).
- Maternal oxygen administration.
- Expectant management or induction of labor: Close observation of mother and fetus with ability to intervene immediately.
- If there is fetal distress, perform C-section.

Up to 20% of placental abruptions can present without vaginal bleeding because bleeding is concealed.

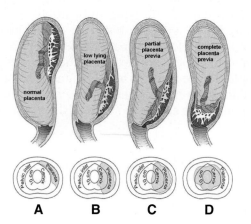

FIGURE 8-6. A. Normal placenta. B. Low implantation. C. Partial placenta previa. D. Complete placenta previa.

(Reproduced, with permission, from DeCherney AH, Nathan L. *Current Obstetric & Gynecologic Diagnosis & Treatment*, 9th ed. New York: McGraw-Hill, 2003.)

Placenta Previa

A condition in which the placenta is implanted in the immediate vicinity of the cervical os. It can be classified into four types:

- **Complete placenta previa:** The placenta covers the entire internal cervical os (see Figure 8-6).
- **Partial placenta previa:** The placenta partially covers the internal cervical os.
- **Marginal placenta previa:** One edge of the placenta extends to the edge of the internal cervical os.
- **Low-lying placenta:** Within 2 cm of the internal cervical os.

INCIDENCE

0.5–1%.

ETIOLOGY

Unknown, but associated with:

- High parity.
- Older mothers.
- Previous abortions.
- Previous history of placenta previa.
- Fetal anomalies.
- Five to ten percent associated with placenta accreta, especially if prior low transverse cesarean section.

Third trimester bleeding:
Painless bleeding = previa
Painful bleeding = abruption

US reveals that a baby is lying transversely. What are you suspicious of? Placenta previa

CLINICAL PRESENTATION

- **Painless,** profuse bleeding in second or third trimester.
- Postcoital bleeding.
- Spotting during first and second trimester that subsides, and then recurs later in pregnancy.

DIAGNOSIS

- **Transabdominal US** (95% accurate).
- **Magnetic resonance imaging (MRI) findings:** Placenta previa is diagnosed on MRI when it is low lying and partially or completely covering the internal os. It is best demonstrated on sagittal images.
- **Double setup exam:** Take the patient to the operating room and prep for a C-section. Do speculum exam: If there is local bleeding, do a C-section; if not, palpate fornices to determine if placenta is covering the os. The double setup exam is performed only on the rare occasion that the US is inconclusive and there is no MRI.

MANAGEMENT

Cesarean delivery is indicated for placenta previa.

Fetal Vessel Rupture

Two conditions cause third-trimester bleeding resulting from fetal vessel rupture: (1) vasa previa and (2) velamentous cord insertion. These two conditions often occur together and can cause fetal hemorrhage and death very quickly.

VASA PREVIA

- A condition in which the unprotected fetal cord vessels pass over the internal cervical os, making them susceptible to rupture when membranes are ruptured.
- **Incidence:** 0.03–0.05%.

VELAMENTOUS CORD INSERTION

- Fetal vessels insert in the membranes and travel unprotected to the placenta. This leaves them susceptible to tearing when the amniotic sac ruptures. The vessels are usually covered by Wharton's jelly in the umbilical cord until they insert into the placenta.
- **Incidence:** 1% of singletons, 10% of twins, 50% of triplets.

CLINICAL PRESENTATION

Vaginal bleeding with fetal distress.

MANAGEMENT

Correction of shock and immediate delivery (usually cesarean delivery).

Uterine Rupture

The disruption of the uterine musculature through all of its layers, usually with part of the fetus protruding through the opening.

COMPLICATIONS

- Maternal: Hemorrhage, hysterectomy, death.
- Fetal: Permanent neurologic impairment, cerebral palsy, death.

RISK FACTORS

Prior uterine scar from a cesarean delivery is the most important risk factor:

- Vertical scar: 10% risk due to scarring of the active, contractile portion of the uterus.
- Low transverse scar: 0.5% risk.
- Can occur in the setting of trauma.

PRESENTATION AND DIAGNOSIS

- Nonreassuring fetal heart tones or bradycardia: Most suggestive of uterine rupture.
- Sudden cessation of uterine contractions.
- "Tearing" sensation in abdomen.
- Presenting fetal part moves higher in the pelvis.
- Vaginal bleeding.
- Maternal hypovolemia from concealed hemorrhage.

MANAGEMENT

- Immediate laparotomy and delivery.
- May require a cesarean hysterectomy if uterus cannot be reconstructed.

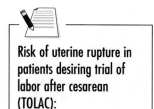

Sinusoidal heart rate pattern = fetal anemia (from any cause).

Risk of uterine rupture in patients desiring trial of labor after cesarean (TOLAC):

- < 1% if previous low transverse cesarean × 1.
- < 2% if previous low transverse cesareans × 2.
- ~10% if previous classical cesarean. Classical uterine scar is a contraindication for TOLAC.

The biggest risk for uterine rupture is a prior cesarean delivery.

Other Obstetric Causes of Third-Trimester Bleeding

Extrusion of cervical mucus ("bloody show"): A consequence of effacement and dilation of the cervix, with tearing of the small vessels leading to small amount of bleeding that is mixed with the cervical mucus. Benign finding. Often used as a marker for the onset of labor.

ABNORMALITIES OF THE THIRD STAGE OF LABOR

A 37-year-old G6P6006 with a history of asthma and chronic hypertension has just undergone a spontaneous vaginal delivery of a 5000-g infant. Her labor course was complicated by chorioamnionitis and preeclampsia. The placenta delivered spontaneously, but profuse vaginal bleeding is noted from the vagina. Pitocin is given, and fundal massage is performed, but the uterus feels soft and boggy. Large clots are removed from the uterus. No vaginal, cervical, or perineal lacerations are noted. Estimated blood loss is 700 cc. What is the most likely cause of the bleeding? What is the next best treatment for the patient?

Answer: Uterine atony is the most likely cause for this patient's postpartum hemorrhage. Prostaglandin F2α (asthma) and methergine (hypertension) are contraindicated due to her medical conditions. The next best agent is misoprostol.

Early Postpartum Hemorrhage (PPH)

- Excessive bleeding that makes patient symptomatic and/or results in signs of hypovolemia.
- Blood loss > 500 mL in vaginal delivery; > 1000 mL for cesarean delivery (difficult to quantify).
- During first 24 hr: **"Early"** PPH.
- Between 24 hr and 6 weeks after delivery: **"Late"** PPH.
- The most common cause of early PPH is uterine atony where the uterus does not contract as expected. Normally, the uterus contracts, compressing blood vessels and preventing bleeding. Other causes of postpartum hemorrhage are summarized in the mnemonic CARPIT.

RISK FACTORS

- Blood transfusion/hemorrhage during a previous pregnancy.
- Coagulopathy.
- Trial of labor after cesarean (TOLAC).
- High parity.
- Large infant/twins/polyhydramnios.
- Midforceps delivery.
- Chorioamnionitis.

MANAGEMENT

1. Manually compress and massage the uterus—controls most cases of hemorrhage due to atony.
2. Start two large-bore IVs and infuse isotonic crystalloids. Type and cross blood. Monitor vitals. Strict inputs and outputs.
3. Carefully explore the uterine cavity to ensure that all placental parts have been delivered and that the uterus is intact.

One unit of blood PRBCs contains ≈ 250 mL/unit

Incidence of excessive blood loss following vaginal delivery is 5–8%.

Most common cause of early PPH = uterine atony.

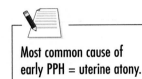

Causes of postpartum hemorrhage—

CARPIT

Coagulation defect
Atony of uterus
Rupture of uterus
Placenta retained
Implantation site bleeding
Trauma to genitourinary tract

4. Inspect the cervix and vagina for trauma/lacerations.
5. If uterus is boggy, suspect atony:
    - Give additional dilute oxytocin.
    - Methergine—contraindicated: HTN.
    - Prostaglandin F2α—contraindicated: Asthma.
    - Misoprostol.
    - ↓ uterine pulse pressure:
        - Uterine artery embolization.
        - Hypogastric artery ligation.
        - Ligation of utero-ovarian ligament.
    - Hysterectomy.
6. Consider coagulopathy if persistent bleeding with above management.
    - Red top tube for clot retraction test. Normal coags if clot forms < 8 min. Coagulopathy if no clot >12 min.
    - Uterine packing until fresh frozen plasma and/or cryoprecipitate available.
    - Hysterectomy (additional surgery) should be avoided in setting of co-agulopathy.

Oxytocin should never be given as undiluted bolus because serious hypotension can result.

Placental Attachment Disorders

The abnormal implantation of the placenta in the uterus can cause retention of the placenta after birth and heavy bleeding.

The cause of the postpartum bleeding should be sought out and treated immediately.

TYPES

- **Placenta accreta:** Placental villi attach directly to the myometrium rather than to the decidua basalis (see Figure 8-7).
- **Placenta increta:** Placental villi invade the myometrium.
- **Placenta percreta:** Placental villi penetrate through the myometrium. May invade the bladder.

Accreta = Attaches
Increta = Invades
Percreta = Penetrates

FIGURE 8-7. Placenta accreta, increta, and percreta.

(Reproduced, with permission, from Cunningham FG, Leveno KJ, Bloom SL, et al. *Williams Obstetrics*, 22nd ed. New York: McGraw-Hill, 2005: 831.)

ETIOLOGY

Placenta accreta, increta, and percreta are associated with:

- Placenta previa.
- Previous cesareans (↑ number, ↑ risk).
- Previous dilation and curettage (D&C).
- Grand multiparity.

MANAGEMENT

All of these conditions result in hemorrhage in the third stage of labor. Treatment of choice: hysterectomy.

Uterine Inversion

This medical emergency most often results from an inexperienced person's pulling too hard when delivering the placenta. It can also be a result of abnormal placental implantation. Morbidity results from shock and sepsis.

INCIDENCE

One in 2200 deliveries.

MANAGEMENT

- Administer anesthesia.
- Large-bore IV.
- Give blood PRN.
- Give uterine relaxants.
- Replace inverted uterus by pushing on the fundus toward the vagina.
- Oxytocin is given after uterus is restored to normal configuration and anesthesia is stopped.

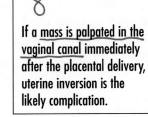

If a mass is palpated in the vaginal canal immediately after the placental delivery, uterine inversion is the likely complication.

Never pull on the cord to deliver the placenta. Gentle traction will be sufficient in a normally implanted placenta.

CHAPTER 9

Infections in Pregnancy

Infant cell-mediated and humoral immunity begins to develop at 9–15 weeks. The initial fetal response to infection is the production of immunoglobulin M (IgM). Passive immunity is provided by transplacental crossing of IgG from the mother. After birth, breast-feeding provides some protection that wanes after 2 months. Infections diagnosed in neonates less than 72 hr of age are usually acquired in utero or during delivery. Infections after this time are acquired after birth (see Table 9-1).

TABLE 9-1. Perinatal Infections

INTRAUTERINE[a]	VIRAL	BACTERIAL	PROTOZOAN
Transplacental	Varicella-zoster	*Listeria*	Toxoplasmosis
	Coxsackievirus	Syphilis	Malaria
	Parvovirus		
	Rubella		
	Cytomegalovirus		
	HIV		
	Hepatitis		
Ascending infection	HSV	GBS	
		Coliforms, GC/ chlamydia	
INTRAPARTUM[b]			
Maternal exposure	HSV	Gonorrhea	
	Papillomavirus	*Chlamydia*	
	HIV	GBS	
	HBV	TB	
External contamination	HSV	*Staphylococcus* coliforms	
NEONATAL			
Human transmission	HSV	*Staphylococcus*	
Respirators and catheters		*Staphylococcus* coliforms	

[a]Bacteria, viruses, or parasites may gain access transplacentally or cross the intact membranes.

[b]Organisms may colonize and infect the fetus during L&D.

GBS, group B Streptococcus; GC, gonococcus; HBV, hepatitis B virus; HIV, human immunodeficiency virus; HSV, herpes simplex virus; TB, tuberculosis.

A 25-year-old G1P0 at 15 weeks gestation reports that she came in contact with a child that had chickenpox 2 days ago. She does not recall ever having chickenpox. What is the next step?

Answer: She should be tested for the presence of varicella antibodies. Many people are immune to chickenpox, but do not recall ever having it. If testing indicates that she lacks the antibodies, she should receive the varicella immunoglobulin within 96 hr. If she has the varicella antibodies, nothing further needs to be done.

- More severe in adults; even more severe in pregnancy.
- Can cause **pneumonia**; treat with IV acyclovir.
- Up to 90% of adults are immune due to symptomatic or asymptomatic infection.
- Confirm presence of antibodies if immunity is uncertain.
- Prevention with **VZIG** (anti-varicella immunoglobulins) within 96 hr is indicated for those who are exposed and susceptible.

Varicella infection can cause maternal pneumonia in pregnancy.

FETAL EFFECTS

- Early pregnancy: Transplacental infection causes congenital malformations.
  - Chorioretinitis.
  - Cerebral cortical atrophy.
  - Hydronephrosis.
  - Cutaneous and bony leg defects.
- Late pregnancy: Less risk of congenital varicella infection.
- Before/during labor:
  - Much higher risk to infant due to absence of protective maternal antibodies.
  - Neonates develop disseminated disease that can be fatal.
  - If maternal infection 5 days before or after delivery, give infant VZIG for passive immunity.

VACCINE

- Live attenuated: **Not** recommended for pregnant women or newborn.
- Not secreted in breast milk, so can give postpartum.

Not usually life threatening, but pulmonary involvement can be serious.

FETAL EFFECTS

Possible neural tube defects (NTDs) due to high fevers if exposed in early pregnancy.

TREATMENT

- Antivirals: Amantadine and rimantadine recommended for prophylaxis.
- Neuraminidase inhibitors for treatment and prophylaxis.
- Category C drugs.

HIGH-YIELD FACTS

Infections in Pregnancy

VACCINE

- Inactivated vaccine recommended for all pregnant women at any gestational age (GA) during flu season.
- Live attenuated intranasal vaccine not recommended for pregnant women.

> Influenza vaccine should be given to all pregnant women at any GA.

PARVOVIRUS (B19)

> A 30-year-old G2P1001 at 24⁶/₇ weeks gestation presents with a bright red rash on both of her cheeks that started yesterday. She reports a fever of 100.4°F (38°C) and feeling lethargic 2 days ago. On physical exam, she is afebrile; has a fine erythematous, lacelike rash on her arms; and no other findings. What is the most likely diagnosis? What is the risk to the fetus?
>
> **Answer:** Flulike symptoms, slapped cheeks, and fine rash is a classic presentation for parvovirus infection. The fetus is at risk for aplastic anemia, which can cause nonimmune hydrops and fetal death.

- Causes **erythema infectiosum** or **fifth disease**.
- Transmitted via respiratory or hand-to-mouth contact.
- Infectivity highest before clinical illness.
- Highest infection in women with school-aged children and day care workers (not teachers).
- Flulike symptoms are followed by bright red rash on the face—**slapped-cheek** appearance. Rash may become lacelike, spreading to trunk and extremities.
- Twenty to thirty percent of adults are asymptomatic.
- IgM is produced 10–12 days after infection and persists for 3–6 months.
- IgG present several days after IgM appears. IgG persists for life and offers natural immunity against subsequent infections.

FETAL EFFECTS

- Abortion, fetal death.
- Nonimmune hydrops: 1% of infected women, due to fetal aplastic anemia.

MANAGEMENT

- After exposure, check IgM and IgG.
- If IgM+, then perform ultrasound (US) for hydrops.
- Middle cerebral artery resistance evaluates for anemia.
- Sample fetal blood for degree of anemia.
- Consider transfusion.
- Delivery based on GA.

PREVENTION

None.

Mild infection in adults caused by an RNA virus.

FETAL EFFECTS

- One of the most teratogenic infections, worse during organogenesis.
- Congenital rubella syndrome:
  - Cataracts, congenital glaucoma (blindness!).
  - **Deafness:** Most common single defect.
- Central nervous system (CNS) defects: Microcephaly, mental retardation.
- Newborns shed virus for many months; susceptible infants and adults at risk.

PRENATAL DIAGNOSIS

Rubella RNA in chorionic villi, amniotic fluid, fetal blood can confirm fetal infection.

VACCINE

Live attenuated vaccine should be avoided 1 month before and during pregnancy.

Most common finding in congenital rubella syndrome: Deafness.

CYTOMEGALOVIRUS (CMV)

- Most common cause of perinatal infection in the developed world.
- Spread via body fluids and person-to-person contact.
- Fetal infection via intrauterine, intrapartum, or postpartum infection (breast-feeding).
- Day care centers are common source of infection.

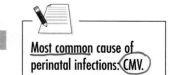

Most common cause of perinatal infections: CMV.

MATERNAL INFECTION

- Most asymptomatic.
- Fifteen percent of adults have mononucleosis-type symptoms (fever, pharyngitis, lymphadenopathy, polyarthritis).
- Primary infection → virus latent → periodic reactivation and shedding.
  - Primary infections cause severe fetal morbidity in fetus.
  - Infections from reactivation have few sequelae.
- Maternal immunity does not prevent:
  - Recurrence.
  - Reactivation.
  - Exogenous infection.
  - Congenital infection.
  - Infection from a different strain.

CONGENITAL INFECTION

Five percent of infected infants have this syndrome:

- Intracranial calcifications.
- Chorioretinitis.
- Microcephaly.
- Mental and motor retardation.

Previous CMV infection does **not** confer immunity.

- Hemolytic anemia.
- Sensorineural deficits.

PRENATAL DIAGNOSIS

- US can show microcephaly, ventriculomegaly, intracranial calcifications.
- Polymerase chain reaction (PCR) detects and quantifies viral DNA in amniotic fluid and fetal blood.

MANAGEMENT

- Routine maternal serologic screen is not recommended.
- Measurement of maternal serum IgM and IgG is used to confirm infection.
- If maternal primary infection confirmed, then invasive prenatal testing with US and amniocentesis.

TREATMENT

No maternal treatment. No fetal treatment or prophylaxis.

GROUP B STREPTOCOCCUS (GBS)

A 27-year-old woman at 37 weeks gestation presents with a 2 day history of fever of 101°F (38.3°C), rupture of membranes, and diffuse abdominal tenderness. What is the most likely diagnosis? What is the gold standard for diagnosis? What is the most common cause? How is it treated?

Answer: Chorioamnionitis (infection of the amniotic fluid, membranes, placenta or decidua—also known as intra-amniotic infection). Amniotic fluid culture is the gold standard for diagnosis. Most common cause is Group B streptococcus. It is treated with IV antibiotics: ampicillin + gentamicin +/- clindamycin.

↳ c̄ endometritis

Asymptomatic carrier state of GBS (*S agalactiae*) in vagina and rectum is common.

COMPLICATIONS

- Preterm labor.
- Premature rupture of membranes (PROM).
- Chorioamnionitis.
- Fetal/neonatal infections.
- Pyelonephritis.
- Endometritis.

NEONATAL SEPSIS

- Low-birth-weight and premature infants have worse outcome than term infants.
- **Early-onset disease:**
  - Neonatal infection < 7 days after birth:
  - Can prevent with intrapartum prophylaxis.
  - Results from vertical transmission.
  - Sepsis can develop within 6–12 hr of birth with signs of respiratory distress syndrome (RDS), apnea, shock.

> Intrapartum GBS prophylaxis prevents early-onset GBS disease. Always treat GBS (with or without symptoms) in pregnant women!

- **Late-onset disease:**
  - Infection 1 week to 3 months after birth.
  - Usually meningitis, not preventable with intrapartum prophylaxis.
  - Infection community acquired or nosocomial.

PREVENTION

See Figure 9-1.

- Culture-based approach:
  - Culture all women for GBS at 35–37 weeks.
  - Intrapartum prophylaxis if GBS positive.
- Risk-based approach: For unknown GBS at the time of labor.
- **Penicillin:** First-line agent.
  - Penicillin allergy: Cefazolin if anaphylaxis risk low.
    - If anaphylaxis risk is high, perform sensitivities for erythromycin and clindamycin.
    - If resistant to above, give vancomycin.

All women should be screened for GBS at 35–37 weeks.

Penicillin: First line for GBS prophylaxis.

TOXOPLASMOSIS

- *Toxoplasma gondii* transmitted by:
  - Eating infected raw or undercooked meat.
  - Infected cat feces.
- Maternal infections are usually asymptomatic.
- Infection confers immunity; pre-pregnancy infection almost eliminates vertical transmission.
- Infected fetus clears the infection from organs, but it may be localized to CNS.
- Severity of fetal infection depends on the GA at the time of the maternal primary infection.

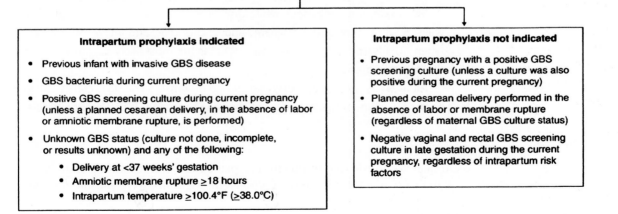

Vaginal and rectal GBS screening cultures at 35–37 weeks' gestation for **ALL** pregnant women (unless patient had GBS bacteriuria during the current pregnancy or a previous infant with invasive GBS disease)

Intrapartum prophylaxis indicated

- Previous infant with invasive GBS disease
- GBS bacteriuria during current pregnancy
- Positive GBS screening culture during current pregnancy (unless a planned cesarean delivery, in the absence of labor or amniotic membrane rupture, is performed)
- Unknown GBS status (culture not done, incomplete, or results unknown) and any of the following:
  - Delivery at <37 weeks' gestation
  - Amniotic membrane rupture ≥18 hours
  - Intrapartum temperature ≥100.4°F (≥38.0°C)

Intrapartum prophylaxis not indicated

- Previous pregnancy with a positive GBS screening culture (unless a culture was also positive during the current pregnancy)
- Planned cesarean delivery performed in the absence of labor or membrane rupture (regardless of maternal GBS culture status)
- Negative vaginal and rectal GBS screening culture in late gestation during the current pregnancy, regardless of intrapartum risk factors

FIGURE 9-1 Intrapartum GBS prophylaxis.

(Reproduced, with permission, from Cunningham FG, Leveno KJ, Bloom SL, et al. *Williams Obstetrics*, 22nd ed. New York, New York: McGraw-Hill, 2005: 1286.)

- **Classic triad** of newborn complications:
  - Chorioretinitis
  - Intracranial calcifications
  - Hydrocephalus
- Can also cause mental retardation and blindness.

MANAGEMENT

- Routine screening not recommended.
- Confirm diagnosis:
  - By seroconversion of IgG and IgM or > 4-fold rise in paired specimen.
  - Avidity IgG testing: If high-avidity IgG found, infection in the preceding 3–5 months is excluded.
  - PCR for *T gondii* in amniotic fluid.

TREATMENT

- Prevents and reduces congenital infection. Does not eliminate the risk.
- Sulfonamides + pyrimethamine, sulfonamides: Presumptive treatment in late pregnancy.
- Spiramycin. ⑥

PREVENTION

- No vaccines.
- Practice good hygiene when handling raw meat and contaminated utensils.
- Clean and peel fruits and vegetables.
- Wear gloves when cleaning cat litter or delegate the duty. Keep cats indoors

BACTERIAL VAGINOSIS (BV)

A 32-year-old G2P1001 at 32 weeks gestation presents with a 4-day history of vaginal discharge. She denies itching, burning, or pain. On physical exam, a homogenous white discharge is noted to coat the vaginal side walls. A wet mount of the discharge shows clue cells, and a fishy odor is noted when KOH is added to the discharge. What is the most likely diagnosis? What is the best treatment?

Answer: Symptoms and diagnosis based on Amsel's criteria is consistent with bacterial vaginosis. The treatment of choice in pregnancy is oral metronidazole.

Clinical syndrome that results from replacement of normal *Lactobacillus* in the vagina with anaerobic bacteria, *Gardnerella vaginalis*, *Mycoplasma hominis*.

DIAGNOSIS

- **Amsel clinical criteria:**
  - Homogenous, white discharge that coats vaginal walls.
  - Clue cells on microscopy.
  - Vaginal pH > 4.5.
  - Whiff test positive: Fishy odor when KOH added to vaginal discharge.

- Nugent criteria: Gram stain.
- Pap smears have low sensitivity for the diagnosis of BV—not used.
- Increased risk of antepartum complications:
  - Preterm birth
  - PROM
  - Preterm labor
  - Chorioamnionitis

TREATMENT

- Does not improve perinatal outcome.
- Oral metronidazole for symptoms.
- Treatment of partners not routinely recommended.

CANDIDIASIS

Yeast infection on the vulva and in the vagina usually caused by *Candida albicans*.

DIAGNOSIS

Pseudohyphae seen on wet prep microscopy.

TREATMENT

- Topical treatment with antifungals preferred.
- Can give oral fluconazole.

SEXUALLY TRANSMITTED INFECTIONS (STIs)

See Chapter 18 for additional information on STIs.

Syphilis

- *Treponema pallidum* spirochetes cross the placenta and cause congenital infection.
  - Any stage of maternal syphilis may result in fetal infection.
- Newborns can have jaundice, hepatosplenomegaly, skin lesions, rhinitis, pneumonia, myocarditis, nephrosis.
- One screening test should be followed by one confirmatory test:
  - Screening tests:
    - Rapid plasma reagin (RPR)
    - Venereal Disease Reasearch Laboratory (VDRL)
  - Confirmatory tests:
    - Fluorescent treponemal antibody absorption test (FTA-ABS)
    - Microhemagglutination assay (MHA-TP)
- US findings: Edema, ascites, hydrops, thickened placenta.
- **Penicillin** is the treatment of choice for all stages of syphilis (same as nonpregnant patients). If patient is penicillin allergic, then she must be desensitized and still treated with penicillin.
- **Jarisch-Herxheimer reaction** occurs with penicillin treatment. It involves uterine contractions and late decelerations in the fetal heart rate as the dead spirochetes occlude the placental circulation.

What are late manifestations of congenital syphilis? Deafness with bone and teeth abnormalities
- Frontal bossing
- Short maxilla
- High palatal arch
- Saddle nose deformity
- Malformed teeth

Penicillin is the only syphilis therapy in pregnancy that prevents congenital syphilis.

Gonorrhea

- Often, the patient has concomitant *Chlamydia* infection.
- In pregnancy, usually limited to lower genital tract (cervix, urethra, peri-urethral glands, and vestibular glands). Acute salpingitis is rare in pregnancy.
- Prenatal screen should be done at the first prenatal visit. Repeat later in pregnancy if high risk factors.
- Diagnosed with nucleic acid PCR.
- **Complications:**
  - Septic abortion
  - Preterm delivery
  - PROM
  - Chorioamnionitis
  - Postpartum infections
- Treat with ceftriaxone.
- Gonorrhea can cause conjunctivitis and blindness in neonates. All newborns are given prophylaxis against conjunctivitis.

Infections associated with preterm delivery:
- Gonorrhea
- Trichomoniasis
- Bacterial vaginosis

Chlamydia

- Most pregnant patients are asymptomatic.
- Can cause delayed postpartum uterine infection.
- Diagnosed with nucleic acid PCR.
- **Neonatal infections:**
  - Ophthalmia neonatorum: Conjunctivitis, blindness.
  - Pneumonia.
- Prenatal screen: Screen at the first prenatal visit. Repeat in T3 if at high risk.
- Treatment: Erythromycin, amoxicillin, azithromycin.

Most common cause of ophthalmia neonatorum: *Chlamydia trachomatis.*

Herpes Simplex Virus

- **Signs and symptoms:** Numbness, tingling, pain (prodromal symptoms), vesicles with erythematous base that heal without scarring.
- **Treatment:** Acyclovir and valacyclovir can shorten the length of symptoms and amount of viral shedding. Shedding not completely eliminated.
  - Safe in pregnancy.
  - Suppression with acyclovir starting at 36 weeks is indicated for those with a history of herpes.
- Neonatal infections can occur via intrauterine (5%), peripartum (85%), and postnatal (10%).
- Newborn infection with three forms:
  - Skin, eye, mouth with localized involvement.
  - CNS disease with encephalitis.
  - Disseminated disease with multiple organ involvement.
- When patient presents in labor:
  - Ask about prodromal symptoms.
  - Examine perineum, vagina, cervix for lesions.
  - If prodromal symptoms or lesions are present, patient should be offered a cesarean delivery to ↓ the risk of vertical transmission.
- Can breast-feed, even when on antivirals. Avoid breast-feeding if herpes lesions on breast that can come in contact with infant.

If herpes lesions or prodromal symptoms are present at the time of labor, a cesarean delivery must be performed to ↓ the risk of vertical transmission.

Hepatitis B Virus

> A 30-year-old G1P0 at 39 weeks gestation is admitted for active labor. Her prenatal course is complicated by an infection with chronic hepatitis B. How should the infant be treated once the delivery takes place?
>
> **Answer:** The infant should receive the first of the hepatitis vaccine series and hepatitis immune globulin soon after birth.

- Chronic infection occurs in 70–90% of acutely infected infants leading to:
  - Cirrhosis
  - Hepatocellular carcinoma
- Screen at first prenatal visit and at delivery with hepatitis B surface antigen (HBsAg).
- Antiviral treatment not recommended during pregnancy.
- ↑ risk of preterm delivery.
- Small amount of transplacental passage.
- Most neonatal infection due to ingestion of infected fluid in the peripartum or with breast-feeding.
- ↑ risk of infectivity with ↑ levels of hepatitis B early antigen (HBeAg).
- Vaccine can be given during pregnancy.
- **Prevention** of neonatal infection: If mother with hepatitis B:
  - Give hepatitis B immunoglobulin (HBIG) to infant upon delivery.
  - Give first of three hepatitis B vaccines upon delivery.
  - Can breast-feed if infant given prophylaxis.

Human Immunodeficiency Virus (HIV)

- HIV screening recommended at first prenatal visit. Some states require a repeat test in T3. Opt-out approach used for HIV testing.
  - **Screening:** Enzyme-linked immunosorbent assay (ELISA).
  - **Confirmatory:** Western blot and/or PCR.
- The vast majority of cases of pediatric AIDS are secondary to vertical transmission from mother to fetus.
- Risk of perinatal transmission ~25%. If zidovudine (ZDV) is given during antepartum, intrapartum, and to neonate, risk of transmission is reduced to 8%.
- Combination antiretroviral therapy (HAART) started in the antenatal period can reduce risk of vertical transmission to 2%.
- Reduce maternal viral load:
  - Antiretroviral therapy should be encouraged in **all** HIV-infected pregnant women regardless of CD4+ count and viral load in order to reduce vertical transmission.
  - CD4+ counts and viral loads should be monitored at regular intervals.
  - Blood counts and liver functions should be monitored monthly while patient is on ZDV.
- Reduce vertical transmission:
  - Give maternal IV ZDV.
  - Reduce duration of ruptured membranes.
  - Recommend cesarean delivery before labor or rupture of membranes if viral load > 1000 copies.
  - Avoid breast-feeding.
  - Give ZDV syrup to newborn for 6 weeks.

HIV Testing

Opt-in approach: Patient must consent to receive the test.

Opt-out approach: Test is routinely done on all patients; patient must decline the test if she does not want it.

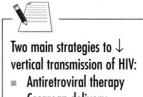

Two main strategies to ↓ vertical transmission of HIV:
- Antiretroviral therapy
- Cesarean delivery

With antiretrovirals and cesarean delivery, vertical transmission of HIV is reduced from 25% to 2%.

Human Papillomavirus (HPV)

Chronic viral infection that can cause genital condyloma, cervical, vaginal, and vulvar cancer.

- Clearance of virus slower during pregnancy.
- Condyloma acuminata, external genital warts, ↑ in number and size in pregnancy.
- If size and location of lesions obstruct vaginal delivery, may need to perform a cesarean delivery.
- Lesions regress spontaneously after delivery.
- Cesarean delivery not routinely recommended.

HPV can cause laryngeal papillomatosis in fetus.

TREATMENT

- Trichloroacetic or bichloroacetic acid applied weekly for external warts.
- Cryotherapy.
- Laser.
- **Not** recommended for pregnancy:
  - Podophyllin resin
  - Podofilox
  - 5-fluorouracil
  - Imiquimod
  - Interferon

NEONATAL INFECTION

Juvenile-onset respiratory laryngeal papillomatosis: Rare benign neoplasm of the larynx.

- Hoarseness, respiratory distress.
- Due to HPV-6 and -11.

Trichomoniasis

- Diagnosis made when **flagellated organisms** seen on **wet prep**.
- **Complications:**
  - Preterm delivery.
  - Preterm premature ruptured membranes.
- Treat with oral metronidazole.

Twin Gestation

Gain 24 pounds by 24 weeks in a multiple gestation pregnancy.

When did cell division occur? Chorionicity is important to determine early in the pregnancy — can be done with ultrasound.

Number of twin pregnancies is on the rise due to ↑ use of assisted reproduction techniques.

Multiple-gestation pregnancy has a high incidence of preterm labor.

Serial US assessments are the only reliable way to document adequate fetal growth and fetal growth restriction.

A size/date discrepancy when measuring uterine fundal height of > 3 cm should prompt US assessment.

Multiple gestation or twins continues to ↑ in the United States secondary to assisted reproductive techniques and an advancing maternal age at childbirth. Maternal and perinatal morbidity are ↑ in multiple gestations, as well as congenital anomalies. Prenatal visits are more frequent with multiple gestations, since they are at increased risk for complications. Many of these women require care by a trained specialist. In twins, normal physiologic changes are increased, compared with a singleton pregnancy. There is an increase in cardiac output, iron requirements, plasma volume, blood volume, glomerular filtration rate, and caloric requirements.

MATERNAL ADAPTATIONS

Maternal physiologic changes are more exaggerated compared to a singleton pregnancy.

- **Cardiac:**
  - ↑ heart rate, ↑ stroke volume, ↑ cardiac output is more secondary to the ↑ myometrial contractility and blood volume.
  - ↑ in uterine volume/weight.
- **Respiratory:** Further ↑ in tidal volume and oxygen consumption.
- **Renal:** ↑ GFR and ↑ in renal size.
- **Nutrition:**
  - Calories: Average to consume 3000–4000 kcal/day compared to 2400 kcal/day in singletons.
  - Weight gain: Avg/week is 1–1.5 pounds; total gain: 35–45 pounds.

TYPES OF TWINS

A 22-year-old P2012 at 15 weeks gestation, consistent with LMP, presents for the first antenatal visit. She reports that fetal movement is present. On physical exam, her fundal height is 20 cm, at the level of the umbilicus. A bedside ultrasound, reveals a twin gestation. Management of her antenatal care should include what important tests/procedures?

Answer: An ultrasound to determine chorionicity and serial ultrasounds to check for fetal growth restriction/discrepancy.

A **zygote** is the result of fertilization of an ovum with a spermatozoan.

- **Dizygotic twins** are the result of two ova fertilized by two different sperm. Risk factors include fertility drugs, race, advanced maternal age, and parity. These are fraternal twins.
- **Monozygotic twins** are the result of a single ovum fertilized by one sperm which subsequently divides. The frequency of 1 in 250 pregnancies (see Figure 10-1). These are indentical twins.
- The timing of cell division within the monozygotic twin determines the amnionicity and chorionicity of twins.
  - Division of the ovum between days 0 and 3: Dichorionic, diamniotic monozygotic twins.
  - Division between 4 and 8 days: Monochorionic, diamniotic monozygotic twins.

Incidence: 1:250 pregnancies

Fetal Sex: same (except meiotic non-disjunction, eg., xo, xy)

Fertilization: 1 sperm, 1 egg

| | Blastomeres | Morula | Blastocyst | Implanted Zygote | Conjoined Embryos |

Day 0 — Day 3 — Day 6-8 — Day 12

Chorion Completed Amnion Completed Implantation — Embryonic Disc Completed

Division of Zygote:

| Before Chorion — Dichorionic Diamnionic | Before amnion After chorion — Monochorionic Diamnionic | After amnion After chorion — Monochorionic Monoamnionic | After amnion After chorion After embryonic disc — Monochorionic Monoamnionic Conjoined |

Placenta: one fused or two separate
(two separate → dichorionic)

FIGURE 10-1. Mechanism of monozygous twinning.

(Reproduced, with permission, from Cunningham FG, Leveno KJ, Bloom SL, et al. *Williams Obstetrics*, 22nd ed. New York: McGraw-Hill, 2005: 914.)

- Division between 9 and 12 days: Monochorionic, monoamniotic monozygotic twins.
- Division after 13 days: Conjoined twins.
- Monochorionic twins have more complications than dichorionic.
- Monoamniotic twins have more complications than diamniotic.

PRENATAL DIAGNOSIS

- Diagnosis and genetic counseling is important because of the ↑ risk of congenital anomalies.
- Both monozygotic and dizygotic twins are at ↑ for structural anomalies.
- Multiple gestation have an increased risk of aneuploidy.
  - First-trimester serum markers not as valid for multiple gestation.
  - Nuchal translucency is the preferred first-trimester marker.

DIAGNOSIS AND MANAGEMENT OF TWINS

- **Physical exam** may show a uterine size/gestational age (GA) difference with size greater than expected from GA.
- **Ultrasound** is used for the following in multiple gestations:
  - Confirm diagnosis.
  - Determine chorionicity.
  - Detect fetal anomalies.

Vaginal delivery of twins can be performed but requires an obstetrician skilled in vaginal twin deliveries; otherwise, cesarean delivery is recommended.

Differential diagnoses for a size/date discrepancy in pregnancy include:

- Twins
- Adnexal mass
- Distended bladder
- Fetal macrosomia
- Hydramnios
- Maternal obesity
- Uncertain LMP
- Molar pregnancy

Multiple gestation pregnancies are at increased risk for complications, such as diabetes mellitus, hypertension, congenital anomalies, and growth restriction

Dizygotic twins are more common that monozygotic twins.

Monochorionic twins have higher complication rates than dichorionic twins, and require more frequent surveillance.

TWINS

Twin-twin transfusion: Deadly complication in monochorionic twin gestations.

- Measure cervical length.
- Evaluate for fetal growth.
- Guide invasive procedures.
- Confirm fetal well-being.
- Determining chorionicity is important:
  - Chorionicity can best be determined in the first or early second trimester by ultrasound (US).
  - Monochorionic twins should undergo US examination to look for fetal growth every 4 weeks, while dichorionic twins can be scanned every 6–8 weeks for growth.
  - Growth restriction rates are higher among the monochorionic in comparison to the dichorionic twin gestation.
  - Monochorionic twins may also be at risk for twin-twin transfusion syndrome.
- Induction of labor of twins should be strongly considered when 38 weeks gestation has been reached, as the rate of stillbirth and growth restriction ↑ after this GA.
- Determining the route of delivery (vaginal versus cesarean) should be based on the experience of the obstetrician and the presentation of both twins.
- Breech presentation of Twin A and cephalic presentation of Twin B may causes interlocking twins, and cesarean delivery should be undertaken in this causes.

TWIN-TWIN TRANSFUSION

- A **serious complication** of monochorionic multifetal gestation in which blood/intravascular volume is shunted from one twin to another.
- The major risk is intrauterine fetal demise, in which one twin develops complications of due to underperfusion and the other due to over perfusion.
- The theoretical cause is *unbalanced vascular anastomoses*.
- US is needed for diagnosis.
- **Treatment** is laser coagulation of the anastomoses.

CHAPTER 11

Abortions and Fetal Death

Always check blood type and Rh on all pregnant patients with vaginal bleeding. Give anti-D immunoglobulin if Rh negative.

An anti-D antibody injection should be given to all pregnant patients that:
- Have vaginal bleeding.
- D (Rh) antigen negative.
- D (Rh) antibody screen negative.

Loss of a fetus of < 20 weeks GA or a fetus born weighing < 500 g = an "abortus."

Majority of spontaneous abortions in the first trimester are a due to chromosomal abnormalities.

FIRST-TRIMESTER BLEEDING

Bleeding in the first trimester can be from many causes that may or may not be related to the pregnancy.

DIFFERENTIAL DIAGNOSIS

- Spontaneous abortion.
- Ectopic pregnancy.
- Hydatidiform mole.
- Benign and malignant lesions (ie, choriocarcinoma, cervical cancer).
- Trauma.

WORKUP

- History: Vaginal bleeding +/- abdominal pain.
- Physical:
  - Vital signs (rule out shock/sepsis).
  - Pelvic exam (note the source of bleeding and cervical dilation).
- Diagnostic tests:
  - Quantitive β-human chorionic gonadotropin (hCG) level.
  - Complete blood count (CBC).
  - Blood type and Rh. An anti-D immunoglobulin injection should be given to all pregnant patients that:
    - Have vaginal bleeding.
    - D (Rh) antigen negative.
    - D (Rh) antibody screen negative.
    - Prevents maternal isoimmunization (generation of antibodies against fetal red blood cells in current or future pregnancies).
- Ultrasound (US) assesses fetal viability and contents of the uterus.

SPONTANEOUS ABORTIONS

Spontaneous abortions are accidents of pregnancy. Etiology of spontaneous abortion are numerous, including chromosomal abnormalities, infections, anatomic, endocrine, immunologic, and environmental factors.

- **Abortion** = intentional or unintentional termination of a pregnancy < 20 gestation or weight of < 500 g.
- Completed spontaneous abortion is the spontaneous expulsion of all fetal and placental tissue from the uterine cavity before 20 weeks gestation.
- Occurs in 30% of all recognized pregnancies.
- Most are unrecognized because they occur before or at the time of the next expected menses (70–80%).

ETIOLOGIES

Chromosomal Abnormalities
- Majority of abnormal karyotypes are numeric abnormalities as a result of errors during gametogenesis, fertilization, or the first division of the fertilized ovum.

- Frequency:
  - Trisomy: 50–60%.
  - Monosomy (45,X): 7–15%.
  - Triploidy: 15%.
  - Tetraploidy: 10%.

Infections

Infectious agents in cervix, uterine cavity, or seminal fluid can cause abortions. These infections may be asymptomatic:

- *Toxoplasma gondii*
- Herpes simplex
- *Ureaplasma urealyticum*
- *Mycoplasma hominis*
- *Listeria monocytogenes*
- Chlamydia
- Gonorrhea

Structural Abnormalities

- Septate/bicornuate uterus: 25–30%.
- Cervical incompetence.
- Leiomyomas (especially submucosal).
- Intrauterine adhesions (ie, from previous curettage).

Endocrine Abnormalities

- Progesterone deficiency.
- Polycystic ovarian syndrome (PCOS).
- Diabetes—uncontrolled.

Immunologic Factors

- Lupus anticoagulant.
- Anticardiolipin antibody (antiphospholipid syndrome).

Environmental Factors

- Tobacco: ≥ 14 cigarettes/day ↑ abortion rates.
- Alcohol.
- Irradiation.
- Environmental toxin exposure.
- Caffeine: > 5 cups/day.
- Trauma.

Top etiologies of spontaneous abortion:
1. Chromosomal abnormalities
2. Unknown
3. Infection
4. Anatomic defects
5. Endocrine factors

Abortions and Fetal Death

See Table 11-1.

Threatened Abortion

A 34-year-old G1P0 at 8 weeks gestation presents to the ED with vaginal bleeding. She denies cramping, trauma, or intercourse. She is afebrile and hemodynamically stable. Physical exam reveals a nontender abdomen. Sterile speculum shows 5 cc of dark blood in the vaginal vault with no active bleeding. The cervix is closed, thick, and high. US shows an 8-week gestation with cardiac activity present. What is the likely diagnosis? What is the best treatment for her condition?

Answer: Threatened abortion. The patient should be managed expectantly. Many patients have a normal pregnancy course; others may have a complete/incomplete/septic abortion.

TABLE 11-1. Types of Spontaneous Abortions

TERMINOLOGY	HISTORY	PASSAGE OF TISSUE?	CERVICAL OS	VIABILITY OF PREGNANCY?	MANAGEMENT
Threatened abortion	Vaginal Bleeding	No	Closed	Uncertain; up to 50% will miscarry	Transvaginal US hCG levels Expectant management
Inevitable abortion	Cramping, bleeding	No	Open	Abortion is inevitable	D&C vs expectant management
Incomplete abortion	Cramping, bleeding (on going)	Some but not all tissue passed	Open	Nonviable	D&C
Complete abortion	Cramping, bleeding previously but now subsided	All tissue passed	Closed	Nonviable	Follow hCG levels to negative
Missed abortion	No symptoms	No	Closed	Nonviable (diagnosed on ultrasound)	D&C vs expectant management
Septic abortion	Fever, abdominal/ pelvic pain, ruptured membranes	Passed/not passed	Open/closed	Viable/not viable	IV antibiotics D&C

(Reproduced, with permission, from Toy EC, et al. *Case Files: Obstetrics and Gynecology,* 3rd ed. New York: McGraw-Hill, 2009: 96.)

HIGH-YIELD FACTS

Abortions and Fetal Death

Threatened abortion is uterine bleeding from a gestation that is < 20 weeks without cervical dilation or passage of tissue.

- Pregnancy may continue, although up to 50% may result in loss of pregnancy.
- It increases the risk of preterm labor and delivery.

DIAGNOSIS

- Speculum exam reveals blood coming from a **closed cervical os, without amniotic fluid or products of conception (POC) in the endocervical canal.**
- US will show an empty uterus if gestation very early, gestational sac, or fetus with cardiac activity. If uncertain of diagnosis, can follow serial hCGs; should ↑ by a minimum of 60% every 48 hr if normal pregnancy (peaks at ~10 weeks).

MANAGEMENT

Observation, pelvic rest.

Inevitable Abortion

An 18-year-old G1P0 at 8 weeks gestation presents to the ED complaining of worsening cramping and vaginal spotting. She denies passage of tissue. Physical exam shows bleeding from the cervical os and a cervical dilation of 3 cm. There are no palpable adnexal masses. Ultrasound shows an intrauterine gestational sac with a viable fetus. What is the most likely diagnosis?

Answer: Vaginal bleeding before 20 weeks gestation, open cervical os, and no expulsion of products of conception is an inevitable abortion.

Inevitable abortion is vaginal bleeding, cramps, and **cervical dilation at < 20 weeks gestation without expulsion of POC.** Expulsion of POC is imminent.

DIAGNOSIS

- Presence of menstrual-like cramps.
- Speculum exam reveals blood coming from an **open** cervical os.
- Fetal cardiac activity may or may not be present on US.

MANAGEMENT

- Surgical evacuation of the uterus if fetal cardiac activity is absent.
- Expectant management if fetal cardiac activity is present.

Incomplete Abortion

Incomplete abortion is the **passage of some, but not all, POC** from the uterine cavity before 20 weeks gestation.

Increased risk of:

- Ongoing bleeding requiring a blood transfusion.
- Ascending infection, septic abortion.

DIAGNOSIS

- Continued cramping and bleeding.
- Enlarged, boggy uterus; dilated internal os.
- POC present in the endocervical canal or vagina.
- POC retained in the uterus may be seen with US.

MANAGEMENT

- Assess hemodynamic status and stabilize (IV fluids, blood transfusion).
- Suction dilation and curettage (D&C) to remove the POC from the uterus. Send POC to pathology.
- Karyotype POC if recurrent abortion.

> Dilated cervix is seen with inevitable and incomplete abortions.

Complete Abortion

A 24-year-old woman presents to the ED with complaints of vaginal bleeding and cramping that is now decreased. She reports that she is 9 weeks pregnant and an ultrasound done 3 days prior showed a viable fetus. Vitals are normal. On physical exam she denies abdominal pain, there is 5 cc of dark blood in the vaginal vault, and the cervix is closed. An ultrasound shows an empty uterus.
Answer: Complete abortion.

Complete abortion is the **complete passage of POC**. The **cervical os is closed** after the abortion is completed.

DIAGNOSIS

- Pain has ceased.
- Uterus is well contracted. Cervical os may be closed.
- US shows empty uterus.

MANAGEMENT

- Send POC to pathology to verify intrauterine pregnancy.
- Between 8 and 14 weeks, curettage is often performed due to ↑ likelihood that the abortion was incomplete.
- Observe patient for further bleeding and signs of infection.

Missed Abortion

Missed abortion is **fetal demise** before 20 weeks of gestation **without expulsion of any POC**.

DIAGNOSIS

- The pregnant uterus fails to grow, and symptoms of pregnancy have disappeared.
- Intermittent vaginal bleeding/spotting/brown discharge and a firm, closed cervix.
- Quantitative β-hCG may decline, platue, or continue to ↑.
- US confirms absent fetal cardiac activity or empty gestational sac.

MANAGEMENT

- Expectant management.
  - Most women will spontaneously deliver a fetal demise within 2 weeks.
  - Risk of incomplete or septic abortion that may require a D&C.
  - Concern for coagulopathy if dead fetus is not delivered. More so for fetal demise in T2 and T3.
- Suction D&C.
- Cervical dilators with prostaglandin E_1 suppositories.

Low-normal range fibrinogen level: Early sign of consumption coagulopathy, especially:
- Low platelets
- Prolonged PT/PTT

Septic Abortion

A 25-year-old G3P1011 at 9 weeks gestation by LMP presents to the ED with fever, lower abdominal pain, and foul-smelling discharge. She reported having a copious amount of clear vaginal discharge 2 days prior. Her temperature is 101.1°F (38.4°C), blood pressure 110/70, pulse 100, and respiratory rate 18. She appears lethargic and ill. She is tender to palpation in the lower abdomen. Sterile speculum exam shows a copious amount of foul-smelling discharge in the vagina. Bimanual exam reveals uterine tenderness and no adnexal masses. The cervix is dilated 1 cm, thick, and high. Complete blood count (CBC) shows a white blood cell count (WBC) of 20K. US shows a 9-week intrauterine pregnancy with cardiac activity present and minimal fluid around it. What is the most likely diagnosis? What is the best treatment for her condition?

Answer: The patient has a septic abortion and should receive broad-spectrum IV antibiotics and a D&C.

- **Infected POC are present.**
- Can be threatened, inevitable, or incomplete type of abortion.
- The infection is usually polymicrobial.
- Infection can spread from endometrium, through myometrium, to parametrium and sometimes to peritoneum.
- Septic shock may occur.

If POC are not removed in a septic abortion, severe sepsis often occurs.

DIAGNOSIS

- Fever, hypotension, tachycardia, generalized pelvic discomfort, uterine tenderness, signs of peritonitis.
- Speculum exam: Malodorous vaginal and cervical discharge.
- Leukocytosis.
- US shows retained POC.

MANAGEMENT

- Vaginal discharge culture, blood culture, check CBC, urinalysis (UA), serum electrolytes, liver function tests (LFTs), blood urea nitrogen (BUN), creatinine, and coagulation panel.
- Broad-spectrum IV antibiotics that has anaerobic bacteria coverage.

Consumptive coagulopathy (DIC) is an uncommon but serious complication of septic abortion.

- D&C after adequate tissue level of antibiotics (2 hr) in a hemodynamically stable patient. If hemodynamically unstable, start IV fluids and antibiotics; perform D&C when patient adequately stabilized.
- Hysterectomy if unable to evacuate the infected uterine contents.

Recurrent Abortion

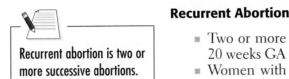

Recurrent abortion is two or more successive abortions.

- Two or more successive clinically recognized pregnancy losses prior to 20 weeks GA constitutes recurrent abortion.
- Women with two successive spontaneous abortions have a recurrence risk of 25–30%.

ETIOLOGY

- Parental chromosomal abnormalities (<u>balanced translocation</u> is the most common).
- Anatomic abnormalities: Uterine didelphys, septate uterus, bicornuate, and unicornuate uterus.
- Acquired defects: Intrauterine synechiae adhesions (Asherman syndrome), leiomyomas.
- Cervical incompetence: Painless cervical dilation leads to second-trimester abortions. Treat with cervical cerclage.
- Endocrinologic abnormalities.
- Infections: *Chlamydia*, *Ureaplasma*, *Listeria*, *Mycoplasma*, *Toxoplasma*, or syphilis.
- Autoimmune conditions (classically, antiphospholipid syndrome [APA] in which thrombosis results in fetal demise).
- Unexplained in a majority of cases.
- Maternal thrombophilia (genetic mutations that increase the risk of thrombi formation).

Women with a history of recurrent abortion have a 23% chance of abortion in subsequent pregnancies that are detectable by US.

MANAGEMENT

Investigate possible etiologies. Potentially useful tests include:

- Karyotype of abortus.
- Parental karyotypes: Balanced translocation in parents may result in unbalanced translocation in the fetus.
- Sonohysterogram, hysteroscopy: Evaluate uterine cavity.
- Luteal-phase endometrial biopsy not very helpful.
- Anticardiolipin and antiphosphatidyl serine antibodies.
- Lupus anticoagulant (antiphospholipid workup).
- Factor V Leiden.

INDUCED ABORTION

DEFINITIONS

- **Induced abortion:** Intentional termination of pregnancy, before 20 weeks gestation.
- **Elective termination of pregnancy:** Intentional termination performed based on the woman's desire.
- **Therapeutic abortion:** Intentional termination performed to maintain maternal health.

Assessment of the Patient

- **US:** Important in confirming gestation age.
  - If there is a discrepancy between dates and uterine size.
  - Ectopic pregnancy suspected.
  - Leiomyomata present—uterus may feel bigger.
  - Critical for T2 abortions for dating—miscalculation of gestational age (GA) can lead to complications.
  - Can help during the procedure.
- **Blood type and Rh type:** If patient is Rh negative, anti-D immunoglobulins should be administered prophylactically.
- Careful patient counseling should be performed.

Indications for Therapeutic Abortion (Not an Exhaustive List)

MATERNAL

- Cardiovascular disease.
- Genetic syndrome (eg, Marfan).
- Hematologic disease (eg, thrombotic thrombocytopenic purpura [TTP]).
- Metabolic (eg, proliferative diabetic retinopathy).
- Neoplastic (eg, cervical cancer; mother needs prompt chemotherapy).
- Neurologic (eg, berry aneurysm; cerebrovascular malformation).
- Renal disease.
- Intrauterine infection.
- Severe preeclampsia/eclampsia.

FETAL

- Major malformation (eg, anencephaly).
- Genetic (eg, spinal muscular atrophy).

Methods of Abortion

- Induction of labor with pharmacologic agents.
- Surgical methods.

PHARMACOLOGIC AGENTS

- Abortions in T1 and T2 can be performed with pharmacologic agents.
- Hypertonic solution instilled in the amniotic cavity: Infrequently used.
- **Prostaglandin E_2, E_1, $F_2\alpha$:**
  - Can be administered orally or vaginally, depending on the type of prostaglandin.
  - Given every 2–6 hr until uterus evacuated.
  - **Advantages:** Easy to use, can be safely used in women with prior cesarean delivery.
  - **Disadvantages:** Diarrhea, fever.
- **Mifepristone (RU 486) and misoprostol:**
  - Antiprogestin mifepristone is followed by misoprotol 48 hours later.
  - Ninety-two percent successful for pregnancy < 49 days gestation (7 weeks).
  - Seventy-seven percent successful for pregnancy 57–63 days gestation (8–9 weeks).

Differential diagnosis for T1 bleeding:
- Spontaneous abortion
- Ectopic pregnancy
- Molar pregnancy
- Vaginal/cervical lesions/lacerations

Differential diagnosis for T3 bleeding:
- Abruptio placenta
- Placenta previa
- Rupture of vasa previa
- Uterine rupture

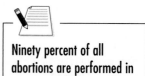

Ninety percent of all abortions are performed in the first trimester.

Suction curettage:
- Most common procedure for abortion in T1.
- Safest surgical abortion method.

Complications are 4 times higher for T2 abortions than T1 abortions. Establishing GA is critical.

Death is a risk of abortion, but it is **10 times less** than the risk of death from giving birth.

The most common method of induced abortion in the United States is D&C.

Medical methods of abortions are best used in the first <u>49 days</u>.

PGF$_{2\alpha}$ is contraindicated for use in asthmatics, as it induces smooth muscle contraction.

Most common reason for T2 abortions: Congenital anomalies.

SURGICAL METHOD

- **Dilation and curettage (D&C):** Used most often in T1. It involves dilating the cervix and using a suction apparatus to remove the contents of the uterus.
- **Dilation and evacuation (D&E):** Used most often in T2. It involves dilation of cervix and extraction of fetal parts using various instruments.
  - **Advantages:** Less emotional stress for patient, avoid hospitalization, greater convenience.
  - **Disadvantages:** Need technical expertise, trauma to the cervix.
- Hysterotomy.
- Hysterectomy: Consider if patient has concurrent fibroids or carcinoma in situ of the cervix.

COMPLICATIONS OF SURGICAL ABORTIONS

- Infection: Most common complication.
- Incomplete removal of POC.
- Disseminated intravascular coagulation (DIC).
- Hemorrhage.
- Cervical laceration.
- Uterine perforation/rupture.
- Psychological sequelae.
- Risk of anesthesia.
- Death.

FETAL DEATH

Death of the fetus > **20 weeks** gestation, **prior to complete expulsion** or extraction from the mother. It can result in a spontaneous abortion or a missed abortion.

ETIOLOGY/RISK FACTORS

Three main classes are fetal, placental, and maternal causes.

Fetal
- Fetal growth restriction: Significant ↑ in the risk of stillbirth. It is associated with:
  - Fetal aneuploidies
  - Fetal infection
  - Maternal smoking
  - Hypertension
  - Autoimmune disease
  - Obesity
  - Diabetes
- Chromosomal and genetic abnormalities: Found in up to 8–13% of fetal death.
- Multiple gestation.

Placental
- Placental abruption is a common cause of fetal death.
  - Maternal cocaine and other illicit drug use.
  - Smoking.
  - Hypertension.
  - Preeclampsia.

- Placental infarction.
- Placental or membrane infection.
- Twin-twin transfusion syndrome.

Maternal
- Non-Hispanic black race.
- Nulliparity.
- Advanced maternal age.
- Obesity.
- Drugs, alcohol, smoking.
- Medical comorbidities:
  - Hypertension
  - Diabetes

> The frequency of chromosomal abnormalities in fetal deaths is 10 times higher than that in live births.

Causes of Fetal Death Based on Trimester

T1 (1–13 WEEKS)

- Chromosomal abnormalities.
- Environmental factors (eg, medications, smoking, toxins).
- Maternal anatomic defects (eg, müllerian defects).
- Endocrine factors (eg, progesterone insufficiency, thyroid dysfunction, diabetes).
- Unknown.

> A carefully performed autopsy is the single most useful step in identifying the cause of fetal death.

T2 (14–27 WEEKS)

- Anticardiolipin antibodies.
- Antiphospholipid antibodies.
- Chromosomal abnormalities.
- Anatomic defects of uterus and cervix.
- Erythroblastosis.
- Placental pathological conditions (eg, circumvallate placentation, placenta previa).

T3 (28 WEEKS–TERM)

- Anticardiolipin antibodies.
- Placental pathological conditions (eg, circumvallate placentation, placenta previa, abruptio placentae).
- Infections (eg, toxoplasmosis, CMV, parvovirus).

> Up to 35% of fetal deaths are associated with the presence of congenital malformation.

TIME NONSPECIFIC

- Trauma.
- Cord accident.
- Maternal systemic disease (eg, diabetes, hypertension).
- Maternal infection (eg, chorioamnionitis).
- Substance abuse (eg, cocaine).

DIAGNOSIS

- In late pregnancy, absent fetal movement detected by the mother is usually the first sign.
- Absent fetal heart tones by Doppler.
- **Real-time US** showing absent fetal heart movement is the **diagnostic method of choice**.

- D&E may be used if fetal death occurs in T2. D&E has ↓ maternal mortality compared to PGE_2 labor induction, but also has the risk of uterine perforation.
- Labor induction if fetal death occurs in T3. Induction of labor with vaginal misoprostol is safe and effective even in patients with a prior cesarean delivery with a low transverse uterine scar.
- Every attempt should be made to avoid a hysterotomy.
- The patient should be encouraged to seek counseling due to emotional stress caused by diagnosis of fetal death and length of time between diagnosis and delivery.

Ectopic Pregnancy

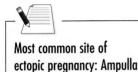

Ectopic pregnancy is the leading cause of pregnancy-related maternal death during T1. Diagnose and treat *before* rupture occurs to ↓ the risk of death!

Most common site of ectopic pregnancy: Ampulla of fallopian tube

Biggest risk factor for ectopic pregnancy: Prior ectopic pregnancy

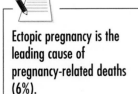

Ectopic pregnancy is the leading cause of pregnancy-related deaths (6%).

Ectopic pregnancy is a pregnancy that is located outside the uterine cavity. The most common site is the **fallopian tubes** (97%), followed by the abdominal cavity, ovary, and cervix. Within the fallopian tubes, the **ampulla** is the most common site, followed by the isthmus and fimbria. Cornual pregnancies that occur in the intramural portion of the fallopian tube are the most dangerous due to ↑ risk of uterine rupture (see Figure 12-1). Rupture of the ectopic pregnancy can lead to rapid bleeding and death.

EPIDEMIOLOGY

- Rate of occurrence: 2% of reported pregnancies.
- Increased risk of recurrance.
- Three to four times more common in women over age 35 compared to those in the 15- to 24-year-old age group.

RISK FACTORS

> A 20-year-old G1P1001 whose last menstrual period (LMP) was 7 weeks ago presents to the ED with right lower quadrant (RLQ) pain and vaginal spotting. She reports that her menses have been regular, except that she is currently 3 weeks late. She has a history of pelvic inflammatory disease, and she smokes one pack of cigarettes per day. Review of systems is positive for nausea and vomiting, Physical exam shows blood pressure 100/70, heart rate 90, and temperature 98.8°F (37.1°C). She has RLQ tenderness without rebound or guarding. Pelvic exam shows 5 cc of dark blood in the vault and right adnexal tenderness. Quantitative β-human chorionic gonadotropin (β-hCG) is 3000 mIU/mL. Ultrasonography (US) shows an empty uterus. What is the most likely diagnosis?
>
> **Answer:** Ectopic pregnancy. All reproductive-age women who present with abdominal pain and bleeding should have a β-hCG done. The quantitative β-hCG is at a level where an intrauterine pregnancy should be visualized in the uterus. Since the uterus is empty, the pregnancy must be in an ectopic location.

- Pelvic inflammatory disease (PID)/history of sexually transmitted infections (STIs) is a major risk factor. This can create scarring of the fallopian tubes.
- Previous ectopic pregnancy.
- Tubal scarring from surgery or tuberculosis.
- Current intrauterine device (IUD) use.
- Congenital malformations of the uterus: Septate uterus.
- Current smoking.
- Assisted reproduction technology: Ovulation-inducing drugs and in vitro fertilization.
- In utero diethylstilbestrol (DES) exposure.

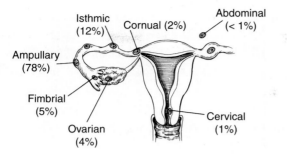

Isthmic (12%)
Cornual (2%)
Abdominal (< 1%)
Ampullary (78%)
Fimbrial (5%)
Ovarian (4%)
Cervical (1%)

FIGURE 12-1. Sites of ectopic pregnancy.

(Reproduced, with permission, from Pearlman MD, Tintinalli JE, eds. *Emergency Care of the Woman.* New York: McGraw-Hill, 1998: 22.)

EXAM

- Pelvic exam may reveal normal or slightly enlarged uterus.
- Vaginal bleeding.
- Pelvic pain.
- Palpable adnexal mass.
- Signs of ruptured ectopic:
  - Hypotension.
  - Tachycardia.
  - Abdominal exam with rebound and guarding.

> Always check a pregnancy test on all reproductive age women with abdominal pain and/or vaginal bleeding.

DIFFERENTIAL DIAGNOSIS

Think of anything that can cause abdominal, adnexal pain, or bleeding in a premenopausal woman:

- Threatened abortion
- Ovarian torsion
- PID
- Acute appendicitis
- Ruptured ovarian cyst
- Tubo-ovarian abscess
- Degenerating uterine leiomyoma

A 26-year-old G2P0010 at 6 weeks gestation by LMP presents to the ED with left-sided abdominal pain and vaginal bleeding. She denies chest pain, dizziness, or shortness of breath. She had performed a urine pregnancy test at home 2 weeks ago, and it was positive, but has not received prenatal care yet. She was treated for pelvic inflammatory disease 1 year ago. The serum β-hCG is 2000 mIU/mL. What is the next step that will help to confirm or exclude the diagnosis of ectopic pregnancy?

Answer: Transvaginal ultrasound is the modality of choice and should be done next. The presence of an intrauterine pregnancy makes the risk of ectopic very low (not zero). The TVUSG may show an empty uterus or findings consistent with an ectopic pregnancy.

If the quantitative β-hCG is ≥ 1200 mIU/mL, and there is no evidence of an IUP, suspect ectopic pregnancy.

- β-hCG of 25 will have a positive urine pregnancy test.
- β-hCG of 1200–2000: IUP detectable with TVUS.
- β-hCG of 5000: IUP detectable with abdominal US.

β-hCG levels **do not** correlate with:
- Size of ectopic
- Potential for rupture
- Location of ectopic
- Gestational age of ectopic

- **Urine pregnancy test (UPT)** to confirm pregnancy: The UPT will be positive, with β-hCG levels > 25 mIU/mL, approximately 1 week after conception.
- **Quantitative serum β-hCG:**
  - Should ↑ by at least 66% every 48 hr in the first 6–7 weeks of gestation after day 9.
  - Value of serial β-hCGs: Stable reliable patients can be followed with serial β-hCG levels. Inadequate rise in β-hCG is suggestive of ectopic or nonviable pregnancy.
- **Progesterone:** Results often not available immediately.
  - > 25 ng/mL: Suggests normal intrauterine pregnancy (IUP).
  - < 5 ng/mL: Suggests abnormal pregnancy (either ectopic or nonviable pregnancy).
  - 5–25 ng/mL: Unclear. Unfortunately, many results fall in this range and are not helpful.
- **US: Diagnostic modality of choice:**
  - Transvaginal sonography (TVUS) is more sensitive than transabdominal approach.
  - Ectopic pregnancy is suspected if a gestational sac is not seen within the uterine cavity with a serum pregnancy test at a threshold value. Threshold for detecting an IUP on TVUS is β-hCG = 1200 mIU/mL (see Figure 12-2).
  - US findings suggestive of ectopic pregnancy:
    - **Absence of intrauterine gestational sac.**
    - Ectopic gestational sac or cardiac activity.
    - Complex adnexal mass.
    - Fluid in the cul de sac: Fluid in the dependent portion of the pelvis can represent blood from the ruptured ectopic pregnancy.

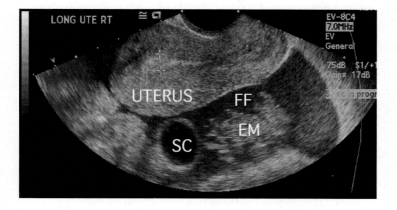

FIGURE 12-2. Transvaginal ultrasound demonstrating an ectopic pregnancy.

Note the large amount of free fluid (FF) in the pelvis. No intrauterine pregnancy was seen. A large complex echogenic mass (EM) was seen in the left adnexa, consistent with an ectopic pregnancy. A simple cyst (SC) is also seen, in the right adnexa.

MANAGEMENT

A 30-year-old G2P1001 at 6 weeks gestation presents to the ED with vaginal spotting and right lower quadrant pain. She denies any medical conditions, any prior surgeries, or any substance abuse. She is afebrile with stable vital signs. She is tender in the right lower quadrant without rebound or guarding. Serum β-hCG is 4000 mIU/mL. US shows an empty uterus with a 2.5-cm hyperechoic ring consistent with an ectopic in the right adnexa. There is a small amount of fluid in the cul de sac. What is the best treatment for this patient?

Answer: Methotrexate. This hemodynamically stable patient has findings consistent with an ectopic pregnancy. She should undergo additional blood work to ensure there are no blood dyscrasias and be able to have regular follow-up. With methotrexate, she avoids risks of surgery and can preserve the fallopian tube.

General

Determine if the patient is hemodynamically stable. Determine if the ectopic pregnancy is ruptured. Administer Anti-D immunoglobulin if patient is D negative.

Medical

Methotrexate (MTX) an option if early ectopic pregnancy and unruptured.

- Antimetabolite.
- Inhibits dihydrofolic acid reductase.
- Interferes with DNA synthesis.
- Treatment of certain neoplastic diseases, rheumatoid arthritis, psoriasis, and ectopic pregnancies.

- Indications:
  - Hemodynamically stable patient.
  - Ectopic pregnancy < 3.5 cm.
  - Patient compliant for follow-up.
  - Intrauterine pregnancy ruled out.
- Relative contraindications:
  - Fetal cardiac activity of ectopic pregnancy.
  - Quantitative β-hCG > 15,000 mIU/mL.
  - Ectopic pregnancy > 3.5 cm.
- Absolute contraindications:
  - Hemodynamically unstable patient: MTX requires time to work.
  - Leukopenia: MTX can further suppress immune system.
  - Thrombocytopenia (< 100K).
  - Active renal/hepatic disease.
  - Active peptic ulcer disease.
  - Possibility of concurrent viable intrauterine pregnancy.
  - Presence of ruptured ectopic pregnancy.
  - Breast-feeding.

Do not coadminister a nonsteroidal anti-inflammatory drug (NSAID) with MTX, as it can potentiate nephrotoxicity.

Surgical

- **Laparotomy** if patient is hemodynamically unstable:
  - Enter into the peritoneal cavity via a large incision on abdominal wall. Place two large bore IVs to administer normal saline and type and cross for blood.
  - Most commonly used for hemodynamically unstable patient.
  - Fast access and minimal equipment needed.
- **Laparoscopy** if patient is hemodynamically stable:
  - Entry into peritoneal cavity via small incisions and visualization of abdominal and pelvic organs with a small camera.
  - Can be diagnostic (only visualize) or operative (perform surgical procedures).
- **Salpingectomy:** Removal of the tube:
  - Partial salpingectomy: Removal of part of the tube.
  - Complete salpingectomy: Removal of the whole tube.
- **Salpingostomy:**
  - Incision on the antimesenteric portion of the tube.
  - Used for unruptured distal tubal ectopic pregnancy.
  - Allows pregnancy to be removed while sparing the tube.
  - Should follow the β-hCG down to zero as some pregnancy tissue may be left behind and continue to grow, which can cause a chronic ectopic.

A partial salpingectomy may cause a future ectopic pregnancy.

SECTION III

High-Yield Facts in Gynecology

CHAPTER 13

Contraception and Sterilization

Contraception is a way to prevent pregnancy using medications, devices, or abstinence. Contraceptives can be used regularly prior to intercourse, at the time of intercourse, or after intercourse. A patient's choice of contraceptive method will be influenced by personal considerations, noncontraceptive benefits, efficacy, safety, cost, and contraceptive method (see Table 13-1).

TABLE 13-1. Comparison of Contraceptive Agents

CATEGORY	AGENTS	MECHANISM	BEST SUITED FOR	DISADVANTAGES AND CONTRAINDICATIONS
Barrier	■ Diaphragm ■ Cervical caps ■ Condoms	■ Mechanical obstruction	■ Not desiring hormones ■ ↓ **STIs**	■ Pelvic organ prolapse ■ Patient discomfort with placing devices on genitals ■ **Lack of spontaneity** ■ Allergies to materials ■ Diaphragm may be associated with more UTIs
Combined hormonal (estrogen and progestin)	■ Combined oral contraceptives ■ Contraception patch ■ Vaginal ring	■ Inhibits ovulation ■ Thickens cervical mucus to inhibit sperm penetration ■ Alters motility of uterus and fallopian tubes ■ Thins endometrium	■ Iron deficiency anemia ■ Dysmenorrhea ■ Ovarian cysts ■ Endometriosis ■ OCP—take pill every day ■ Patch—less to remember but may have more nausea ■ Ring—less to remember, but may have vaginal irritation and discharge	■ Known thrombogenic mutations ■ Prior thromboembolic event ■ Cerebrovascular or coronary artery disease ■ Cigarette smoker over age of 35 ■ Uncontrolled hypertension ■ Diabetic retinopathy, nephropathy, peripheral vascular disease ■ Undiagnosed vaginal bleeding ■ Migraines with aura ■ Benign or malignant liver tumors, active liver disease, liver failure ■ Known or suspected pregnancy
Progestin-only oral	■ Minipill	■ Thickens cervical mucous to inhibit sperm penetration ■ Alters motility of uterus and fallopian tubes ■ Thins endometrium	■ **Breast-feeding**	■ Dependent on taking pill each day at same time ■ Patient needs to remember to take pill

TABLE 13-1. Comparison of Contraceptive Agents *(continued)*

CATEGORY	AGENTS	MECHANISM	BEST SUITED FOR	DISADVANTAGES AND CONTRAINDICATIONS
Injectables	◾ Depo-medroxy progesterone acetate	◾ Inhibits ovulation ◾ Thins endometrium ◾ Alters cervical mucous to inhibit sperm penetration	◾ Breast-feeding ◾ Desires long-term contraception ◾ Iron deficiency anemia ◾ **Sickle cell disease** ◾ **Epilepsy** ◾ Dysmenorrhea ◾ Ovarian cysts ◾ Endometriosis	◾ ↑ Depression ◾ ↑ Osteopenia/ osteoporosis ◾ Weight gain
Implants (subdermal in arm)	◾ Etonorgestrel (progestin)	◾ Inhibits ovulation ◾ Thins endometrium ◾ Thickens cervical mucous to inhibit sperm penetration	◾ Breast-feeding ◾ Desires long-term contraception (lasts 3 yr) ◾ Iron deficiency anemia ◾ Dysmenorrhea ◾ Ovarian cysts ◾ Endometriosis	◾ Current or past history of thrombosis or thromboembolic disorders ◾ Hepatic tumors (benign or malignant), active liver disease ◾ Undiagnosed abnormal vaginal bleeding ◾ Known or suspected carcinoma of the breast or personal history of breast cancer ◾ Hypersensitivity to any of the components ◾ **May ↑ irregular vaginal bleeding**
IUD	◾ Levonorgestrel IUD	◾ Thickens cervical mucous ◾ Thins endometrium	◾ Desires long-term reversible contraception (5 yr) ◾ Stable, mutually monogamous relationship ◾ Menorrhagia ◾ Dysmenorrhea	◾ Current STI or recent PID ◾ Unexplained vaginal bleeding ◾ Malignant gestational trophoblastic disease ◾ Untreated cervical or endometrial cancer ◾ Current breast cancer ◾ Anatomical abnormalities distorting the uterine cavity ◾ Uterine fibroids distorting endometrial cavity

TABLE 13-1. Comparison of Contraceptive Agents *(continued)*

Category	Agents	Mechanism	Best Suited For	Disadvantages and Contraindications
IUD	▪ Copper-T	▪ Inhibits sperm migration and viability ▪ Changes transport speed of ovum ▪ Damages ovum	▪ Desires long-term reversible contraception (10 yr) ▪ Stable, mutually monogamous relationship ▪ Contraindication to contraceptive steroids	▪ Current STI ▪ Current PID within past 2 months ▪ Unexplained vaginal bleeding ▪ Malignant gestational trophoblastic disease ▪ Untreated cervical or endometrial cancer ▪ Current breast cancer ▪ Anatomical abnormalities distorting the uterine cavity ▪ Uterine fibriods distorting endometrial cavity ▪ Wilson disease *Cu!* ▪ May cause more bleeding or dysmenorrhea
Permanent sterilization	▪ Bilateral tubal occlusion	▪ Mechanical obstruction of tubes	▪ Does not desire more children	▪ Contraindications to surgery ▪ May want children in the future

IUD, intrauterine device; PID, pelvic inflammatory disease; STI, sexually transmitted infection; UTI, urinary tract infection.
(Reprinted, with permission, from Toy EC, et al. *Case Files: Obstetrics and Gynecology*, 3rd ed. New York: McGraw-Hill, 2009: 283.)

General methods of preventing pregnancy include:

- Barrier
- Hormonal
- Intrauterine device (IUD)
- Sterilization
- Abstinence

Barrier Methods

FEMALE CONDOM

- Rarely used because of expense and inconvenience (it must not be removed for 6–8 hr after intercourse).
- It offers labial protection, unlike the male condom.
- Efficacy: 79%.

MALE CONDOM

TYPES

- Latex (most common, inexpensive).
- Polyurethane (newest, sensitive, expensive).

- Animal skins (sensitive, least protection against sexually transmitted infections [STIs]).

EFFICACY

86–97%, depending on proper use.

DRAWBACKS

- Must be placed properly before genital contact.
- ↓ sensation.
- May rupture.

DIAPHRAGM

A flexible ring with a rubber dome that must be fitted by a gynecologist. It creates a barrier between the cervix and the lower portion of the vagina. It must be inserted with spermicide and left in place after intercourse for 6–8 hr.

EFFICACY

80–94%.

COMPLICATIONS

- If left in for too long, may result in *Staphylococcus aureus* infection (which may cause **toxic shock syndrome**).
- May ↑ risk of urinary tract infection (UTI).

CERVICAL CAP

A smaller version of a diaphragm that fits directly over the cervix. It is more popular in Europe than in the United States.

EFFICACY

- In women who have not given birth: 80–90%.
- In women who have given birth: 60–70%.

SPERMICIDE

Foams, gels, creams placed in vagina up to 30 min before intercourse. Do not reduce the risk of STIs.

TYPES

Nonoxynol-9 and octoxynol-3 are active ingredients of spermicide, which disrupt the sperm cell membrane; effective for only about 1 hr.

EFFICACY

74–94%.

SPONGE

A polyurethane sponge containing nonoxynol-9 that is placed over the cervix. It can be inserted up to 24 hr before intercourse. Production has been discontinued in the United States.

EFFICACY

84%.

The **only** contraceptive method that protects against STIs is the male and female condoms.

Inconsistent condom use accounts for most failures.

Efficacy rates for spermicides are much higher when combined with other barriers (eg, condoms, diaphragms).

P450 inducers will decrease the efficacy of oral contraceptives (OCPs) (eg, phenytoin, rifampin, griseofulvin, carbamazepine, alcohol, barbiturates) due to increased clearance.

Hormonal patch may be less effective in obese (≥ 200 lbs) women.

Side bar (left column)

Types of estrogens:
Estradiol: Reproductive life
Estriol: Pregnancy
Estrone: Menopause

Tension headaches are **not** a contraindication for oral contraceptive agents. Migraine headaches with aura can ↑ risk of stroke in patients who take combination hormonal contraception.

The inactive pills in the COC simulate hormone withdrawal of the normal menstrual cycle, which results in menses.

COC: Estrogen and progesterone combined. Main mechanisms:
- Prevents ovulation
- Alters uterine and fallopian tube motility
- Thickens cervical mucus to prevent sperm penetration
- Causes endometrial atrophy

RISK

Toxic shock syndrome.

Hormonal Agents

A 37-year-old G2P2 woman desires a reversible form of contraception. Her history reveals that she smokes cigarettes, suffers from migraines with auras, has uncontrolled hypertension (HTN), and has a first-degree relative with a history of breast cancer. She requests combination oral contraceptive pills (COCs). How do you counsel this patient?

Answer: The patient should not be placed on COCs due to her risk factors for developing venous thromboembolism and strokes. Contraindications for OCP use include: female smokers > 35 years old, uncontrolled HTN, diabetes with vascular disease, migraines with aura, and benign or malignant liver tumors, liver disease, history of breast cancer, and pregnancy.

COMBINATION ORAL CONTRACEPTIVES (COCs)

EFFICACY

- 95–99.9% (variability due to compliance).
- Contain estrogen and progestin; types include fixed dosing and phasic dosing:
  - **Fixed dosing:** Requires the same dose every day of cycle.
  - **Phasic dosing:** Gradual ↑ in amount of progestin as well as some changes in the level of estrogen.

MECHANISM OF ACTION

- **Estrogen** suppresses follicle-stimulating hormone (FSH) and therefore prevents follicular emergence. Maintains stability of endometrium.
- **Progesterone** prevents luteinizing hormone (LH) surge and therefore inhibits ovulation.
  - Thickens cervical mucus to pose as a barrier for sperm.
  - Alters motility of fallopian tube and uterus.
  - Causes endometrial atrophy.

SIDE EFFECTS

- Nausea.
- Headache.
- Bloating.

BENEFITS

- ↓ risk of ovarian cancer by 75%.
- ↓ risk of endometrial cancer by 50%.
- ↓ bleeding and dysmenorrhea.
- Regulates menses.
- Reduces the risk of pelvic inflammatory disease (PID) (thicker mucus), fibrocystic breast change, ovarian cysts, ectopic pregnancy, osteoporosis, acne, and hirsutism.
- ↓ risk of anemia.

RISKS

- ↑ risk of venous thromboembolism/stroke (3/10,000).
- ↑ risk of myocardial infarction (in smokers > 35 years old).
- Depression in some.
- Migraines.

CONTRAINDICATIONS

- Known thrombogenic mutations.
- Prior thromboembolic events.
- Cerebrovascular or coronary artery disease (current or remote).
- Cigarette smoking over age 35.
- Uncontrolled HTN.
- Diabetic retinopathy, nephropathy, peripheral vascular disease.
- Known or suspected breast or endometrial cancer.
- Undiagnosed vaginal bleeding.
- Migraines with aura.
- Benign or malignant liver tumors, active liver disease, liver failure.
- Known or suspected pregnancy.

PROGESTION-ONLY ORAL CONTRACEPTIVES

EFFICACY

Comparable to COCs (95–99%), but must be taken at same time each day (within 3 hr).

MECHANISM OF ACTION

- Thickens mucous to prevent sperm penetration.
- Alters motility of uterus and fallopian tubes.
- Causes thinning of endometrial glands.
- Contain only progestin: There is LH suppression and therefore no ovulation. The main differences from combination pills are:
  - A mature follicle is formed (but not released).
  - No placebo is used.
- Progestin-only pills are best for:
  - Lactating women (progestin, unlike estrogen, does *not* suppress breast milk).
  - Women for whom estrogen is contraindicated (eg, estrogen-sensitive tumors).

SIDE EFFECTS

- Breakthrough bleeding.
- Nausea (10–30% of women).

Always check a β-hCG to rule out pregnancy before prescribing the acne medicine isotretinin (very teratogenic!).

What is the treatment for idiopathic hirsutism? OCP

Oral contraception mechanism in a nutshell:
- Estrogen inhibits FSH.
- Progestin inhibits LH.

Estrogen suppresses breast milk, so combination pills are not used for nursing mothers. Progestin-only pills are used.

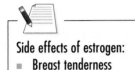

Oral contraceptives' link to an ↑ in breast cancer is not proven.

Side effects of estrogen:
- Breast tenderness
- Nausea
- Headache

Side effects of progestin:
- Depression
- Acne
- Weight gain
- Irregular bleeding

Why is estrogen a procoagulant? Estrogen ↑ factors VII and X and ↓ antithrombin III.

Progestin-only pill requires strict compliance and requires taking the pill at the same time every day.

> A 20-year-old G0 desires long-term reversible contraception. She has a history of grand mal seizures for which she takes an anticonvulsant. She still has seizures once about every 6 months. What is the best contraceptive method for her?
>
> **Answer:** Medroxyprogesterone acetate injection can ↑ the seizure threshold and ↓ the number of seizures. It also ↓ the number of sickle cell crises in patients with sickle cell disease. It improves anemia, ↓ dysmenorrhea and ovarian cysts, and improves symptoms of endometriosis.

Medroxyprogesterone acetate (DMPA) IM injection given every 3 months.

EFFICACY

99.7%.

MECHANISM OF ACTION

Sustained high progesterone level to block LH surge (and hence ovulation). Thicker mucus and endometrial atrophy also contribute. There is no FSH suppression.

INDICATIONS

- Especially suitable for women who either cannot tolerate COCs or who are unable to take COCs as prescribed.
- DMPA can provide noncontraceptive benefits in:
  - Seizure disorder: ↓ the number of seizure episodes.
  - Sickle cell disease: ↓ the number of sickle cell crises.

SIDE EFFECTS

- Bleeding irregularity/spotting.
- Unknown when menstruation/fertility will resume after treatment cessation (can remain infertile for up to 9 months).
- ↑ hair shedding.
- Mood changes.
- ↓ high-density lipoprotein (HDL).
- ↓ libido.
- Weight gain.
- Osteopenia/osteoporosis. Reverse when stop using DMPA.

CONTRAINDICATIONS

- Known/suspected pregnancy.
- Undiagnosed vaginal bleeding.
- Breast cancer.
- Liver disease.
- Osteoporosis/osteopenia.

IMPLANTABLE HORMONAL AGENTS

Etonorgestrel (progestin) containing rod inserted in the subcutaneous tissue of the arm. It should be replaced every 3 years.

EFFICACY

99.8%.

MECHANISM OF ACTION

- Suppression of LH surge and inhibition of ovulation.
- Thickened mucus.
- Endometrial atrophy.

INDICATIONS

- Contraindication/intolerance to oral contraceptives.
- Smokers > 35 years old.
- Women with diabetes mellitus, HTN, coronary artery disease (CAD).

SIDE EFFECTS

- Irregular bleeding
- Acne
- ↓ libido
- Adnexal enlargement
- Possible difficult removal

CONTRAINDICATIONS

- Thrombophlebitis/embolism
- Known/suspected pregnancy
- Liver disease/cancer
- Breast cancer
- Concomitant anticonvulsant therapy

TRANSDERMAL (ORTHO EVRA)

- Efficacy similar to COC.
- Better compliance.
- May come off and need replacement.

VAGINAL RING (NUVARING)

- Must be changed every 3 weeks.
- Must be inserted at the same time.
- ↓ efficacy if out > 3 hr.

Intrauterine Device

Insertion of a T-shaped device into the endometrial cavity with a nylon filament protruding through the cervix into the vagina to facilitate removal.

EFFICACY

97–99.1%.

MECHANISM OF ACTION

- Copper T:
  - Copper causes a sterile inflammatory reaction, creating a hostile environment.
  - Inhibits sperm migration and viability.
  - Damages ovum, changes ovum transport speed.
  - Used for 10 yr.
- Levonorgestrel IUD:
  - Thickens cervical mucous
  - Thins endometrium
  - Used for 5 yr
  - Spermicidal

INDICATIONS

- Oral contraceptives contraindicated/not tolerated.
- Smokers > 35 years old.
- Levonorgestrel IUD can be used for menorrhagia.

CONTRAINDICATIONS

- Multiple sexual partners.
- Recent history of PID.
- Immunocompromised (eg, HIV, sickle cell disease).
- Known/suspected pregnancy.
- Wilson disease.
- Copper allergy.
- Absolute contraindications: Current or suspected pregnancy, undiagnosed abnormal vaginal bleeding, suspected gynecologic malignancy, acute infection (cervical, uterine, or salpingeal), history of PID, immunosuppressed patients, severe anatomical uterine distortion.

COMPLICATIONS

- PID.
- Uterine perforation.

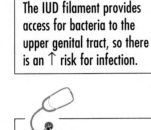

The IUD filament provides access for bacteria to the upper genital tract, so there is an ↑ risk for infection.

Non-user-dependent methods like the IUD, subdermal implant, and injections have lower failure rates than OCPs.

Contraindication for IUD placement: Women with multiple sex partners

- Ectopic pregnancy.
- Menorrhagia with Copper T.
- IUD expulsion.
- *Actinomyces* infection.

Ectopic pregnancy is a dangerous complication of IUD use.

Postcoital/Emergency Contraception

 A 19-year-old G0P0 woman presents to the office concerned that she may have an undesired pregnancy after engaging in unprotected sex with her boyfriend 2 days ago. The patient does not remember the date of her last menstrual period. What therapy can you offer this patient?
Answer: Emergency contraception is effective when initiated within 72 hr of intercourse. It consists of high-dose progestin, high-dose OCPs, or insertion of a Copper T IUD.

Copper and levonorgestrel IUD reduce the risk of ectopic pregnancy compared to no contraceptives, but not as much as OCPs.

UP TO 3 DAYS AFTER INTERCOURSE

Levonorgestrel (Plan B): One 0.75-mg tablet taken within 72 hr of coitus. A second 0.75-mg tablet is taken 12 hr after the first dose. Efficacy: 89%.

UP TO 5 DAYS AFTER INTERCOURSE

Copper T IUD: Can be left in the uterine cavity and provide contraception for up to 10 yr. Efficacy: Nearly 100%.

What are the two methods of emergency postcoital contraception? Up to 3 days after intercourse: levonorgestrel (plan B). Up to 5 days after: Copper T IUD.

STERILIZATION

Sterilization is an elective surgery that leaves a male or female unable to reproduce. With about 1 million procedures per year in the United States, sterilization is the most popular form of birth control. There are 1–4 pregnancies per 1000 sterilizations.

- Male type: Vasectomy.
- Female type: Tubal occlusion.
- It is estimated that 10–12% of men who undergo vasectomies and 13–25% of women who undergo tubal ligations may experience regret after permanent sterilization. Higher regret rate is associated in women younger than age 25, women not married at the time of their tubal ligation, or women whose tubal ligation was performed less than a year after delivery.

What are options for emergency contraception? IUD within 5 days or low-dose progesterone within 72 hr.

Vasectomy

- Excision of a small section of both vas deferens, followed by sealing of the proximal and distal cut ends (office procedure done under local anesthesia). Ejaculation still occurs.
- Sperm can still be found proximal to the surgical site, so to ensure sterility one must use contraception for 12 weeks or 20 ejaculations and then have two consecutive negative sperm counts.

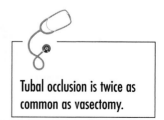

Tubal occlusion is twice as common as vasectomy.

Bilateral Tubal Occlusion

Procedures can be performed (Figure 13-1) either postpartum (during cesarean section or immediately after vaginal delivery) or interval (remote from a pregnancy). An interval tubal occlusion should be performed in the <u>follicular phase</u> of the menstrual cycle in order to avoid the time of ovulation and possible pregnancy.

LAPAROSCOPIC TUBAL OCCLUSION

Eighty to ninety percent of tubal occlusions are done laparoscopically. All methods occlude the fallopian tubes bilaterally.

ELECTROCAUTERY

This involves the cauterization of a 3-cm zone of the isthmus. It is the most popular method (very effective but most difficult to reverse).

CLIPPING

The Hulka-Clemens clip (also Filshie clip), similar to a staple, is applied at a 90-degree angle on the isthmus. It is the most easily reversed method but also has the highest failure rate.

BANDING

A length of isthmus is drawn up into the end of the trocar, and a silicone band, or Fallope ring, is placed around the base of the drawn-up portion of fallopian tube.

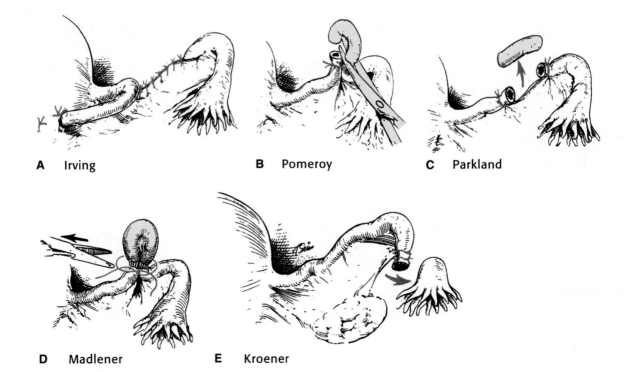

FIGURE 13-1. Various techniques for tubal sterility.

(Reproduced, with permission, from Cunningham G, et al. *Williams Obstetrics*, 21st ed. New York: McGraw-Hill, 2001: 1556.)

Hysteroscopic Occlusion (Essure)

- Small polyester/nickel/titanium/steel coil implant is placed in the proximal fallopian tube.
- Minimally invasive.
- Two-year data shows 99.8% efficacy.
- Alternative contraception needed until tubal occlusion proved by hysterosalpingogram 3 months after implant placed.
- **Mechanism of action:** Scarring forms around implant over 3 months and prevents sperm to enter the fallopian tube.

Essure is the <u>most effective</u> method of permanent sterilization available

Postpartum Tubal Occlusion

- **Pomeroy method:** A segment of isthmus is lifted and a suture is tied around the approximated base. The resulting loop is excised, leaving a gap between the proximal and distal ends. This is the most popular method.
- **Parkland method:** A window is made in the mesosalpinx and a segment of isthmus is tied proximally and distally and then excised.
- **Madlener method:** Similar to the Pomeroy but without the excision, a segment of isthmus is lifted and crushed and tied at the base.
- **Irving method:** The isthmus is cut, with the proximal end buried in the myometrium and the distal end buried in the mesosalpinx.
- **Kroener method:** Resection of the distal ampulla and fimbriae following ligation around the proximal ampulla.
- **Uchida method:** Epinephrine is injected beneath the serosa of the isthmus. The mesosalpinx is reflected off the tube, and the proximal end of the tube is ligated and excised. The distal end is not excised. The mesosalpinx is reattached to the excised proximal stump, while the long distal end is left to "dangle" outside of the mesosalpinx.

Be sure to follow-up on pathology report after tubal ligation to ensure that tissue excised was fallopian tubes.

Selection of patient for tubal ligation is important:
- Little to no history of pelvic adhesions
- Little to no history of significant PID
- Body habitus

Partial or Total Salpingectomy

Removal of part or all of the fallopian tube.

Luteal-Phase Pregnancy

A luteal-phase pregnancy is a *pregnancy diagnosed after tubal sterilization but conceived before.* Occurs around 2–3/1000 sterilizations. It is prevented by either performing sensitive pregnancy tests prior to the procedure or performing the procedure during the follicular phase.

Reversibility of Tubal Obstruction

Around one-third of tubal ligations can be reversed such that pregnancy can result. **Pregnancies after tubal ligation reversal are ectopic until proven otherwise.**

Complications of Tubal Occlusion

- Failure of procedure (patient still fertile).
- **Poststerility syndrome:** Pelvic pain/dysmenorrhea, menorrhagia, ovarian cyst.
- **Fistula formation:** Uteroperitoneal fistulas can occur, especially if the procedure is performed on the fallopian tubes < 2–3 cm from the uterus.
- Infection.
- Operative complications most commonly from anesthesia.

Other Methods of Sterilization

COLPOTOMY

Utilizes entry through the vaginal wall near the posterior cul-de-sac and occludes the fallopian tubes by employing methods similar to those performed in laparoscopy and laparotomy.

HYSTERECTOMY

Removal of the uterus, either vaginally or abdominally; rarely performed for sterilization purposes. Failure rate is < 1%. **Pregnancy after hysterectomy = ectopic pregnancy = emergency.**

ABSTINENCE

Continuous Abstinence

Abstaining from vaginal intercourse at any time. It is the only 100% effective way to prevent pregnancy.

Natural Family Planning (NFP)

A form of birth control based on the timing of sex during a woman's menstrual cycle. It can be an effective, low-cost, and safe way to prevent an unwanted pregnancy. The success or failure of this methods will depend on the patient's ability to recognize the signs that ovulation is about to occur and abstain from having sex or use another form of contraception during the fertile period.

There are four methods of NFP:

1. Basal body temperature method
2. Ovulation/cervical mucus method
3. Symptothermal method
4. Lactational amenorrhea

> NFP has a 75–99% success rate in preventing pregnancy, depending on patient compliance.

BASAL BODY TEMPERATURE

The woman must take and record her basal body temperature every morning as soon as she wakes up. Her temperature should ↑ by 0.3–1°F for 3 consecutive days when she has a progesterone surge, indicating that she is ovulating. The couple can abstain if they do not desire pregnancy or have intercourse if they are trying to conceive.

OVULATION/CERVICAL MUCUS METHOD (BILLINGS METHOD)

The woman checks for the presence and change of cervical mucus at the opening of the vagina to determine if she is fertile. Most women will secrete mucus as they move closer to ovulation. At time of ovulation, a woman's mucus becomes more clear, profuse, wet, stretchy, and slippery, and is referred to as the "peak day" of fertility. After the peak day, the mucus will become thick again and go away. If couple does not desire pregnancy, they are advised to abstain from sex at the first signs mucus until 4 days after the peak day.

Symptothermal Method

Combination of previous two methods. In addition to taking the temperature and checking for mucus changes every day, the woman checks for other signs of ovulation: abdominal pain or cramps, spotting, and changes in the position and firmness of the cervix. This method requires that you abstain from sex from the day you first notice signs of fertility until the third day after the elevation in temperature. This method can be more effective than either of the other two methods because it uses a variety of signs.

Lactational Amenorrhea

The use of breast-feeding to space pregnancies through exclusive breast-feeding, which means no pacifiers, no bottles, and nursing on demand. This may be difficult for working mothers, so it may not be as reliable for child spacing.

ADVANTAGES OF NFP

- No side effects, allergies, breakthrough bleeding, bloating, or hormonal impact on libido.
- Low cost.
- Reversible.
- Improved knowledge and understanding of woman's fertility and normal cycle.
- Improve communication: The woman should communicate her fertility status to her partner.
- No impact on breast-feeding—no risk to baby.

DISADVANTAGES OF NFP

- Abstinence isn't always easy.
- Requires a committed and cooperative couple.
- No protection against STIs.
- Takes time to learn fertility awareness.

CHAPTER 14

Menstruation

- Puberty is the transition from childhood to the final stage of maturation that allows for reproduction.
- Puberty is believed to begin with **disinhibition** of the pulsatile gonadotropin-releasing hormone (GnRH) secretion from the hypothalamus (mechanism is unknown).

Secondary Sex Characteristics

Development of the secondary sexual characteristics proceeds in the following order:

1. **Thelarche** (breast budding). Average age 10 years. Due to increase in estradiol.
2. **Pubarche** (axillary and pubic hair growth). Average age 11 years. Due to increase in adrenal hormones.
3. **Menarche** (first menses). Average age 12 years. Due to increase in estradiol.

Tanner Stages

The Tanner stages of development refer to the sequence of events of breast and pubic hair development.

- **Stage 1:** Prepubertal child.
- **Stages 2–4:** Development stages.
- **Stage 5:** Adult.

Precocious Puberty

Appearance of the secondary sexual characteristics before 8 years of age is referred to as precocious puberty and requires investigation into the etiology.

ETIOLOGY (NOT AN EXHAUSTIVE LIST)

- Idiopathic: Most common.
- Tumors of the hypothalamic-pituitary stalk: Prevent negative feedback.
- Inflammation of the hypothalamus: ↑ GnRH production.
- 21-hydroxylase deficiency.
- Estrogen-secreting tumors.
- Excess exogenous estrogen.
- McCune – Albright syn

The menstrual cycle is the cyclical changes that occur in the female reproductive system (see Figure 14-1 and Table 14-1). The hypothalamus, pituitary, ovaries, and uterus interact to allow ovulation approximately once per month (average 28 days [+/–7 days]). The following description is based on a 28-day menstrual cycle.

- Many follicles are stimulated by follicle-stimulating hormone (FSH), but *the follicle that secretes more estrogen than androgen will be released.*

What is the order of pubertal landmarks?
Thelarche, pubarche, menarche

CHARACTERISTIC	AGE	HORMONE
Thelarche	10	Estradiol
Pubarche	11	Adrenal hormones
Menarche	12	Estradiol

A female age 13 or older without any breast development has estrogen deficiency and needs evaluation.

HIGH-YIELD FACTS

Menstruation

TABLE 14-1. Summary of Menstrual Cycle

Menstruation: Withdrawal of progesterone causes endometrial sloughing.
Follicular phase: ■ FSH causes follicle maturation and estrogen secretion. ■ Estrogen causes endometrial proliferation.
Ovulation: LH surge causes oocyte to be released.
Luteal phase: Corpus luteum secretes progesterone, which causes: ■ Endometrial maturation. ■ ↓ FSH, ↓ LH.

This dominant follicle releases the most estradiol so that its positive feedback causes an LH surge.

■ Average menses = 4 days. More than 7 days is abnormal.
■ Blood loss in menstruation averages 30–50 mL and should not form clots; > 80 mL is an abnormally high amount of blood loss.

Prostaglandins released from the endometrium cause dysmenorrhea.

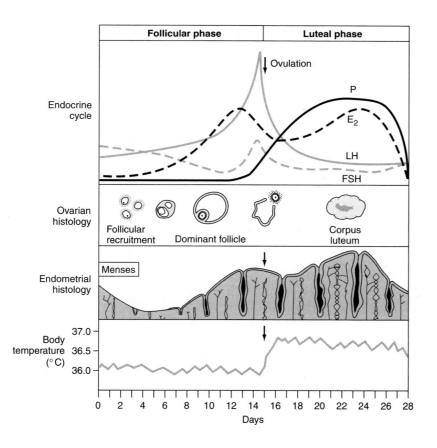

FIGURE 14-1. The menstrual cycle.

(Modified, with permission, from Fauci AS, Braunwald E, Isselbacher KJ, et al. *Harrison's Principles of Internal Medicine*, 14th ed. New York: McGraw-Hill, 1998: 2101.)

Ovulation takes place 24–36 hr after LH surge and 12 hr after LH peak.

The follicular phase is highly variable. The luteal phase is usually about 11 days due to the length of time the corpus luteum is able to secrete progesterone.

The corpus luteum is maintained after fertilization by hCG, released by the embryo.

Days 1–14: Follicular Phase (time for interval tubal)

- The follicular phase begins on the first day of menses. All hormone levels are low. Without any negative feedback, **GnRH** from the hypothalamus causes **FSH** release from the pituitary.
- **FSH** stimulates maturation of granulosa cells in the ovary. The granulosa cells secrete **estradiol** in response.
- **Estradiol** inhibits luteinizing hormone (**LH**) and **FSH** due to negative feedback. In the meantime, the **estradiol** secretion also causes the endometrium to proliferate.
- **LH** acts on the theca cells to ↑ secretion of **androgens** (which are converted to estradiol), prepare the cells for progesterone secretion, and cause further granulosa maturation.

Day 14: Ovulation

- A critical level of estradiol triggers an LH surge.
- The **LH surge** causes the oocyte to be released from the follicle. The ruptured follicle then becomes the corpus luteum, which secretes progesterone.

Days 14–28: Luteal Phase

- The corpus luteum secretes progesterone for only about 11 days in the absence of human chorionic gonadotropin (hCG).
- **Progesterone** causes the endometrium to mature in preparation for possible implantation. It becomes highly vascularized and ↑ glandular secretions (see Table 14-2).
- **Progesterone** also causes inhibition of **FSH** and **LH** release.
- If fertilization does not occur, the corpus luteum involutes, **progesterone** and **estradiol** levels fall, with subsequent endometrial sloughing (menses). The hypothalamic-pituitary axis is released from inhibition, and the cycle begins again.

TABLE 14-2. Ovarian Hormone Effect on Uterus

	OVARIAN PHASE	DOMINANT HORMONE	UTERINE PHASE
Before ovulation	Follicular	Estrogen	Proliferative
After ovulation	Luteal	Progesterone	Secretory

CHAPTER 15

Premenstrual Syndrome/ Premenstrual Dysphoric Disorder

Premenstrual syndrome (PMS) and premenstrual dysphoric disorder (PMDD) have many symptoms that overlap with anxiety and depression. A differentiation should be made because each has a different treatment. PMS and PMDD both have similar symptoms, but PMDD has markedly severe symptoms. The symptoms of PMS **do not impair** daily activities; however, the symptoms of PMDD **do affect** the activities of daily living. The symptoms occur in the luteal phase for both conditions.

> Pathognomonic for PMS: Symptoms during luteal phase.

DEFINITION

- Refers to a group of mild to moderate symptoms.
- Both physical and behavioral.
- Occur in luteal of the menstrual cycle.
- May interfere with work and personal relationships.
- Symptoms followed by a symptom-free period.
- Monitor for 2–3 months because symptoms can be variable month to month.

PREMENSTRUAL SYNDROME DIAGNOSTIC CRITERIA

A 26-year-old woman complains of feeling sad and confused before her menses. She reports having headaches and breast pain. She feels better when she is alone, but she is able to work and take care of her 2 children. Once she begins menses, she no longer has these symptoms. What is the most likely diagnosis. What is the best way to make the diagnosis?

Answer: PMS. This patient has affective and somatic complaints that resolve with menses. She is able to continue her daily activities despite the symptoms. Best diagnostic method is keeping a prospective symptom diary for 2 months.

- At least one of the following affective and somatic symptoms during the 5 days before menses:
  - Affective symptoms:
    - Depression
    - Angry outburst
    - Irritability
    - Anxiety
    - Confusion
    - Social withdrawal
  - Somatic symptoms:
    - Breast tenderness
    - Abdominal bloating
    - Headache
    - Extremity swelling
- Relieved within 4 days of onset of menses.
- No recurrence until cycle day 13.
- Symptoms occur in two prospectively monitored cycles.
- Exclude other diagnoses—depression and anxiety may present all throughout the cycle.

PREMENSTRUAL DYSPHORIC DISORDER DIAGNOSTIC CRITERIA (DSM-IV CRITERIA)

A 17-year-old G0 complains of being sad 4 days right before she starts menstruating. She reports low energy, fatigue, hopelessness, anxiety, mood swings, bloating, breast tenderness, headache, and sleep disturbances during these days. These symptoms disappear 2 days after the start of menses. They occur on a monthly basis. She reports that she misses school on a monthly basis because she cannot get out of bed for 3 days. What is the most likely diagnosis? What is the best objective test to confirm the diagnosis?

Answer: PMDD. This patient has symptoms consistent with PMS, but with markedly severe symptoms that affect daily activities. She should monitor her symptoms in relation to her menses and record them prospectively.

- Symptoms with prospectively monitored cycles.
- Five symptoms of PMS including one affective symptom:
  - Feeling sad, hopeless, or having self-deprecating thoughts.
  - Anxiety or tension.
  - Mood lability and crying.
  - Persistent irritability, anger, ↑ interpersonal conflicts.

Diagnosis of PMS should be made from recording symptoms on a prospective calendar.

TESTS

Prospective calendar of symptoms in relation to menses.

TREATMENT

No drugs are currently FDA approved for the treatment of PMS or PMDD, but several drugs are helpful when used off label. There are also some dietary and lifestyle modifications that have been helpful. Treatment can be recommended based on severity of symptoms.

The therapy with most evidence for effectiveness for PMS/PMDD: SSRIs and ovulation blocking agents.

- **Supportive therapy:**
  - Reassurance and information counseling.
  - Relaxation therapy for severe symptoms has been shown to help.
- **Aerobic exercise** reduces affective symptoms, especially depression.
- **Dietary supplementation:**
  - Calcium is helpful.
  - Vitamin E ↓ mastalgia.
  - Carbohydrate-rich foods ↑ tryptophan, a precursor to serotonin.
- **Selective serotonin reuptake inhibitors (SSRIs):**
  - Fluoxetine and sertraline have been well studied and shown to help.
  - Can be administered throughout the menstrual cycle or just with symptoms during the last 2 weeks of the cycle.
- **Other:**
  - Spironolactone: Diuretic helps with the symptoms of fluid retention.
  - Nonsteroidal anti-inflammatory drugs (NSAIDs).

Calcium and aerobic exercise help PMS/PMDD symptoms.

- Oral contraceptives:
  - May help with physical symptoms, but not mood.
  - Monophasic, continuous best.

Leuprolide et al —— Gonadotropin-releasing hormone (GnRH) agonists: Severe PMS.
- Bilateral salpingo-oophorectomy: Reserved for those who are therapeutic with GnRH agonists only, and do not want to continue taking GnRH agonists on a daily basis, and want definitive treatment.

CHAPTER 16

Infertility

The monthly conception rate is 20% in a group of normal fertile couples. Infertility ↑ with increasing age of the female partner.

- Female factors account for 40–50% of infertile couples.
- Male factors account for 23% of infertile couples.
- In 40% of infertile couples, there are multiple causes.

DEFINITION: INFERTILITY

Infertility is defined as a failure to conceive after 1 yr of unprotected intercourse.

- The inability to conceive **after 12 months** of unprotected sexual intercourse.
- Affects 15% of couples.

TYPES

- **Primary infertility:** Infertility in the absence of previous pregnancy.
- **Secondary infertility:** Infertility after previous pregnancy.

FEMALE FACTORS AFFECTING INFERTILITY

- Multifactorial: 40%.
- Unexplained: 28%.
- Anovulation: 18%.
- Tubal disease: 14%.
- Endometriosis: 9%.

MALE FACTORS AFFECTING INFERTILITY

- Abnormal sperm function.
- Abnormal sperm production.
- Obstruction of ductal system (seminiferous tubules to urethral oriface).

INFERTILITY WORKUP

See Table 16-1.

Calcium channel blockers and furantoins can impair sperm number and function.

Male Factor

SEMEN ANALYSIS

Performed after at least 48 hr of abstinence, with examination of the sperm within a maximum of 2 hrs from time of ejaculation (for those who prefer to collect at home). Two properly performed semen analyses should be obtained at least 4 weeks apart. The analysis reflects sperm production that occurred 3 months ago.

CHARACTERISTICS

- Volume: Normal > 2 mL.
- Semen count: Normal > 20 million/mL.

TABLE 16-1. Evaluation of Infertile Couple

Male factor: Semen analysis.
Ovulation factor: Serum progesterone, day 3 FSH, prolactin, endometrial biopsy.
Cervical factor: Postcoital test.
Uterine factor: Ultrasonography, hysterosonogram, hysterosalpingogram, hysteroscopy.
Tubal factor: Hysterosalpingogram, laparoscopy.
Endometriosis: Laparoscopy.

- Motility: Normal > 50% with forward movement.
- Morphology: Normal > 40%.

TREATMENT FOR ABNORMAL SEMEN ANALYSIS

- Depends on the cause.
- Refer to urologist.
- Smoking and alcohol cessation.
- Avoid lubricants with intercourse.
- Clomiphene 25 mg/day for 25 days, with 5 days of rest (for the male partner). Binds estrogen receptors: ↑ pituitary gonadotropins
- Artificial insemination (with partner or donor sperm):
  - Intrauterine insemination: Sperm injected through cervix.
  - Intracytoplasmic sperm injection.
- If semen analysis is normal, continue workup of other factors.

Most male infertility is idiopathic.

Ovulatory Factor

A 28-year-old woman G0 has been unable to conceive with her husband over the last year. Her periods are irregular. She has a BMI of 30, displays coarse facial hair and a dark velvety pigmentation on the back of her neck. What is the likely diagnosis in this patient? What is the reason she is unable to conceive?

Answer: Polycystic ovarian syndrome (PCOS) affects approximately 5% of all women, and is a leading cause of infertility. The patient is anovulatory and will need clomiphene, an ovulation induction agent, in order to conceive.

METHODS OF ASSESSING OVULATION

- **History of regular monthly menses** is a strong indicator of normal ovulation.
- **Basal body temperature (BBT):** Body temperature rises about 0.5°–1°F during the luteal phase due to the ↑ level of progesterone. Elevation of BBT is a good indicator that ovulation is taking place.
- Serum progesterone: May be low if the corpus luteum is not producing enough.
- **Day 3 FSH:** Elevated if patient is anovulatory.
- **Endometrial biopsy:** Determines histologically the presence/absence of ovulation.

Initial workup for infertility:
- BBT
- Semen analysis
- Hysterosalpingogram

- **Pituitary insufficiency:** Treat with intramuscular luteinizing hormone/follicle-stimulating hormone (LH/FSH) or clomiphene.
- **Hyperprolactinemia:** Administer bromocriptine, a dopamine agonist, which supresses prolactin.
- **PCOS:** Treat with clomiphene +/– metformin, weight loss.
- **Other causes:** Hyper/hypothyroid, androgen excess, obesity/starvation, galactorrhea, stress.

Uterine Factors

A 30-year-old female G0 is undergoing an evaluation of her uterus as part of the workup for infertility. What procedure is diagnostic and therapeutic in the evaluation of the uterus?

Answer: Hysteroscopy is diagnostic and therapeutic.

If ovulation analysis and semen analysis are normal, analysis of the internal architecture of the uterus and fallopian tubes is performed to determine if there is an anatomic obstruction causing infertility. In most cases, an internal architecture study is part of the initial workup.

- **Hysteroscopy:**
  - A hysteroscope is an telescope that is connected to a video unit with a fiber-optic light source.
  - It is introduced through the cervix and allows visualization of the uterine cavity.
  - It is diagnostic and therapeutic. It can view the abnormality and treat it at the same time.
  - Hysteroscopy is useful in:
    - Asherman syndrome (lyse intrauterine adhesions).
    - Endometrial polyps (polypectomy).
    - Congenital uterine malformations (eg, excise a uterine septum).
    - Submucosal fibroids (resect).
- **Hysterosalpingogram:**
  - Radiopaque dye is injected into the cervix and uterus. Dye passes through the fallopian tubes to the peritoneal cavity. It should outline the inner uterine contour and both fallopian tubes when imaged with fluoroscopy.
  - Allows visualization of uterus and fallopian tubes.
  - Performed during follicular phase (avoid possibility of pregnancy).
  - There is a risk of salpingitis from the injection.
  - An interventional radiologist can use catheters to open the fallopian tubes that are occluded proximally.
- **Sonohysterogram:**
  - Fluid is instilled in the endometrial cavity concurrently with a pelvic ultrasound.
  - Outlines intrauterine pathology (ie, polyps, submucosal fibroids).
  - Can be done with an ultrasound in an office setting.
- **Ultrasound:**
  - In office study.
- **Laparoscopy:**
  - A telescope is placed through the skin of the abdominal wall into the peritoneal cavitiy.

- Can visualize outside of the uterus to assist in diagnosis of some mullerian malformations.

CAUSES AND TREATMENTS FOR UTERINE FACTOR INFERTILITY

- Submucosal fibroid: Resection, myomectomy.
- Intrauterine septum: Hysteroscopic resection of septum.
- Uterine didelphys: Metroplasty—a procedure to unify the two endometrial cavities.
- Asherman syndrome: Hysteroscopic lysis of intrauterine adhesions.

Tubal Factor

A 30-year-old female G0 has been having unprotected intercourse for 18 months without getting pregnant. She reports regular menstrual cycles. She had two episodes of pelvic inflammatory disease (PID) in the past. What is the best diagnostic modality to evaluate this patient? What will be the best treatment for her infertility? → *in follicular phase!*

Answer: Hysterosalpingogram will help determine if there is tubal blockage due to PID. If tubal blockage is present, the most effective treatment is in vitro fertilization.

EVALUATION

- Hysterosalpingogram
- Laparoscopy

CAUSES AND TREATMENTS FOR TUBAL FACTOR INFERTILITY

- Adhesions:
  - Lysis of adhesions via laparoscope.
  - Microsurgical tuboplasty.
  - Neosalpingostomy (blocked tubes are opened).
  - Tubal reimplantation for intramural obstruction.
  - In vitro fertilization (IVF).
- Tubal blockage: Tubal flushing.
- If the evaluation up to this point is within normal limits, then a diagnostic laparoscopy should be done.

Peritoneal Factors

Laparoscopy is diagnostic and therapeutic.

CAUSES AND TREATMENTS FOR PERITONEAL FACTOR INFERTILITY

- **Adhesions:** Lysis of adhesions via laparoscopy.
- **Endometriosis: Excision or ablation of implants.**

Damage from tubal surgery can result in ectopic pregnancy. Most reproductive endocrinologists recommend in vitro fertilization if tubal factor is present.

ASSISTED REPRODUCTIVE TECHNOLOGIES

Assisted reproductive technologies (ARTs) include clinical and laboratory techniques that are used to achieve pregnancy in infertile couples. ARTs are employed when correction of the underlying cause of infertility is not feasible.

Definition

Directly retrieving eggs from ovary followed by manipulation and replacement. **Generally employed for inadequate spermatogenesis.** The following are examples. Aside from intrauterine insemination, ARTs can utilize patient or donor egg and /or sperm.

Intrauterine Insemination

- Washed sperm is injected into the uterus.
- Must have a normal tube for fertilization to take place.

In Vitro Fertilization (IVF) and Embryo Transfer

- Egg cells are fertilized by sperm outside the uterus.
- Consists of ovarian stimulation, egg retrieval, fertilization, selection, and embryo transfer into uterus.
- Success rate of IVF is about 20%.
- Expensive.

IVF ↑ the chances of multiple gestation.

Intracytoplasmic Sperm Injection (ICSI)

- Subtype of IVF.
- Injection of spermatozoan into oocyte cytoplasm.
- Revolutionized treatment of infertility in men with severe oligospermia (low number), azoospermia (absence of live sperm), asthenospermia (low motility), teratospermia (abnormal morphology).
- Pregnancy rate: 20% per cycle.
- Multiple pregnancy rate: 28–38%.
- Not influenced by cause of abnormal sperm.
- Can use spermatozoa from testicular biopsies.
- Expensive.

Gamete Intrafallopian Transfer (GIFT)

- Egg and sperm are placed in a normal fallopian tube for fertilization.
- Success rate is about 25%.

Zygote Intrafallopian Transfer (ZIFT)

- Zygote created via fertilization in vitro and placed in fallopian tube, where it proceeds to uterus for natural implantation.
- Success rate is about 30%.

Artificial Insemination with Donor Sperm

- Success rate is 75% in six cycles.
- Donor sperm is used for ARTs.

CHAPTER 17

Amenorrhea

The causes of amenorrhea are quite varied. The hypothalamic-pituitary-ovarian (HPO) axis is involved in the regulation of the menstrual cycle, the uterus responds to the HPO axis, and normal cervix and vagina allow the outflow of menstrual blood. If there is an abnormality in any one of these components, the result will be amenorrhea.

Absence of menses for more than 35 days to 6 months is defined as **oligomenorrhea.**

- **Primary amenorrhea:** Absence of menses by age 16 with normal growth and secondary sexual characteristics. Usually genetic or anatomic causes. Also, absence of menses by age 14 in a girl with no secondary sexual characteristics.
- **Secondary amenorrhea:** Absence of menses for ≥ 6 months in a woman who previously had normal menses. Usually caused by underlying medical condition.

When evaluating a patient with primary amenorrhea, note presence/absence of breasts and uterus.

The causes of primary amenorrhea have been traditionally classified based on where the abnormality takes place along the HPO axis. It is more clinically useful to group the causes of primary amenorrhea on the basis of whether secondary sexual characteristics (breasts) and female internal genitalia (uterus) are present or absent. The external female genitalia are normal for these patients, but noting breast and uterus development on physical exam can indicate the diagnostic tests that will be most helpful.

Breasts Absent, Uterus Present

Patients without breasts and with a uterus have no ovarian estrogen. It is important to distinguish the disease processes because it can have an impact on fertility.

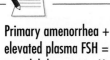

Primary amenorrhea + elevated plasma FSH = gonadal dysgenesis. Most common cause of primary amenorrhea.

- Gonadal dysgenesis (hypergonadotropic hypogonadism): *pit is good* Most common cause of primary amenorrhea. Most commonly due to chromosomal deletion or disorder. Ovaries are replaced by a band of fibrous tissue called *gonadal streak*. Due to the absence of ovarian follicles, there is no synthesis of ovarian steroids. Due to low levels of estrogen, breast development does not occur. Follicle-stimulating hormone (FSH) and luteinizing hormone (LH) levels are markedly elevated because the ↓ levels of estrogen do not provide negative feedback. Estrogen is not necessary for müllerian duct development or wolffian duct regression, so the internal and external genitalia are phenotypically female.
- **Turner syndrome (45,X):** In addition to primary amenorrhea and absent breasts, these patients have other somatic abnormalities: short stature (most prevalent), webbing of the neck, short fourth metacarpal, and cubitus valgus, cardiac abnormality, renal abnormalities, and hypothyroidism. At puberty, the patient is given estrogen and progesterone to allow for secondary sexual characteristics. Patients also receive growth hormone.
- **Structurally abnormal X chromosome:** May have the same abnormalities as Turner syndrome patients.
- **17α-hydroxylase deficiency:** Can occur in 46,XX. Patients have ↓ cortisol and adrenal/gonadal sex steroid secretion. They have hypertension, hypernatremia, and hypokalemia due to excess mineralocorticoid. These *aldo*

HIGH-YIELD FACTS

Amenorrhea

patients need replacement with sex steroids and cortisol. Despite low levels of sex steroids, pregnancies have been achieved with in vitro fertilization/embryo transfer. Those with karyotype 46,XY and 17α-hydroxylase deficiency will have no breasts or female internal genitalia.

- **Hypothalamic-pituitary disorders:** Low levels of estrogen are due to low gonadotropin release.
  - **Lesions:** Anatomic lesions of the hypothalamus or pituitary can result in low gonadotropin production.
    - Congenital: Stenosis of aqueduct, absence of sellar floor.
    - Acquired: Prolactinoma, chromophobe adenoma, craniopharyngiomas.
  - **Inadequate gonadotropin-releasing hormone (GnRH) release (hypogonadotropic hypogonadism):** Will have normal levels of gonadotropins if stimulated with GnRH. These patients should receive estrogen-progesterone supplementation to induce breast development and allow for epiphyseal closure. Human menopausal gonadotropins or pulsatile GnRH is administered for fertility. Clomiphene does not work due to low levels of endogenous estrogen.
    - **Kallmann syndrome:** Anosmia associated with low gonadotropins.
  - **Isolated gonadotropin deficiency (pituitary disease):** Associated with:
    - Prepubertal hypothyroidism.
    - Kernicterus.
    - Mumps encephalitis.
    - Thalassemia major: Iron deposits in the pituitary.
    - Retinitis pigmentosa.

> **17α hydroxylase deficiency:**
> 46,XX: Breast absent, uterus present
> 46,XY: Breast absent, uterus absent.

Breasts Present, Uterus Absent

An 18-year-old G0, presents with complaints of never having started menses. Her siblings started menses at age 12. She denies use of drugs, heavy exercise, or significant weight loss. She is 5'5" and 130 lb. Her blood pressure is 110/60. She has Tanner stage IV breasts, but no axillary or pubic hair. She has a blind vaginal pouch. What is the most likely diagnosis?

Answer: Androgen insensitivity. Breasts are present; uterus and axillary/pubic hair is absent in androgen insensitivity.

- **Androgen insensitivity (testicular feminization):** This condition results from the absence of androgen receptors or lack of responsiveness to androgen stimulus. These patients have an XY karyotype and normally functioning male gonads that produce normal male levels of testosterone and dihydrotestosterone. The müllerian ducts regress due to the presence of antimüllerian hormone, and the wolffian ducts do not develop because they are not stimulated by testosterone. Patients with this condition have no male or female internal genitalia, have normal female external genitalia, and have either a short or absent vagina. These patients have normal breasts and scant or absent axillary and pubic hair. Intra-abdominal testes or those in the inguinal canal have an ↑ risk of developing a malignancy (gonadoblastoma or dysgerminoma), usually after age 20. The gonads should be removed after puberty to allow for breast development and adequate bone growth. Estrogen is then given. These patients are raised as females.

> **Androgen insensitivity:**
> Patients look female externally. No pubic hair. Remove gonads after puberty to avoid risk of malignancy (gonadoblastoma or dysgerminoma).

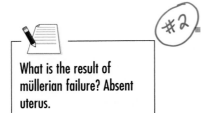

What is the result of müllerian failure? Absent uterus.

Müllerian agenesis: Second most common cause of primary amenorrhea.

Normal breast and pubic hair + no menses + cyclic pelvic pain + bulging blue mass at the introitus = hematocolpos from imperforate hymen.

(#2) **Müllerian agenesis (Mayer-Rokitansky-Kuster-Hauser syndrome):** In this condition, the patients have no uterus and have a shortened vagina, but have normally ovulating ovaries, normal breast development, and normal axillary and pubic hair. These patients have associated renal and skeletal abnormalities and should be screened with an ultrasound or MRI. They have normal endocrine function and do not need supplemental hormones. They may undergo surgical reconstruction of the vagina or use vaginal dilators to make the vagina functional (see Table 17-1).

Breasts Absent, Uterus Absent

17α-hydroxylase deficiency: These patients are XY, have testes, but lack the enzyme needed to synthesize sex steroids. They have female external genitalia. Antimüllerian hormone causes the regression of the müllerian ducts. Low testosterone levels do not allow the development of internal male genitalia. There is insufficient estrogen to allow breast development. Those with karyotype 46, XX, will have no breasts, but a uterus will be present.

Breasts Present, Uterus Present

- This is the second largest category of individuals with primary amenorrhea (chromosomal/gonadal dysgenesis #1). These women should be evaluated similar to those with secondary amenorrhea.
- **Imperforate hymen; transverse vaginal septum.** These patients present with cyclic pelvic pain due to menstrual blood not having an egress. A hematocolpos (accumulation of menstrual blood in the vagina from an imperforate hymen) can be palpated as a perirectal mass on physical exam. The treatment is to excise obstruction.

TABLE 17-1. **Comparison of Androgen Insensitivity and Müllerian Agenesis**

	ANDROGEN RESISTANCE	MÜLLERIAN AGENESIS
Karyotype	XY	XX
Breast	Present	Present
Uterus	Absent	Absent
Pubic/axillary hair	Absent	Normal
Testosterone	Normal male levels	Female levels
Further evaluation	Need gonadectomy	Renal/skeletal abnormalities

HIGH-YIELD FACTS

Amenorrhea

EVALUATION OF PRIMARY AMENORRHEA

HISTORY

- Other stages of puberty reached? Lack of any pubertal development suggests ovarian/pituitary cause.
- Family history.
- Height compared to other family members.
- Neonatal/childhood health problems.
- Symptoms of virilization.
- Recent stress, weight change, exercise.
- Drugs: Heroin/methadone can affect hypothalamus.
- Galactorrhea: Antipsychotics, Reglan (metoclopramide) can cause hyperprolactinemia.
- Headaches, vision problems, fatigue, polyuria, polydipsia: Hypothalamic/pituitary disorders.

PHYSICAL EXAM

- Height, weight, growth chart, arm span.
- Blood pressure:
  - Turner syndrome with coarctation of aorta.
  - Adrenal disorders.
- Breast development (Tanner staging): Marker of ovary function and estrogen action.
- Genital exam:
  - Clitoral size.
  - Tanner staging of pubic hair.
  - Hymen.
  - Vaginal depth.
  - Vaginal or rectal exam to evaluate internal organs.
- Skin: Hirsutism, acne, striae, acanthosis nigracans, vitiligo.
- Turner stigmata: Low hairline, web neck, shield chest, widely spaced nipples.

STUDIES

- Confirm presence of uterus: Ultrasound, rarely MRI.
- Uterus absent: Karyotype, serum testosterone: Müllerian anomalies have 46,XX with normal female levels of testosterone. Androgen insensitivity has 46,XY with male levels of testosterone.
- Uterus present. No other anatomic findings:
  - β-hCG to rule out pregnancy.
  - FSH
    - High: Indicative of primary ovarian failure. Karyotype: Turner syndrome (46,X); 17α-hydroxylase deficiency—(46, XX) electrolytes, ↑ progesterone, ↑ deoxycorticosterone, ↓ 17α-hydroxyprogesterone. Remove testes if Y chromosome present.
    - Low/normal: Functional hypothalamic amenorrhea, GnRH deficiency, hypothalamic/pituitary disorders. Head CT or MRI to evaluate for infiltrative disease or adenoma. Prolactin, thyroid-stimulating hormone (TSH). Testosterone and dehydroepiandrosterone sulfate (DHEA-S) if signs of hyperandrogenism.
    - Normal: With normal breast and uterus. Focus workup on secondary amenorrhea.

Check FSH to distinguish between gonadal failure and hypogonadotropic hypogonadism. FSH is high with gonadal failure and low with hypogonadotropic hypogonadism.

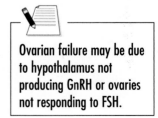

Ovarian failure may be due to hypothalamus not producing GnRH or ovaries not responding to FSH.

The most common cause of secondary amenorrhea is pregnancy. Always check a pregnancy test in a reproductive-age woman.

A 30-year-old Hispanic G2P2002, with last menstrual period (LMP) 8 weeks ago complains of no menses for the past 2 months. She usually has menses regularly every 28 days, lasting for 5 days. She denies any medical or surgical history. She has had two term spontaneous vaginal deliveries. She uses combination oral contraceptive pills (OCPs) regularly, and has not missed any pills recently. What is the next step in management of this patient?

Answer: The most common cause of amenorrhea in a reproductive-age woman is pregnancy, so a urine or serum β-hCG should be checked. Contraception use does not prevent pregnancy 100% of the time.

Think about the causes in terms of the HPO axis.

Causes

- Pregnancy.
- Hypothalamus (35%).
- Pituitary (19%).
- Ovary (40%).
- Uterus (5%).
- Other (1%): Cervical, endocrine.

HYPOTHALAMIC

Low levels of gonadotropins, estrogen, absent withdrawal bleed with progesterone.

The most common cause of amenorrhea in adolescent girls is anorexia nervosa.

- **Lesions:** Craniopharyngiomas, granulomatous disease, encephalitis sequelae.
- **Drugs:** OCPs act at the level of the hypothalamus and pituitary. Postpill amenorrhea can occur up to 6 months after stopping the pill.
- **Stress and exercise.**
- **Weight loss/anorexia nervosa:** Those who are malnourished have a ↓ reproductive ability. Weight gain will allow menses to resume.
- **Functional hypothalamic amenorrhea:** ↓ GnRH secretion, without other causes.

PITUITARY (HYPOESTROGENIC AMENORRHEA)

- **Neoplasms:** Chromophobe adenomas are the most common non-prolactin-secreting pituitary tumors. Prolactinomas will be discussed in a later section. Treatment may involve suppression with medication (prolactinomas) or excision.
- **Lesions:** The pituitary gland can be damaged from anoxia, thrombosis, or hemorrhage. May be associated with ↓ secretion of other pituitary hormones like adrenocorticotropic hormone (ACTH), TSH, LH, and FSH. The patients may have hypothyroidism and adrenal insufficiency.
  - **Sheehan syndrome:** Pituitary cell destruction occurs due to hypotensive episode during pregnancy (usually due to catastrophic hemorrhage). Treatment includes replacement of pituitary hormones.
  - **Simmonds disease:** Pituitary damage unrelated to pregnancy.

A 35-year-old G3P3003 complains of absence of menses for 8 months. She reports menarche at age 12 with menses every 40–50 days until recently. She complains of an ↑ of 20 lb in her weight over the last year. She denies any family history or use of medications or drugs. She used clomiphene to become pregnant with her last two pregnancies. She is 5'4", weight 220 lb, BP 120/80. She has hair on her upper lip and chin. She has acne and oily skin on her face. What is the most likely diagnosis? If left untreated, what is this patient at ↑ risk for?

Answer: Polycystic ovarian syndrome (PCOS). Diagnosis of PCOS is established with two out of three of the following: a history of oligomenorrhea/amenorrhea, features of hyperandrogenism (acne, hirsutism), and multiple cysts seen on ultrasound. This patient is at ↑ risk for endometrial hyperplasia or cancer if left untreated.

A 35-year-old G2P2002 with LMP one year ago presents with hot flashes and vaginal dryness. Her serum FSH is very high and in the menopausal range. What is the most likely diagnosis?

Answer: Premature ovarian failure. Symptoms are similar to those in menopause and FSH is a comfirmatory test.

- **Premature ovarian failure (POF):** Depletion of oocytes resulting in amenorrhea before the age of 40.
    - May be due to radiation or systemic chemotherapy.
    - Autoimmune conditions can be present.
    - Fragile X permutation.
    - Turner syndrome.
    - Treatment may include hormone replacement. Need strategies for bone protection.
- **Surgical:** Bilateral salpingo-oophorectomy.
- **Polycystic ovaries:** Hyperandrogenism.
    - **Diagnosis:** Established if two out of three of the following are present:
        - Polycystic ovaries on ultrasound.
        - Signs of androgen excess (hirsutism, acne).
        - Oligomenorrhea/amenorrhea.
    - **Signs:**
        - Hirsutism.
        - Acne.
        - Oligomenorrhea/amenorrhea.
        - Obesity.
        - Acanthosis nigricans (gray, brown velvety skin discoloration present most commonly on neck and axilla).
        - Premature pubarche and/or precocious puberty.
    - Aim treatment toward hirsutism (cosmetic methods, spironolactone, Vaniqa [eflornithine]) and infertility (ovulation induction with clomiphene). Start cyclic or continuous OCPs/hormone therapy to prevent endometrial hyperplasia/endometrial cancer and regulate menses.

Premature ovarian failure:
- Age < 40
- Amenorrhea
- Elevated FSH

PCOS is the most common cause of hirsutism.

Treatment of choice for PCOS: OCPs

Progestin challenge test: Give oral progestin for 10 days. If the endometrium has been primed with estrogen from ovaries or peripheral fat, the withdrawal of progestin after 10 days will cause endometrial sloughing with resultant menses. No menses indicates absence of ovaries, estrogen deficiency, or outflow obstruction.

Asherman syndrome is intrauterine adhesions (IUAs) or fibrosis, secondary to curettage and scarring. It can cause secondary amenorrhea.

The most common cause of Asherman syndrome is curettage performed during pregnancy or shortly thereafter.

UTERINE

- **Asherman syndrome:** Intrauterine adhesions can obliterate the endometrial cavity and cause amenorrhea.
  - Most frequent cause is endometrial curettage associated with pregnancy.
  - Adhesions may form after myomectomy, metroplasty, or cesarean delivery.
  - Confirm the diagnosis with hysterosalpingogram (HSG) or hysteroscopy.
  - Treat via hysteroscopic resection of adhesions. Estrogens administered to stimulate regrowth of endometrium.
- **Endometrial ablation:** This procedure may have been performed for menorrhagia.
- **Infection:** Endometritis or tuberculosis.

CERVICAL

Stenosis due to loop electrosurgical excision procedure (LEEP) or cold-knife cone. Treat with cervical dilation.

ENDOCRINE

Can cause secondary amenorrhea.

- Hyper/hypothyroidism.
- Diabetes mellitus.
- Hyperandrogenism (neoplasm, exogenous androgens).

Evaluation

HISTORY

- Recent stress, weight change, new diet or exercise habits, illness.
- Acne, hirsutism, deepening of voice.
- Symptoms of hypothalamic-pituitary disease:
  - Headaches.
  - Galactorrhea.
  - Visual field defects.
  - Fatigue.
  - Polyuria, polydipsia.
- Symptoms of estrogen deficiency:
  - Hot flashes.
  - Vaginal dryness.
  - Poor sleep.
  - ↓ libido.
- Obstetric emergency with hemorrhage (Sheehan syndrome).
- Medications:
  - Initiation or discontinuation of OCPs.
  - Androgenic drugs.
  - High-dose progestins.
  - Metoclopramide, antipsychotics: cause ↑ prolactin leading to amenorrhea.

PHYSICAL EXAM

- Body mass index (BMI): > 30 kg/m² in women with PCOS.
- Signs of systemic illness/cachexia, anorexia.
- Genital tissue with signs of estrogen deficiency: POF.
- Breast exam for galactorrhea.
- Neurologic exam for visual fields: Pituitary adenoma.
- Skin:
  - Hirsutism, acne, acanthosis nigricans: PCOS.
  - Thin/dry skin, thickened skin: Thyroid disorders.

STUDIES

- Serum prolactin, TSH, FSH. FSH is high in POF. Consider karyotype.
- DHEA-S and testosterone if signs of hyperandrogenism.
- Estrogen status:
  - Serum estradiol.
  - Progestin withdrawal test with Provera (medroxyprogesterone) 10 mg for 10 days. If bleeding occurs, then adequate estrogen is present in the body.

TREATMENT

Treatment is individualized based on the etiology of amenorrhea.

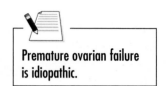

Absence of vaginal bleeding after progesterone challenge is due to very low levels of estrogen.

Premature ovarian failure is idiopathic.

HIGH-YIELD FACTS

Amenorrhea

Hyperandrogenism

- **Hirsutism:** Presence of hair in locations where it is not normally found in a woman, specifically in the midline of the body (upper lip, chin, back, intermammary region).
- **Virilization:** Presence of signs of masculinization in a woman (temporal balding, deeper voice, clitoral enlargement, ↑ muscle mass).
- **Hypertrichosis:** A generalized ↑ in the amount of body hair in its normal location.
- **Vellus hairs:** Fine hairs found on most parts of the body. They are barely visible.
- **Terminal hairs:** Coarse, darker hairs found, for example, in the axilla and pubic region. Androgens facilitate the conversion of vellus to terminal hairs.

SOURCES OF ANDROGENS

> Ovary makes testosterone. Adrenal gland makes DHEA-S.

Androgens are produced in the ovary and the adrenal gland. The ovary primarily makes testosterone. It also secretes androstenedione and dehydroepiandrosterone (DHEA) to a smaller degree. Androstenedione and DHEA are converted to testosterone in peripheral tissue. The adrenal gland makes dehydroepiandrosterone sulfate (DHEA-S) and DHEA. To produce a biologic effect, the enzyme 5α-reductase in the peripheral tissue converts testosterone to more potent 5α-dihydrotestosterone (DHT).

Adrenal Production of Androgens

- The **zona fasciculata** and the **zona reticularis** of the adrenal cortex produce androgens, as well as cortisol. ACTH regulates production.
- A third layer of the adrenal cortex, the **zona glomerulosa**, produces aldosterone and is regulated by the renin-angiotensin system.
- All three hormones—cortisol, androgens, and aldosterone—are derived from cholesterol. Androgen products from the adrenal are found mostly in the form of DHEA and DHEA-S. Elevation in these products represents ↑ adrenal androgen production.

Ovarian Production of Androgens

In the ovaries, first, luteinizing hormone (LH) stimulates the theca cells to produce androgens (androstenedione and testosterone). Then, follicle-stimulating hormone (FSH) stimulates granulosa cells to convert these androgens to estrone and estradiol. When LH levels become disproportionately greater than FSH levels, androgens become elevated.

A 35-year-old G3P3003 complains of increasing facial hair that began 2 years ago. She reports menses every 30 days lasting for 4 days, denies taking any medications. She reports her sister has similar symptoms. On physical exam, the patient is normotensive. She has moderately dark hair on her upper lip and chin. No other abnormal distribution of hair. She has normal female genitalia. Serum levels of testosterone and DHEA-S are normal. What is the most likely diagnosis?

Answer: Idiopathic hirsutism. Gradual onset of hirsutism with normal menses, testosterone and DHEA-S indicate idiopathic hirsutism.

This condition manifests with signs of hirsutism, regular menses, and normal levels of testosterone and DHEA-S. This disorder is due to ↑ activity of 5α-reductase activity in the periphery. Antiandrogens that block the peripheral activity of testosterone or inhibit the enzyme 5α-reductase can be used to treat the hirsutism.

ADRENAL ETIOLOGIES

Cushing Syndrome and Cushing Disease

- **Cushing syndrome:** An adrenal tumor produces ↑ levels of cortisol with clinical findings—hirsutism, menstrual irregularity, central obesity, moon face, buffalo hump, abdominal striae, weakness, and muscle wasting. Exogenous or endogenous cortisol can be the cause. Confirm diagnosis with dexamethasone suppression test.
- **Cushing disease** (pituitary disease) is a subset of Cushing syndrome. A benign pituitary adenoma causes an ↑ in the secretion of adrenocorticotropic hormone (ACTH) which results in ↑ cortisol levels. It accounts for 70% of Cushing syndromes. Virilization and hirsutism are associated with this condition because the ACTH stimulates androgen production as well.
- **Paraneoplastic syndromes,** in which tumors (usually small cell lung cancer) produce ectopic ACTH, also cause ↑ cortisol. These account for 15% of Cushing syndromes.
- **Adrenal tumors** (adenoma or carcinoma) account for the remaining 15% of Cushing syndromes. In general, adenomas produce only cortisol, so no hirsutism or virilization is present. Carcinomas, by contrast, often produce androgens as well as cortisol, so they may present with signs of hirsutism and virilization. DHEA-S is markedly elevated, and hirsutism and virilization has a rapid onset. Computed tomography (CT) or magnetic resonance imaging (MRI) can confirm the diagnosis.

Congenital Adrenal Hyperplasia (CAH)

- Caused by a congenital defect in an enzyme that produces cortisol.
  - **21-hydroxylase deficiency:** The most common form of congenital adrenal hyperplasia. The condition has various levels of severity. Affected

Rapid onset of hirsutism or virilization = tumor (ovarian or adrenal).

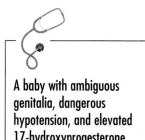

A baby with ambiguous genitalia, dangerous hypotension, and elevated 17-hydroxyprogesterone. *Think: 21-Hydroxylase deficiency*

Most common cause of ambiguous genitalia in a newborn: CAH due to 21-hydroxylase deficiency.

individuals lack an enzyme crucial to cortisol and mineralocorticoid production. Therefore, the ↑ precursors of cortisol are shunted to androgen production. Elevated serum 17-hydroxyprogesterone is used as a marker for establishing the diagnosis of 21-hydroxylase deficiency. In the severe form, affected females have ambiguous genitalia at birth, along with severe salt wasting and cortisol insufficiency. Late-onset 21-hydroxylase deficiency presents with varying degrees of virilization and hirsutism in females after puberty.

- **11β-hydroxylase deficiency:** Associated with ↓ cortisol, but ↑ mineral corticoids and androgens. A typical patient with this enzyme deficiency has severe hypertension with virilization/hirsutism (which results in pseudohermaphroditism of female babies). 11-deoxycortisol levels are high in 11β-hydroxylase deficiency (see Table 18-1).

OVARIAN ETIOLOGIES

Polycystic Ovarian Syndrome (PCOS)

The most common cause of hirsutism and irregular menses is PCOS.

- PCOS is a common condition (affecting 5% of reproductive-age women) and is diagnosed by the presence of two out of three clinical findings: hyperandrogenism, oligomenorrhea/amenorrhea, and multiple cysts on ultrasound.
- An abnormal release of gonadotropin-releasing hormone (GnRH) causes a persistently elevated LH. The LH:FSH ratio is often > 3:1. There are ↑ levels of androgens produced from the adrenal gland and the ovary. These women also have higher levels of estradiol that is not bound to sex hormone–binding globulin (SHBG), although the total estradiol level is not elevated. There is ↑ estrone due to adipose conversion of androgens.
- These patients also have acanthosis nigricans, obesity, insulin resistance, and infertility. In the future, they are at ↑ risk for diabetes mellitus, hypertension, cardiovascular disease, endometrial cancer, and ovarian cancer. The risk of endometrial and ovarian cancer is reduced with the use of oral contraceptive pills (OCPs).

A 24-year-old obese woman with facial hair complains of amenorrhea. LH:FSH ratio is elevated. *Think: PCOS.*

Stromal Hyperthecosis

- LH stimulates theca cells in the ovary resulting in stromal hyperplasia. Theca cells produce large amounts of testosterone.
- Presents with gradual onset, anovulation, amenorrhea, and hirsutism.
- Testosterone secretion is progressively ↑ as a woman ages, resulting in virilization and bilaterally enlarged ovaries up to 5-7 cm in diameter.

TABLE 18-1. Clinical Findings in Congenital Adrenal Hyperplasia

	21-HYDROXYLASE DEFICIENCY	11β-HYDROXYLASE DEFICIENCY
Androgens	High	High
Cortisol	Low	Low
Mineralacorticoids	Low → hypotension	High → hypertension
Marker	↑ 17-hydroxyprogesterone	↑ 11-deoxycortisol

Theca Lutein Cysts

- Theca cells produce androgens, and granulosa cells transform the androgens to estrogens.
- Theca lutein cysts produce abnormally high levels of androgens, in excess of the amount that can be converted to estrogens.
- Diagnosis is made by ovarian biopsy.

Luteoma of Pregnancy

- A benign tumor that grows in response to human chorionic gonadotropin (hCG).
- Virilization may occur in both the mother and the female fetus.
- The tumor usually disappears postpartum, as do maternal clinical features.

A baby with ambiguous genitalia is born to a mother who complains of ↑ facial hair growth over last few months. *Think: Luteoma of pregnancy.*

Androgen-Secreting Ovarian Neoplasms

A 25-year-old G0 complains of dark hair on her upper lip and chin, thinning hair on her head, and deepening of her voice that took place over 2 months. She denies medications. She is normotensive. She has hair growth as stated above and has temporal balding. Her pelvic exam is within normal limits except for clitoromegaly. What is the most likely diagnosis? What is the next step in management?

Answer: Due to the rapid presentation of virilization, this is most likely an adrenal or ovarian tumor. Drawing serum total testosterone and DHEA-S will help differentiate the source. Pelvic US will confirm the presence of an ovarian mass. A CT or MRI will confirm the presence of an adrenal mass.

- Sertoli-Leydig cell tumors and hilar (Leydig) cell tumors are rare conditions in which the neoplasms secrete androgens.
- Sertoli-Leydig cell tumors are distinguished from hilar cell tumors in that Sertoli-Leydig tumors usually present in young women with palpable masses and hilar cell tumors are found in postmenopausal women with nonpalpable masses.
- Neoplasms present with rapid signs of virilization.

HISTORY

- Pregnancy: Theca lutein cysts, luteoma of pregnancy.
- Timing of hirsutism, virilization: Rapid onset suggestive of ovarian or adrenal tumors. Gradual suggestive of idiopathic etiology.

PHYSICAL EXAM

- Note distribution of terminal hair.
- Note signs of virilization.
- Bimanual exam: Pelvic mass.

- Hirsutism, menstrual irregularity, central obesity, moon face, buffalo hump, abdominal striae, weakness, and muscle wasting: Cushing syndrome.

If cortisol levels are low after an overnight dexamethasone suppression test, Cushing syndrome is excluded from the differential.

High dose will suppress Cushing's

STUDIES

- Serum total testosterone (ovarian), DHEA-S (adrenal): Distinguish ovarian vs. adrenal source.
- Ultrasound: Confirm ovarian mass.
- CT/MRI: Confirm adrenal mass.
- Dexamethasone suppression test: Distinguish the etiology of the ACTH stimulation.
- Serum 17-hydroxyprogesterone: Elevated in 21-hydroxylase deficiency.
- Serum 11-deoxycortisol: Elevated in 11β-hydroxylase deficiency.

TREATMENT

- Ovarian and adrenal tumors:
  - Sertoli-Leydig cell tumors: Unilateral salpingo-oophorectomy if not completed childbearing.
  - Hilar cell tumors: Usually in postmenopausal women. Total abdominal hysterectomy (TAH), bilateral salpingo-oophorectomy (BSO).
  - Adrenal adenoma or carcinoma: Surgical removal.
  - Stromal hyperthecosis: TAH, BSO.
- Late onset 21-hydroxylase deficiency:
  - Androgen excess and menstrual irregularities can be treated as PCOS.
  - Infertility: Supplement with glucocorticoids to suppress androgens and allow ovulation.
- PCOS:
  - Weight loss.
  - OCPs for acne and menstrual irregularity. Estrogen component in the OCP ↑ SHBG; SHBG binds androgens; free androgen levels are then ↓. Progestins in the OCP inhibits 5α-reductase activity in the skin.
  - Cyclic progesterone for menstrual irregularity.
  - Infertility: Ovulation induction with clomiphene and metformin.
- Skin disorders:
  - Peripheral antiandrogens: Spironolactone, finasteride, cyproterone acetate.
  - Androgenic acne responds quickly to treatment. Hirsutism moderately responsive; alopecia least responsive to treatment.
- Idiopathic hirsutism:
  - Peripheral androgen activity inhibitor. May take 3 months to work (length of hair life cycle).
  - Electrolysis.
  - OCPs, medroxyprogesterone acetate.
  - Ketoconazole: Risk of hepatitis.
  - Spironolactone: Blocks androgen receptors, ↓ ovarian testosterone production, inhibits 5α-reductase.
  - Finasteride (5α-reductase inhibitor), flutamide (nonsteroidal antiandrogen): Similar effectiveness to spironolactone.

Treatment of choice for idiopathic hirsutism: Spironolactone.

236

CHAPTER 19

Hyperprolactinemia and Galactorrhea

DEFINITIONS

- **Hyperprolactinemia:** Elevated levels of the hormone prolactin (PRL).
- **Galactorrhea:** Watery or milky fluid secreted from the breast that is not in relation to pregnancy.
- **Prolactinoma:** Prolactin-secreting pituitary tumor.

ETIOLOGY

A 35-year-old G2P2002 complains of milky discharge from her breasts for 6 months. She also reports no menses for 6 months. She used to have menses every 28 days, lasting for 4 days. She has started to have hot flashes in the last 4 months. She denies the use of any medications. She is normotensive. No masses are palpated on the breast exam, but a milky discharge is expressed from both breasts. Her vagina is dry. Her serum β-human chorionic gonadotropin (β-hCG) is negative. What is the most likely diagnosis? What studies should be ordered next?

Answer: This patient has galactorrhea, amenorrhea, and low estrogen most likely due to hyperprolactinemia. Serum prolactin and thyrotropin-stimulating hormone (TSH) should be drawn to initiate the evaluation.

- PRL is a peptide hormone produced by the anterior pituitary gland and is important for lactation. The main function of PRL is to stimulate growth of mammary tissue as well as produce and secrete milk into the alveoli. ↑ secretion of prolactin, hyperprolactinemia, may lead to galactorrhea. PRL secretion is stimulated by thyrotropin-releasing hormone (TRH) and serotonin; it is inhibited by dopamine.
- Hyperprolactinemia inhibits the pulsatile release of gonadoropin-releasing hormone (GnRH), resulting in amenorrhea/oligomenorrhea, anovulation, inappropriate lactation and galactorrhea.
- **Causes** of hyperprolactinemia:
  - Drugs: Tranquilizers, tricyclic antidepressants (TCAs), antipsychotics, antihypertensives, narcotics, oral contraceptive pills (OCPs).
  - Hypothyroidism: ↓ negative feedback of thyroxine (T_4) on the hypothalamic-pituitary axis causing an ↑ in TRH. TRH stimulates PRL secretion.
  - Hypothalamic: Craniopharyngioma, sarcoidosis, histiocytosis, leukemia. Interferes with portal circulation of dopamine.
  - Pituitary: Prolactinoma. Microadenoma (< 1 cm), macroadenoma (> 1 cm). See the following section on prolactinoma.
  - Hyperplasia of lactotrophs: Present very similarly to those having microadenomas.
  - Empty sella syndrome: Intrasellar extension of subarachnoid space which causes compression of the pituitary gland and an enlarged sella turcica.
  - Acromegaly: Pituitary gland secretes growth hormone as well as PRL.

- **✱** ■ Acute/chronic renal disease: ↓ metabolic clearance of PRL.
  - ■ Chest surgery or trauma: Breast implants, herpes zoster at breast dermatome.

PROLACTINOMA

- One-tenth of people in the general population have an incidental prolactinoma.
- Fifty percent of women with hyperprolactinemia have a prolactinoma.
- Most prolactinomas are microadenomas.
- Majority of microadenomas do not enlarge.
- Hyperprolactinemia with or without a microadenoma follows a benign clinical course and treatment is not necessary unless estrogen levels are low or pregnancy is desired.
- Microadenoma growth is **not** stimulated by:
  - Pregnancy
  - OCPs
  - Hormone replacement

HISTORY

- Amenorrhea/oligomenorrhea.
- Galactorrhea.
- Headaches.
- Bitemporal visual field deficit.

PHYSICAL EXAM

- Visual field testing if macroadenoma is present. Macroadenomas can exert pressure on the optic chiasm.
- Breast exam.

STUDIES

- PRL level.
- TSH, triiodothyronine (T_3), T_4: Evaluate for hypothyroidism if PRL is elevated.
- Magnetic resonance imaging (MRI): Most sensitive for diagnosis of pituitary masses and empty sella syndrome due to greater soft tissue contrast.

TREATMENT

- **Drugs:** Stop the suspected drug, and repeat PRL after 1 month. If medication cannot be stopped and PRL level above 100 ng/mL, image the sella turcica to determine the presence of macroadenoma.
- Patient with galactorrhea and normal menses: **No further therapy** if normal PRL, normal TSH.

Fifty percent of women with hyperprolactinemia will have a prolactinoma. If PRL is > 200 ng/mL, nearly 100% will have prolactinoma.

Most macroadenomas enlarge with time. Most microadenomas do not.

The most common symptoms of hyperprolactinemia are galactorrhea and amenorrhea.

Sixty percent of women with galactorrhea have hyperprolactinemia. Ninety percent of women with galactorrhea, amenorrhea, and low estrogen have hyperprolactinemia.

MRI: Modality of choice to diagnose pituitary adenomas or empty sella syndrome.

Bromocriptine is the drug of choice for women with PRL-secreting microadenoma who want to conceive.

Cabergoline is the drug of choice for reducing PRL levels and shrinking tumors.

Pregnancy ↑ the likelihood that PRL levels will ↓ or become normal overtime.

Bromocriptine induction of pregnancy is not associated with ↑ congenital abnormalities, spontaneous abortion, or multiple gestation.

Cabergoline is more effective and better tolerated than bromocriptine.

- **Bromocriptine:** Dopamine receptor agonist.
  - For patients with macroadenoma: Can reduce tumor mass.
  - For those that desire to conceive, are anovulatory, with hyperprolactinemia: Discontinued after conception as it crosses the placenta. Not known to be teratogen.
  - For those with galactorrhea only: Inhibits secretion of PRL.
  - Side effects: Severe orthostatic hypotension (fainting, dizziness), nausea, vomiting.
  - Administered orally or vaginally (reduced side effect of nausea and vomiting).
  - Long-term treatment is required.
- **Cabergoline:** Long-acting dopamine receptor agonist. Less frequent and less severe side effects.
- **Transsphenoidal microsurgical resection:**
  - Recommended only if macroadenoma and fail medical therapy.
  - Risk of diabetes insipidus, iatrogenic hypopituitarism.
  - Fifty percent cure for microadenomas, 25% cure for macroadenoma.
- **Radiation:** Adjunctive treatment following incomplete removal of large tumors.
- **Osteoporosis treatment/prophylaxis:** Low levels of estrogen resulting from hyperprolactinemia can result in bone loss.

Abnormal Uterine Bleeding

Menorrhagia: Bleeding too long or too much. History of clots most consistent with diagnosis of anemia.

How much blood loss is necessary to define menorrhagia? > 80 mL

Two main mechanisms for hemostasis during menstruation are hemostatic plug formation and vasoconstriction.

Metrorrhagia: The metro never comes according to schedule (bleeding at frequent, irregular intervals).

Patient with postcoital bleeding should be evaluated for cervical cancer and cervicitis.

DEFINITIONS

Menstrual abnormalities include:

- **Polymenorrhea:** Uterine bleeding occurring at regular intervals of < 21 days.
- **Menorrhagia:** Prolonged (> 7 days) or excessive (> 80 mL) uterine bleeding occurring at regular intervals (synonymous with **hypermenorrhea**).
- **Oligomenorrhea:** Uterine bleeding occurring at intervals > 35 days.
- **Metrorrhagia:** Bleeding occurring at frequent, irregular intervals.
- **Menometrorrhagia:** Combination of both menorrhagia and metrorrhagia; uterine bleeding that is prolonged or excessive, frequent, and irregular.
- **Dysfunctional uterine bleeding:** Bleeding that occurs after organic, systemic, and iatrogenic causes have been ruled out. Two types: anovulatory and ovulatory.

ABNORMAL UTERINE BLEEDING: REPRODUCTIVE AGE

A 24-year-old G0P0 presents to the office with a menstrual period every 3–4 months. Her periods are heavy, lasting 7–9 days. Her body mass index (BMI) is 40. She complains of severe acne since puberty. Recently, she was diagnosed with diabetes mellitus type 2. Her genitourinary (GU) exam was normal, with no palpable masses. What initial lab tests should be ordered in the evaluation of this patient?

Answer: β-hCG, follicle-stimulating hormone (FSH), thyrotropin-stimulating hormone (TSH), prolactin (PRL). These tests cover the top differential diagnosis of pregnancy, premature ovarian failure, thyroid dysfunction, and hyperprolactinemia as the cause of abnormal uterine bleeding (AUB). If all of the results are normal, further workup can be done.

A normal menstrual cycle occurs every 21–35 days (28 ± 7 days) with menstruation for 2–7 days. The normal blood loss is less than 80 mL total (average 35 cc), which represents 8 or fewer soaked pads per day with usually no more than 2 heavy days. AUB is any disturbance of the above. It can occur at any age and has many causes.

Most cases of reproductive age bleeding are related to pregnancy, structural uterine pathology, anovulation, coagulopathy or neoplasia. Less common causes include trauma and infection.

ETIOLOGY

- **Organic:**
  - Reproductive tract disease.
  - Accidents of pregnancy (threatened, incomplete, missed abortion; ectopic pregnancy; trophoblastic disease).
  - Malignancy: Most commonly endometrial and cervical cancers. Estrogen producing ovarian tumors like the granulosa-theca cell tumors may present with excessive uterine bleeding.

- Infection: Endometritis presents with episodic intermenstrual spotting. Cervicitis and severe vaginal infections can present with bleeding.
- Structural causes (fibroids, polyps, adenomyosis).
- Foreign bodies: Tampons retained in the vagina or intrauterine devices for contraception can cause bleeding.
- Endometriosis: Occasionally presents as premenstrual spotting.
- Traumatic vaginal lesions.
- **Systemic:**
  - von Willebrand disease can cause ↑ bleeding due to coagulopathy.
  - Prothrombin deficiency.
  - Leukemia.
  - Sepsis.
  - Idiopathic thrombocytopenic purpura.
  - Hypersplenism.
  - Thyroid dysfunction: Hypothyroidism causes anovulation and is frequently associated with menorrhagia and intermenstrual bleeding.
  - Cirrhosis: Excessive bleeding secondary to the reduced capacity of the liver to metabolize estrogens.
- **Iatrogenic:**
  - Anticoagulation medications.
  - Oral or injectable steroids used for contraception.
  - Hormone replacement therapy (HRT).
  - Tranquilizers and psychotropic drugs: Interfere with neurotransmitters responsible for inhibition and release of hypothalamic hormones, leading to anovulation and AUB. PRL
- **Dysfunctional uterine bleeding (DUB):**
  - **Ovulatory:** After adolescence and before perimenopausal years. Usually menorrhagia and/or intermenstrual bleeding. Due to abnormal endometrial hemostasis for any reason. The diagnosis of ovulatory DUB is made by endometrial biopsy (EMB). On the fourth day of flow, the EMB reveals both proliferative and secretory endometrium.
  - **Anovulatory: Predominant cause of DUB.** There is continuous estradiol production without corpus luteum formation or progesterone production. This steady state of estrogen stimulation results in constant endometrial proliferation without progesterone-mediated maturation and shedding. Fragments of overgrown endometrium sheds sporadically. Anovulation can manifest in:
    - Polycystic ovarian syndrome (PCOS).
    - Obesity.
    - Adolescents (perimenarchal).
    - Perimenopause.

HISTORY

- Ask the patient about the frequency, interval, duration, and amount of bleeding.
- Ask the patient if and when the menstrual pattern changed.
- Ask about the presence of clots.
- Provide the patient with a calendar to record her bleeding episodes and its duration.
- Ask the patient how many full sanitary napkins she uses on average. This is very subjective so beware.
- Menorrhagia present since menarche?

Most common cause of hospital admission for menorrhagia in adolescents = von Willebrand disease.

Tumors (benign and malignant) often present with menorrhagia or metrorrhagia.

DUB is a diagnosis of exclusion—not regular, not predictable, and not associated with PMS. It is diagnosed only when all organic causes are ruled out.

Signs of PCOS
- Oligomenorrhea
- Hirsutism
- Obesity
- Cystic ovaries

Irregular bleeding is often associated with anovulation.

- Family history of bleeding?
- Epistaxis, gum bleeding, postpartum bleeding, surgical bleeding.
- Cold intolerance.

PHYSICAL EXAM

- Bimanual may reveal bulky uterus/discrete fibroids.
- Obesity, hirsutism, acanthosis nigricans (PCO).
- Exopthalmos, goiter, delayed DTRs, dry skin/hair (thyroid disorder).
- Visual field deficits, galactorrhea (hyperprolactinemia).
- Petechia (coagulopathy).

DIAGNOSTIC TESTS

Hysteroscopy can be used to diagnose and treat the uterine abnormality at the same time.

- Pap smear.
- Pregnancy test: Sensitive hCG.
- Hemoglobin, serum Fe, serum ferritin.
- TSH.
- FSH.
- Prolactin.
- Coagulation panel: von Willebrand factor for adolescents with menorrhagia.
- EMB for women ≥ 35 yrs of age or with history of unopposed estrogen.
- Pelvic ultrasound.
- Sonohysterogram (pelvic US combined with intrauterine saline infusion to outline the uterine cavity).
- Hysteroscopy

TREATMENT

A 28-year-old G2P2002 presents to the ED complaining of excessive uterine bleeding for the past week that has worsened over the past 24 hr, shortness of breath, and dizziness. She appears pale; HR 110, BP 90/65. She is sweating profusely and is very restless. Sterile speculum exam shows active bright red bleeding and a normal cervix. What is the best treatment for this patient?

Answer: Dilation and curettage (D&C) is the treatment of choice for a patient with heavy bleeding and hemodynamic instability. Its effect is immediate.

- Address organic, systemic, iatrogenic causes as indicated.
- Medical management: First-line treatment. Used for women who desire future fertility or those who will reach menopause within a short period of time.
  - Nonsteroidal anti-inflammatory drugs (NSAIDs) (tranexamic acid/ mefenamic acid).
  - Iron supplements.
  - Hormones: OCP is the mainstay for anovulatory bleeding. Combination pill or estrogens are used in the acute management of DUB. Progestin intrauterine device (IUD) can be used for DUB.

- D&C: Indicated mainly for women with heavy bleeding leading to hemodynamic instability. Once the acute episode of bleeding is controlled, the patient can be placed on medical management.
- Endometrial ablation: Used as an alternative to hysterectomy when other medical modalities fail or when there are contraindications to their use. It should **not** be used in women who wish to maintain their reproductive capacity.
- Myomectomy.
- Hysterectomy: Reserved for women with other indications for hysterectomy, such as leiomyomas or uterine prolapse. Hysterectomy should be used to treat persistent ovulatory DUB **only** after all medical therapy has failed.

POSTMENOPAUSAL BLEEDING (PMB)

A 55-year-old female with LMP 5 years ago presents with a chief complaint of vaginal spotting. She reports painful intercourse and burning in the vagina. Her spotting is not related to sexual activity. She denies any medical conditions and is not on any medications. Pelvic exam reveals a dry vagina with ↓ rugae. What is the most likely diagnosis for this patient?

Answer: Bleeding due to atrophy is the most common cause for postmenopausal bleeding.

Postmenopausal bleeding is defined as bleeding that occurs after 1 year of amenorrhea. All vaginal bleeding in postmenopausal women must be evaluated. Postmenopausal bleeding can be due to atrophy or endometrial carcinoma, along with various other causes.

ETIOLOGY

- Vaginal/endometrial atrophy (most common): Hypoestrogenism causes atrophy of the endometrium and vagina. In the uterus, the collapsed, atrophic endometrial surfaces contain little or no fluid to prevent intracavitary friction. This results in microerosions of the surface epithelium which is prone to light bleeding or spotting.
- Postmenopausal HRT: Many postmenopausal women who take HRT develop vaginal bleeding; the frequency depends upon the regimen used.
- Endometrial hyperplasia:
  - Endogenous estrogen production from ovarian or adrenal tumors or exogenous estrogen therapy are possible causes.
  - Obese women have high levels of endogenous estrogen due to the conversion of androstenedione to estrone and the aromatization of androgens to estradiol, both of which occur in peripheral adipose tissue.
- Adenomyosis:
  - Confirmed by pathologic examination following hysterectomy.
  - Symptomatic adenomyosis occurs after menopause only in the presence of postmenopausal HRT.
- Post radiation therapy:

Most common cause of postmenopausal bleeding: atrophy of genital tract. Most common lethal cause: endometrial cancer.

HRT for menopausal woman with uterus must contain progestin with estrogen to prevent endometrial hyperplasia / carcinoma.

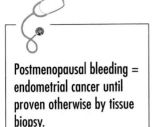

Postmenopausal bleeding = endometrial cancer until proven otherwise by tissue biopsy.

Vaginal bleeding + foul-smelling discharge = cervical cancer.

- A late effect of radiation therapy.
  - Radiation devascularizes tissue, causes sloughing, and bleeding.
  - Vaginal vault necrosis causes uncontrolled bleeding and pain.
- Iatrogenic anticoagulant effect.
- Neoplasia:
  - Endometrial cancer.
  - Cervical cancer. Vaginal bleeding occurs because the cancer outgrows its blood supply. The necrotic and denuded tissue bleeds easily and causes a malodorous discharge.
  - Vulvar cancer.
  - Estrogen-secreting ovarian tumor.
  - Leiomyomata uteri.
  - The diagnosis of a **uterine sarcoma** should be considered in postmenopausal women with rapidly growing leiomyomata.
- Polyps: Endometrial growths of unknown etiology. Growth of polyps can be stimulated by estrogen therapy or tamoxifen. They may be benign, premalignant, or malignant.
- Infection: Uncommon cause of postmenopausal bleeding.
- Trauma.

HISTORY

- Ask the patient about the frequency, duration, and amount of bleeding, and when it started.
- Ask the patient about any associated signs/symptoms like weight loss, fever.
- History of trauma.
- Ask the patient which medications she takes—hormones, anticoagulants, tamoxfien, over the counter, herbal supplements.
- Ask the patient about her past medical history.
- History of bleeding in relation to sexual activity.
- Family history of bleeding, gynecologic cancer, breast cancer.

Differential diagnosis for thickened endometrial stripe in a postmenopausal woman:
- **Endometrial cancer**
- **Endometrial hyperplasia**
- **Leiomyoma**
- **Polyp**

PHYSICAL EXAM

- Note any suspicious lesions, lacerations, discharge, or foreign bodies.
- Classic signs of atrophy include pale, dry vaginal epithelium that has lost its rugae.
- Assess the size, contour, and tenderness of the uterus.

STUDIES

- Vaginal probes and wet mount for infections.
- Pap smear for cervical dysplasia, neoplasia.
- Endometrial biopsy for endometrial hyperplasia or cancer.
- Transvaginal ultrasound to assess endometrial stripe. If endometrial stripe is < 4 mm, endometrial sampling may be deffered unless the patient has persistent bleeding. Rationale is thin lining due to atrophy.
- Diagnostic D&C.
- Hysteroscopy.

Endometrial stripe > 4–5 mm in a patient with PMB should prompt an evaluation.

A 65-year-old overall healthy woman, menopausal for 15 years, presents with vaginal bleeding. She reports 3 days of dark red spotting that has now resolved. An office endometrial biopsy shows endometrial hyperplasia with atypia. What is the best treatment for this patient?

Answer: Hysterectomy with possible staging. Hyperplasia with atypia is thought of as a precursor to endometrial cancer. The cancer may have been missed due to sampling error. The safest procedure for this patient is a hysterectomy, which will allow the pathologist to evaluate the full extent of the uterine disease.

Treatment of postmenopausal bleeding is dependent on the cause:

- Local estrogen cream is used to treat vaginal atrophy and postradiation effect limited to the vaginal region.
- Hysteroscopy, endometrial ablation, or hysterectomy can be offered if symptoms are due to benign lesions like polyps and fibroids.
- Endometrial hyperplasia without atypia can be managed with progestin and ongoing monitoring.
- Endometrial hyperplasia with atypia should be treated as if there is underlying cancer. Small chance that cancer was missed due to sampling error. Hysterectomy is the treatment of choice.
- If carcinoma, consult gynecologic oncology to determine the best treatment (chemotherapy, radiation, or surgery).

Pelvic Pain

> A 35-year-old G2P2, with a history of uterine fibroids, complains of pain lasting 20 minutes, three to four times a week. The pain began 1 year ago. She takes Tylenol for the pain with minimal relief. The exam reveals the uterus to be enlarged, about 16 weeks, in size. She has tenderness directly over the uterus. Her cervix and adnexa are nontender to palpation. Her pregnancy test is negative. What is her most likely diagnosis? What diagnostic test should be ordered? Would you offer the patient surgical or medical treatment?
>
> **Answer:** The most likely diagnosis is fibroid uterus with degeneration. Imaging: pelvic ultrasound. Treatment: nonsteroidal anti-inflammatory drugs (NSAIDs). Medical therapy is instituted first, as conservative management. If pain persists, despite medical therapy, a surgical intervention may be considered.

Pelvic pain accounts for 12% of hysterectomies, 20% of diagnostic laparoscopies, and 40% of repeat office visits.

Mittelschmerz is pelvic pain associated with ovulation. It occurs at the time an egg is released from the ovary.

Chronic pelvic pain — Think of LEAPING pain

Leiomyoma
Endometriosis/Endometritis
Adhesions/Adenomyosis
Pelvic inflammatory disease (PID)
Infections other than PID
Neoplasia
Gastrointestinal

Chronic pelvic pain (CPP) is discomfort in the pelvis lasting for 6 months or longer. The diagnosis and management for the pain is tailored to the organ system involved.

DEFINITION AND CRITERIA

- Pelvic discomfort that is noncyclic and lasts > 6 months.
- Symptoms cause significant distress or impairment in social, occupational, or other important areas of functioning (eg, missed work, homebound, depression, sexual dysfunction).
- Pain that is below the umbilicus, but between the hips.

ETIOLOGIES

- LEAPING:
  - Leiomyoma.
  - Endometriosis/Endometritis.
  - Adhesions/Adenomyosis./Ashermans
  - Pelvic inflammatory disease (PID).
  - Infections other than PID.
  - Neoplasia.
  - Gastrointestinal (inflammatory bowel disease, diverticulosis, or irritable bowel syndrome (IBS).
- Psychological/psychiatric.
- Musculoskeletal.
- Fibromyalgia.
- Urinary tract infection (UTI)/interstitial cystitis.
- Mittelschmerz.

WORKUP

- **Detailed history** (focusing on above etiologies):
  - Temporal pattern: Timing and duration of symptoms.
  - Pain characteristics: Pain may be constant, intermittent, or with monthly menses (cyclic).
  - Associated symptoms/relieving factors: Pain may be associated with positional changes, fever, or nausea/vomiting.
  - Past surgeries: Adhesions form after previous surgeries. Adhesions are fibrous tissue that forms between two internal organs and may be a source of pain.
  - Last menstrual period (LMP) and menstrual history.

- Gastrointestinal (GI) complaints such as nausea, vomiting, diarrhea, or constipation associated with the pain.
- Sexual history: Dyspareunia.
- Social history (marital discourse, depression, stress, history of physical or sexual abuse): Pelvic pain has been known to be associated with psychiatric factors and childhood sexual abuse.
- **Physical exam:** Look for:
  - Masses on abdominal and pelvic exam may suggest an enlarged ovary or a uterine fibroid.
  - Cervical motion tenderness: If present may indicate an infection, such as PID or endometritis. In some cases, may reveal endometriosis.
  - Vulva-tenderness may suggest vulvodynia.
  - Anal tenderness: May suggest hemorrhoids, abscesses, or a fistula.
  - Bladder pain: May suggest interstitial cystitis; anterior vagina may be tender on palpation.
- Mittelschmerz.
- **Labs:**
  - Complete blood count (CBC) with differential: An elevated white blood cell count (WBC) may indicate an infection.
  - Pregnancy test.
  - RPR, if positive then a confirmatory test such as a VDRL or FTA-ABS, HIV, gonorrhea/chlamydia cultures.
  - Urinalysis (UA) and urine culture.
  - Fecal occult blood.
- **Imaging studies:**
  - Pelvic sonogram: Best to evaluate ovarian cyst/neoplasms or uterine fibroids.
  - For further evaluation: Computed tomography (CT)/magnetic resonance imaging (MRI)—best to evaluate for abdominopelvic masses or malignancies.
- **Referrals**
  - Gastroenterology referral for colonoscopy to evaluate for diverticulosis, irritable bowel syndrome, or inflammatory bowel disease.
  - Cystoscopy to evaluate for interstitial cystitis.
  - Psychiatry referral to evaluate for psychosomatic pain and for depression.

> PID is the most common cause of chronic pelvic pain in women less that 30 years old. Endometriosis is the most common cause in women greater than 30 years old.

> Laparoscopy is the final, conclusive step in diagnosing pelvic pain, but it should only be done once psychogenic and gastrointestinal etiologies have been evaluated.

ACUTE PELVIC PAIN

A 22-year-old G0, with an LMP 13 days ago, presents to the ED complaining of right lower quadrant pain in the past 2 days. She reports that Advil is no longer relieving the pain. She is afebrile, with a pulse of 80 and a temperatur of 98.2. Her abdomen is soft, but very tender with rebound and guarding. A pregnancy test is negative. An ultrasound reveals a normal-size left ovary and a 4-cm right ovary, with a small amount of fluid in the cul-de-sac (pouch of Douglas). What is her diagnosis? How will you treat her?

Answer: A ruptured corpus luteal cyst is the diagnosis. She recently ovulated, since her period was 2 weeks ago. She needs surgical treatment. This is acute pain, with signs of an acute abdomen on exam. Since she is hemodynamically stable, she should have a diagnostic laparoscopy to diagnose and treat, instead of a laparotomy.

> **Differential for acute pelvic pain—**
> **A ROPE**
> **A**ppendicitis/**A**bscess/
> **A**bortion
> **R**uptured ovarian cyst
> **O**varian torsion
> **P**ID (tubo-ovarian abscess)
> **E**ctopic pregnancy

Pelvic Pain

Acute pelvic pain is any pain in the pelvic cavity that lasts < 6 months.

ETIOLOGIES

- Gynecologic—may require surgery, if pain is severe:
  - Ruptured ovarian cyst.
  - Adnexal torsion.
  - Tubo-ovarian abscess, PID.
  - Endometriosis.
  - Dysmenorrhea.
- Obstetric:
  - Ectopic pregnancy.
  - Abortion.
- GI/genitourinary (GU):
  - Diverticulitis or diverticulosis.
  - Appendicitis.
  - Inflammatory bowel disease (IBD), or irritable bowel syndrome (IBS).
  - UTI.

WORKUP

- **History:** Include temporal characteristics (cyclic, intermittent, or non-cyclic), location, and severity of pain.
- **Physical exam:** Look for localized/point tenderness, cervical motion tenderness, adnexal tenderness, and abdominal tenderness. The latter three may be signs of PID. Look for signs of an acute abdomen such as guarding, rebound, or severe tenderness.
- **Labs:**
  - Pregnancy test.
  - CBC with differential.
  - UA and culture, if indicated.
  - Cultures (nucleic acid DNA amplification) tests for chlamydia and gonococcus.
- Pelvic sonogram: Look for ovarian cysts/neoplasm, ovarian torsion, an intrauterine/ectopic pregnancy, uterine fibroids, or a tubo-ovarian abscess.

TREATMENT

- Depends on the etiology of the pain.
- Start with conservative management, if not acute, NSAIDs (ie, motrin, naproxen).
- Surgical therapy: Consider if acute pain (signs of an acute abdomen) or if workup of chronic pain persists despite a thorough workup (after eliminating an GI or psychiatric etiology).
- Surgery: May consist of a diagnostic laparoscopy or an exploratory laparotomy.

An elevated WBC may be due to infection (PID or appendicitis), inflammation/necrosis related to adnexal torsion, a degenerating leiomyoma, PID, or appendicitis.

All women of reproductive age, regardless of reported sexual history or contraception, should undergo a pregnancy test during evaluation of abdominal or pelvic pain.

An ovarian ruptured cyst is the most common cause of acute pelvic pain.

A female with new-onset pelvic pain and a negative pregnancy test has an echogenic adnexal mass on ultrasound. What is the diagnosis? A ruptured corpus luteal cyst.

Endometriosis and Adenomyosis

A 32-year-old G0P0 presents to the infertility clinic with a 3-yr history of infertility. She states that her menses began at age 13 and occurs on regular 28-day intervals. She complains of severe monthly pain 1 week before each menses and pain with intercourse. She denies a history of sexually transmitted diseases. Her husband has a child from a previous marriage. On rectovaginal exam, she has uterosacral nodularity and a fixed, retroflexed uterus. What diagnostic test would be the most appropriate at this point to make the diagnosis? What findings would you see on a tissue biopsy?

Answer: The patient has classical symptoms of endometriosis, especially dysmenorrhea and dyspareunia. Endometriosis is a common condition associated with infertility. Laparoscopy is the diagnostic test of choice. The tissue biopsy would show endometrial glands, stroma, and hemosiderin-laden macrophages. Most common site: ovary and pouch of Douglas.

DEFINITION

Ectopic endometrial glands and stroma ectopically growing outside of the uterus, often causing pain and/or infertility.

INCIDENCE

- Ten to fifteen percent of reproductive-aged women.
- Occurs primarily in women in their 20s and 30s. Common in nulliparous woman.
- Accounts for 20% of chronic pelvic pain.
- One-third to one-half of women affected with infertility, have endometriosis.

PATHOPHYSIOLOGY

- The ectopic endometrial tissue is physiologically functional. It responds to hormones and goes through cyclic changes, such as menstrual bleeding.
- The result of this ectopic tissue is "ectopic menses," which causes bleeding, peritoneal inflammation, pain, fibrosis, and, eventually, adhesions.

SITES OF ENDOMETRIOSIS

Common
- Ovary (bilaterally): 60%.
- Peritoneum over uterus.
- Anterior and posterior cul-de-sacs.
- Broad ligaments/fallopian tubes/round ligaments.
- Uterosacral ligaments.
- Bowel.
- Pelvic lymph nodes: 30%.

Endometriosis is the most likely cause of infertility in a menstruating woman over the age of 30, without a history of pelvic inflammatory disease.

A 37-year-old woman complains of hemoptysis during the menstrual period. *Think: Endometriosis of the nasopharynx or lung.*

HIGH-YIELD FACTS

Endometriosis and Adenomyosis

Less Common
- Rectosigmoid: 10–15%.
- Cervix.
- Vagina.
- Bladder.

Rare
- Nasopharynx.
- Lungs.
- Central nervous system (CNS).
- Abdominal wall.
- Abdominal surgical scars or episiotomy scar.
- Arms/legs.

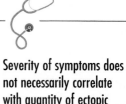

Severity of symptoms does not necessarily correlate with quantity of ectopic endometrial tissue, but may correlate with the depth of penetration of the ectopic tissue.

THEORIES OF ETIOLOGY

Though the mechanisms and etiology are unknown, there are four theories commonly cited. It is likely that multiple theories may explain the diverse nature of this disorder:

- **Retrograde menstruation:** Endometrial tissue fragments are retrogradely transported through the fallopian tubes and implant there or intra-abdominally with a predilection for the ovaries and pelvic peritoneum.
- **Mesothelial (peritoneal) metaplasia:** Under certain conditions, peritoneal tissue develops into functional endometrial tissue, thus responding to hormones.
- **Vascular/lymphatic transport:** Endometrial tissue is transported via blood vessels and lymphatics. This can explain endometriosis in locations outside of the pelvis (ie, lymph nodes, pleural cavity, kidneys).
- **Altered immunity:** There may be deficient or inadequate natural killer (NK) or cell-mediated response. This can explain why some women develop endometriosis, whereas others with similar characteristics do not.
- **Iatrogenic dissemination:** Endometrial glands and stroma can be implanted during a procedure (eg, c-section). Endometriosis can be noted in the anterior abdominal wall.

Long-term complications of endometriosis:
- Prolonged bleeding causes scarring (adhesions).
- Adhesions cause infertility, and small bowel obstruction, pelvic pain, and difficult surgeries.

GENETIC PREDISPOSITION

- A woman with a first-degree relative affected with endometriosis has a 7% chance of being similarly affected as compared with 1% in unrelated persons.
- With a positive family history, a patient may develop endometriosis at an earlier age than the family member.

Congenital anomalies that promote retrograde menstruation may be a common associated finding in adolescents.

CLINICAL PRESENTATION

- Pelvic pain (that is especially worse during menses, but can be chronic):
  - Secondary dysmenorrhea (pain begins up to 48 hr prior to menses).
  - Dyspareunia (painful intercourse) as a result of implants on pouch of Douglas; occurs commonly, with deep penetration.
  - Dyschezia (pain with defecation): Implants on rectosigmoid.
- Infertility.
- Intermenstrual bleeding.
- Cyclic bowel or bladder symptoms (hematuria).
- Up to one-third of women may be asymptomatic.

Chronic pelvic pain may be a result of endometriosis associated with adhesions.

SIGNS

- Fixed retroflexed uterus, with scarring posterior to uterus.
- Tender uterus or presence of adnexal masses.
- "Nodular" uterosacral ligaments or thickening and induration of uterosacral ligaments.
- Ovarian endometriomas: Tender, palpable, and freely mobile implanted masses that occur *within the ovarian capsule* and bleed. This creates a small blood-filled cavity in the ovary, classically known as a "chocolate cyst."
- Blue/brown vaginal implants (rare).

> Classic findings of endometriosis: Dysmenorrhea, dyspareunia, and dyschezia.

DIAGNOSIS

- **Laparoscopy or laparotomy:** Ectopic tissue *must be biopsied for definitive diagnosis.* The gold standard for diagnosis is laparoscopy with biopsy proven hemosiderin laden macrophages. The colors of endometrial implants vary widely:
  - Red implants—new.
  - Brown implants—older.
  - White implants—oldest (scar tissue).
- **Tissue biopsy (cardinal features):** Positive findings contain endometrial glands, stroma, and hemosiderin-laden macrophages.
- Maximum time on estrogen suppression should be 6 months due to adverse effects.

> The classic findings on physical exam are nodularities on the uterosacral ligament and a fixed retroverted uterus.

CLINICAL COURSE

- Thirty-five percent are asymptomatic.
- Symptomatic patients may have increasing pain and possible bowel pain and possible bowel complications.
- Often, there is improvement with pregnancy secondary to temporary cessation of menses.
- May be associated with infertility.

TREATMENT

Medical (temporizing). The primary goal is to induce amenorrhea and cause regression of the endometriotic implants.

- All of these treatments suppress estrogen:
  - Gonadotropin-releasing hormone (GnRH) agonists (leuprolide): Suppress follicle-stimulating hormone (FSH); create a pseudomenopause.
  - Depo-Provera (progesterone [+/– estrogen]): Creates a pseudopregnancy (amenorrhea).
  - Danazol: An androgen derivative that suppresses FSH/luteinizing hormone (LH), thus also causing pseudomenopause.
  - Oral contraceptives (OCPs): Used with mild disease/symptoms.

> The pulsatile fashion of endogenous GnRH stimulates FSH secretion. GnRH agonists cause down regulation of pituitary receptors and supress FSH secretion. This creates a pseudo-menopause state.

Surgical

- Conservative (if reproductivity is to be preserved): Laparoscopic lysis and ablation of adhesions and implants.
- Definitive: Total abdominal hysterectomy and bilateral salpingo-oophorectomy (TAH/BSO).
- A GnRH agonist can be used in conjunction with surgical treatment. It is associated with osteoporosis and should be used for only six months.

A 39-year-old G4P4 comes to the clinic complaining of increasing menorrhagia, dysmenorrhea, and an enlarging uterus. On physical exam, the uterus is 14 weeks in size, boggy, slightly tender, and mobile. What would be the next best step in management?

Answer: Unfortunately there is no proven medical therapy for adenomyosis. GnRH agonists can be used to cause a menopause-like state with complete cessation of ovarian function and menses, causing the abnormal tissue to shrink. NSAIDs and OCPs improve dysmenorrhea and regulate the heavy menses.

Ectopic endometrial tissue does not function like normal uterine endometrium. Thus, it is nonresponsive to hormones in the normal manner as compared to endometriosis.

DEFINITION

Ectopic endometrial glands and stroma are found *within the myometrium*, resulting in a symmetrically enlarged and globular uterus.

INCIDENCE

- Occurs in 30% of women.
- Usually in parous women in their 30s to 50s. Rare in nulliparous women.
- Often coexists with uterine fibroids and to a lesser extent with endometriosis.

Pelvic ultrasounds should be performed to differentiate between adenomyosis and uterine fibroids.

SIGNS AND SYMPTOMS

Common
- **Pelvic pain (usually noncyclical).**
- Symmetrical uterine enlargement.
- Dysmenorrhea that progresses with duration of disease. Dysmenorrhea in adenomyosis doesn't occur as cyclically as it does in endometriosis.
- Menorrhagia: 50% of women are asymptomatic. The diagnosis is usually made incidentally by the pathologist, when examining a surgical specimen.

The diagnosis of adenomyosis is suggested by characteristic clinical manifestations after endometriosis and leiomyomas have been ruled out.

DIAGNOSIS

Either ultrasound or MRI can be used to differentiate between adenomyosis and uterine fibroids.

TREATMENT

- **No proven medical therapy for treatment.**
- GnRH agonist, NSAIDs, and OCPs may be used for pain and bleeding.
- Hysterectomy: Definitive therapy if childbearing is complete. The diagnosis is usually confirmed after histologic examination of the hysterectomy specimen.
- Endometrial ablation will not improve adenomyosis symptoms.

Adenomyosis is described as an enlarged, globular, "boggy" uterus on physical exam.

- **Adenomyosis:**
  - Found in <u>older</u>, <u>multiparous</u> women.
  - Tissue is not as responsive to hormonal stimulation.
  - Noncyclical pain.
- **Endometriosis:**
  - Found in <u>young</u>, <u>nulliparous</u> women.
  - Tissue is responsive to hormonal stimulation.
  - Cyclical pain.

CHAPTER 23

Differential Diagnoses of Pelvic Masses

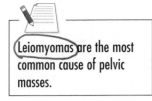

Leiomyomas are the most common cause of pelvic masses.

Pregnancy tests should be done in all women of reproductive age with a pelvic mass on physical exam.

Ovarian masses < 5 cm that are not suspicious for malignancy and asymptomatic are often observed, rather than treated surgically.

Masses in the pelvis may be cystic or solid and can occur at any age. They can originate from the cervix, uterus, or adnexa, or from other organ systems.

DIFFERENTIAL DIAGNOSES

- Physiologic/functional cyst (follicular, corpus luteal, or theca lutein).
- Pregnancy (ectopic pregnancy).
- Infection/inflammation (tubo-ovarian abscess [TOA], diverticular abscess, appendicitis).
- Benign: Fibroid, ovarian neoplasms (most common—cystic teratoma), endometriomas.
- Malignant: Ovaries, fallopian tubes, colon, cervix, metastatic.

DIAGNOSTIC TESTS FOR VARIOUS CAUSES OF PELVIC MASSES

The primary diagnostic tests are: Physical exam, pelvic ultrasound, and a negative pregnancy test.

- **Pregnancy:** Pregnancy test.
- **Ovarian cysts:** Physical exam (+ ultrasound [US] if needed for confirmation).
- **Leiomyoma** (discussed below): Physical exam (+ US, hysteroscopy if needed for confirmation).
- **Ovarian neoplasm** (discussed below): US, computed tomography (CT) scan, CA-125 level, surgical exploration if high level of suspicion due to age, family history.
- **Endometrial neoplasm** (discussed below): Endocervical curettage (ECC), dilation and curettage (D&C).
- **Endometrioma** (discussed below): Laparotomy/laparoscopy.
- **TOA:** History of pelvic inflammatory disease (PID) with a palpable adnexal mass on exam (Figure 23-1).

FUNCTIONAL OVARIAN CYSTS

A 24-year-old G0 with a LMP one week prior, presents to the ED with complaints of sudden severe right-sided pelvic pain. She also complains of feeling "weak" and dizziness. A urine pregnancy test is negative. What should be your next step in management?

Answer: Ultrasound. This patient presents with symptoms common for a ruptured ovarian cyst, which may require surgical intervention.

Follicular Cysts

Follicular cysts are the most common functional ovarian cysts.

PHYSIOLOGY

Failure of rupture or incomplete resorption of the ovarian follicle results in a cyst. Just like the original follicle, the ovarian cyst is granulosa cell lined and contains a clear to yellow estrogen-rich fluid.

FIGURE 23-1. Tubo-ovarian abscess.

Endovaginal sonogram of a patient with pelvic pain, vaginal discharge, and fever. The sonogram demonstrates echogenic fluid (F) in the cul-de-sac and a large cystic mass with internal echoes (arrows) in the left adnexa. This patient was known to have pelvic inflammatory disease and was successfully treated with antibiotics. (Reproduced, with permission, from Callen PW. *Ultrasonography in Obstetrics and Gynecology*, 5th ed. Philadelphia, PA: Saunders; 2007.)

SIGNS AND SYMPTOMS

- Usually asymptomatic when small (< 5 cm). The larger the size, the more pain they cause and the higher the risk of ovarian torsion.
- Polymenorrhea/oligomenorrhea.
- Unilateral abdominal and pelvic pain.
- Acute pelvic pain (ie, rebound and guarding) often signifies rupture of the ovarian cyst.

DIAGNOSIS

- Physical exam: Pelvic and abdominal exams.
- US confirms the diagnosis and is also helpful to see whether the cyst is ruptured. May show an ovarian cyst or fluid in the cul-de-sac, which is consistent with a ruptured cyst.

TREATMENT

- No treatment is necessary for most cysts, since they usually resolve spontaneously within 2 months.
- Oral contraceptives (OCPs) may aid in the resolution of the ovarian cyst, in the symptomatic patient.
- If the cyst is unresolved after 2 months, laparotomy/laparoscopy is indicated to evaluate/rule out neoplasia/endometriosis.
- Chronically symptomatic cysts can be managed with OCPs if no other underlying cause (eg, neoplasia) is found.

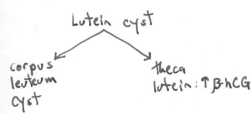

Lutein cyst
corpus leuteum cyst
theca lutein : ↑ β-hCG

- Surgical resection can be considered for symptomatic cysts ≥ 5 cm or for clinical evidence of acute pain, most likely secondary to an ovarian cyst rupture.
- Large ovarian cysts (> 5 cm) increase the risk of ovarian torsion, which is a medical emergency.

Lutein Cysts

There are two types of lutein cysts: **corpus luteum cysts** and **theca lutein cysts.**

CORPUS LUTEUM CYST

- The corpus luteum is enlarged and can produce progesterone for weeks longer than normal, and may delay menses.
- **Corpus hemorrhagicum** is formed when there is hemorrhage into a corpus luteum cyst.
- If this ruptures, the patient will present with acute lower-quadrant pain and vaginal bleeding and may develop signs of shock and hemoperitoneum.
- These cysts rarely grow > 5 cm.

SIGNS AND SYMPTOMS

- Unilateral adnexal tenderness and pain.
- Poly/oligomenorrhea.

DIAGNOSIS

History and pelvic exam, US.

TREATMENT

- Observe for 2 months. Can start OCPs.
- If symptomatic: Analgesics, OCPs, laparotomy/laparoscopy if ruptured, with an acute abdomen.

THECA LUTEIN CYST

↑ levels of human chorionic gonadotropin (hCG) can cause **follicular overstimulation** and lead to theca lutein cysts, which are often multiple and bilateral.

TUBO-OVARIAN ABSCESS (TOA)

An abscess involving the ovary and fallopian tube that most often arises as a consequence of pelvic inflammatory disease (PID).

PHYSIOLOGY

- Primary TOA may arise as a complication of an ascending infection of the reproductive tract.
- Secondary TOA may develop as a result of bowel perforation (appendicitis, diverticulitis) from intraperitoneal spread of infection.
- TOA can also develop in association with pelvic surgery or malignancy.

HIGH-YIELD FACTS

Differential Diagnoses

SIGNS AND SYMPTOMS

- Pelvic and/or abdominal pain.
- Leukocytosis.
- Fever.
- Vaginal discharge.
- Palpable mass.

DIAGNOSIS

- Physical exam: Pelvic and abdominal.
- US confirms the diagnosis and allows the opportunity to assess for other abscesses.

TREATMENT

- Antimicrobial therapy.
- Laparoscopic or US-guided drainage if no response to antibiotics.

TOA are different from other abscesses in that they respond quickly to antibiotic treatment.

ENDOMETRIOMAS

Endometriomas arise as a result of ectopic endometrial tissue in the ovary. They are commonly referred to as "chocolate cysts" due to the thick, brown, tarlike fluid that they contain.

PHYSIOLOGY

Endometriomas arise in women who have endometriosis. Endometriosis is a condition in which endometrial glands and stroma occur outside the uterine cavity and are located on the ovary.

An endometrioma = chocolate cyst.

SIGNS AND SYMPTOMS

- Pelvic pain
- Dysmenorrhea
- Dyspareunia

DIAGNOSIS

- Clinical diagnosis can be made in women with a history of endometriosis, pelvic pain, and an ovarian cyst. As many as 50% of women with endometriosis will develop an endometrioma.
- Definitive diagnosis is made by laparoscopy and a biopsy containing hemosiderin laden macrophages.

TREATMENT

- **Only surgical; medical therapy is not effective treatment for an endometrioma.**
- Conservative surgery (ovarian cystectomy): Entire cyst (endometrioma) can be excised by laparoscopy of laparotomy. Aspiration has proven to be ineffective.
- Definitive surgery (oophorectomy): Alternative to cystectomy. Endometriomas are less likely to recur after oophorectomy, and it is a good option for women who have completed childbearing.

BENIGN CYSTIC TERATOMAS

> A 25-year-old G1P1 presents for an annual well-woman exam. She reports that within the last 3 months, she has had intermittent, dull pain. She is afebrile and on examination, her left ovary palpates to 5-cm with mild tenderness, and the right ovary is normal size and nontender. An ultrasound performed in the office reveals a 5-cm, left hypoechoic unilocular cyst containing calcifications and internal debris. What is the most likely diagnosis? What is the best treatment for this patient?
>
> **Answer:** Diagnosis—benign cystic teratoma. Treatment—laparoscopy with an ovarian cystectomy.

- Benign mature cystic teratomas (dermoid cysts) are the most common ovarian germ cell tumor (OGCT).
- OGCTs arise primarily in young women age 12–30 and account for 70% of tumors in the age group.

PHYSIOLOGY

- Cystic teratomas contain tissue of ectodermal, mesodermal, and endodermal origin. The tissue is mature (benign) and may include skin, bone, teeth, and hair.
- The diverse tissue found within a teratoma is believed to develop from the genetic material in a single oocyte. The tissue is mature (benign) and may include skin, bone, teeth, and hair.
- Oocytes that are able to develop into teratomas undergo an arrest in development after meiosis I.
- Almost all mature cystic teratomas have a 46,XX karyotype.
- Malignant transformation develops in only 1–3% of cases.

DIAGNOSIS

- US is the primary imaging tool used for diagnosis.
- Cystic teratomas can have a consistency ranging from completely cystic to completely solid.

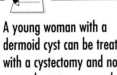

A young woman with a dermoid cyst can be treated with a cystectomy and not an oophorectomy—and the ovary can be preserved.

TREATMENT

- Excision of the teratoma by laparotomy or laparoscopy.
- An ovarian cystectomy is preferred in premenopausal females, < 40 years old.
- If there is no viable ovarian tissue, or if the patient is > 40, then an oophorectomy can be used.

MALIGNANCIES

Malignant ovarian tumors are the leading cause of death from reproductive tract cancer. The lifetime risk of developing ovarian cancer is 1.6%. This risk is ↑ to 5% with one affected first-degree relative.

PATHOLOGY

Origins of the three main types of ovarian tumors:

- Epithelium: Repeated stimulation (ie, ovulation) of the ovarian surface epithelium is hypothesized to result in malignant transformation. These tumors include serous, mucinous, endometrioid, clear cell, and transitional cell.
- Sex-cord stroma: These include granulosa cell, Sertoli cell, Sertoli-Leydig, and steroid.
- Germ cells: These include teratoma, dysgerminoma, yolk-sac, and embryonal choriocarcinoma.

[handwritten margin notes:]
serous
mucinous
endometrioid
clear cell
transitional-cell
granulosa cell
Sertoli-cell
sertoli-Leydig
steroid
teratoma
dysgerminoma
yolk-sac
embryonal choriocarcinoma

RISK FACTORS

- Family history in first-degree relative.
- Age (> 50).
- Nulliparity.
- History of breast cancer.
- Slight ↑ with hormone replacement after menopause.

SIGNS AND SYMPTOMS

- GI symptoms: Abdominal pressure, fullness, swelling, or bloating.
- Urinary urgency.
- Pelvic discomfort or pain.
- Often ovarian neoplasms are **asymptomatic.**

DIAGNOSIS

- An elevated serum CA-125 (> 35 units) indicates an ↑ likelihood that an ovarian tumor is malignant.
- Ultrasound is helpful in distinguishing between masses that are likely to be malignant and benign (see Table 23-1).
- Definitive diagnosis is tissue biopsy.

> Ovarian cancers present with vague GI symptoms (fullness, early satiety, bloating) at a more advanced cancer stage, at the time of the initial diagnosis.

TREATMENT

- Complete surgical staging must be conducted for all women with ovarian cancer.
- In a woman with early-stage ovarian cancer an abdominal hysterectomy with bilateral salpingo-oophorectomy, omentectomy, lymphadenectomy, and peritoneal washings would be performed.
- With more advanced disease, aggressive removal of all visible disease improves survival.
- Ovarian cancer is one of the few cancers in which "surgical debulking" even in the presence of distant metastasis is helpful.

TABLE 23-1. Pelvic Sonographic Findings Suggestive of Malignancy

Solid component of mass, not hyperechoic, nodularity
Multiloculated (fluid trapped in different compartments)
Thick septations (thick walls between compartments)
Presence of ascites
Peritoneal masses, **matted bowels, enlarged nodes**

- Postoperative platinum-based chemotherapy is indicated in all high-grade ovarian cancer.

PROGNOSIS

- Seventy-five percent of women are diagnosed with advanced disease after regional or distant metastases have occurred.
- Overall 5-yr survival:
  - 17% with distant mets.
  - 36% with local spread.
  - 89% with early disease.

CA-125 is elevated in 80% of women with epithelial ovarian cancer overall but in only 50% of women with early disease.

LEIOMYOMAS (FIBROIDS)

A 40-year-old woman presents complaining of heavy menstrual periods that are very painful. Occasionally, she has bleeding in between period. She also complains of pelvic pain and pressure. On exam, the uterus measures 16 weeks in size, irregular, and in the midline. The adnexa are not palpable. What is your next step in management?

Answer: This patient likely has uterine fibroids. A pelvic exam and imaging such as US will help to confirm the diagnosis.

Leiomyomas are most commonly of the subserous type.

Leiomyomas are localized, benign, **smooth muscle tumors** of the uterus, which are hormonally responsive.

EPIDEMIOLOGY

- Clinically found in 25–33% of reproductive-age women and in up to 50% of black women.
- They are almost always multiple.
- The most common indication for hysterectomy.

Rarely do leiomyomas (fibroids) progress to malignancy (leiomyosarcoma).

SEQUELAE

Changes in uterine fibroids over time include:

- Hyaline degeneration.
- Calcification.
- Red degeneration (painful interstitial hemorrhage, often with pregnancy).
- Cystic degeneration—may rupture into adjacent cavities.

A rapidly enlarging myoma = a leiomyosarcoma

UTERINE LOCATIONS OF LEIOMYOMAS

- **Submucous:** Just below endometrium; tend to bleed.
- **Intramural:** Within the uterine wall.
- **Subserous:** Just below the serosa/peritoneum.
- **Cervical:** In the cervix.
- **Parasitic:** The fibroid obtains blood supply from another organ (ie, omentum).
- **Interligamentous:** The fibroid grows laterally into the broad ligament.

Submucosal and intramural types of fibroids usually present as menorrhagia. Subserosal fibroids, which become pedunculated, may present with acute pain and torsion.

SYMPTOMS

- **Asymptomatic** in > 50% of cases.
- **Bleeding** +/– anemia: One-third of cases present with bleeding. Bleeding is usually menorrhagia, caused by:
  - Abnormal blood supply.
  - Pressure ulceration.
  - Abnormal endometrial covering.
- **Pain**: Secondary dysmenorrhea.
- **Pelvic pressure**: May be due to enlarging fibroids.
- **Infertility.**

DIAGNOSIS

- **Physical exam** (bimanual pelvic and abdominal exams): Fibroids are usually <u>midline</u>, enlarged, irregularly shaped, and mobile.
- **Sonography** (may also be visualized by x-ray, magnetic resonance imaging [MRI], CT, hysterosalpingogram [HSG], hysteroscopy.
- Pap, ECC, endometrial biopsy, hysteroscopy, and D&C can be done to rule out malignancy.

TREATMENT

- **No treatment** is indicated for asymptomatic women, as this hormonally sensitive tumor will likely shrink with menopause/pregnancy/not menstruating.
- Pregnancy is usually **uncomplicated**. Some fibroids may grow in size during pregnancy. Bed rest and narcotics are indicated for pain with red degeneration.
- Treatment is usually initiated when:
  - Tumor is > 14 weeks' gestation size.
  - Hematocrit falls.
  - Tumor compresses adjacent structures.
  - Symptoms limit lifestyle.
- Gonadotropin-releasing hormone (GnRH) agonists can be given for up to 6 months to shrink tumors (ie, before surgery) and control bleeding:
  - **Myomectomy**: Surgical removal of the fibroid in infertile patients with no other reason for infertility. A myomectomy is for women who desire to retain their uterus for childbearing.
  - **Hysterectomy**: Indicated for symptomatic women who have completed childbearing.

Pregnancy with fibroids carries ↑ relative risk:
- Abruption: 3.87
- First-trimester bleeding: 1.82
- Dysfunctional labor: 1.85
- Breech: 3.98
- C-section: 6.39

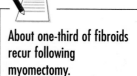

The most common location for a uterine fibroid = subserosal

About one-third of fibroids recur following myomectomy.

The treatment for *asymptomatic* fibroids at <u>11 weeks'</u> size is observation.

Definitive treatment for fibroids = hysterectomy

Cervical Dysplasia

CERVICAL DYSPLASIA

Cervical dysplasia describes abnormal cells of the cervix that can be precursors to cancer. Papanicolaou (Pap) smears are performed regularly to assess for cervical dysplasia. Further workup and treatments include colposcopy, cone biopsy, and the loop electrosurgical excision procedure (LEEP) as well as cryotherapy or laser therapy. Approximately 80% of cervical dysplasia is related to human papillomavirus (HPV) infection, and a new vaccine against this virus can be offered to young women.

Cervical dysplasia and cervical cancer lie on a continuum of conditions. Cervical dysplasia can take one of three paths:

1. Progress to cancer.
2. Remain the same and not progress.
3. Regress to normal.

Squamous cell carcinoma of the cervix is nonexistent in women who have had no sexual contact.

RISK FACTORS FOR CERVICAL DYSPLASIA AND CERVICAL CANCER

- Human papillomavirus (HPV) infection:
  - Eighty percent of cases.
  - Risk highest if infected > 6 months.
  - Types 16, 18, 31, 33, 45—high oncogenic potential.
- ↑ sexual activity (↑ risk of viral/bacterial infections):
  - Multiple sexual partners.
  - Intercourse at early age (< 17 yr).
- Low socioeconomic status.
- Genetic predisposition.
- Cigarette smoking (cocarcinogen substances).
- Alcohol, 2–4 drinks/wk, can ↑ sexual behavior which leads to HPV infection.
- Oral contraceptives (OCPs), particularly with use > 5 yr (condoms ↓ risk in these women).
- Young women whose mothers took diethylstilbestrol (DES) during pregnancy.
- Immunodeficiency.

HPV typical associations:
- Types 6 and 11: Anogenital warts
- Types 16 and 18: Cancer

HUMAN PAPILLOMAVIRUS (HPV)

- HPV is a sexually transmitted infection. Infection can occur through infected intact skin, mucous membranes, or bodily fluids from an infected partner.
- Abstinence, condoms, and decreasing the number of sexual partners can lower the risk of contracting HPV.
- Most HPV infections are subclinical (asymptomatic), but many can manifest by causing cervical abnormalities, such as cervical intraepithelial lesions (I, II, and III).
- There are more than 100 genotypes of HPV.
- HPV types 16 and 18 cause 70% of cervical cancers.

Risk factors for cervical dysplasia—
OSHA Ends Dirt, Garbage, and Chemicals:
Oral contraceptives
Sex
HPV
Alcohol
Education/poverty
Diethylstilbestrol (DES)
Genetics
Cigarettes

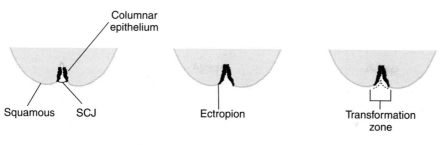

FIGURE 24-1. Sites of cervical cancers.

SQUAMOCOLUMNAR JUNCTION (SCJ)

- Located on the cervix, this is the border between the squamous lining of the vagina and the columnar cells of the uterus.
- Most cervical cancers arise at this site.
- Position is variable (see Figure 24-1).
- In nulliparous women, it is usually located at the external cervical os.
- In pregnancy, it migrates out and is visible to the naked eye.
- The area near the ectocervix where, columnar cells undergo metaplasia and become squamous cells, is referred to as the **transformation zone (TZ).**
- The TZ is the area between the columnar and squamous epithelium.
- The TZ must be biopsied to rule out cancer or precancer.

> Cervical dysplasia almost always occurs at the TZ or SCJ.

PAP SMEAR

> A 21-year-old G2P2 female desires contraception. She has been sexually active for 4 yrs, with three lifetime partners. Her monthly menses are irregular. Before prescribing oral contraceptive pills, what tests need to be performed?
>
> **Answer:** A pregnancy test, then a Pap smear.

> The adolescent cervix is more susceptible to carcinogenic stimuli.

A cytologic **screening test** for cervical neoplasia.

TECHNIQUE

- A speculum is placed in the vagina to expose the uterine cervix (no digital exams or lubricants in the vagina prior to the Pap).
- Cells are scraped from the ectocervix with a spatula, then from the endocervix using an endocervical brush.
- The cells are smeared on a glass slide, fixative spray is applied, and the cells are examined.
- New technique: Cervix is scraped and swabbed as above, but the sample is placed in liquid medium (thin prep).

SUCCESS RATE

- ↓ incidence and mortality rate of invasive cervical cancer by 90%.
- Eighty percent sensitivity.
- Ninety percent specificity.

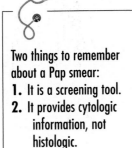

Two things to remember about a Pap smear:
1. It is a screening tool.
2. It provides cytologic information, not histologic.

An abnormal screening test (pap smear) needs a diagnostic test for confirmation (colposcopy, biopsies).

Adolescents should not receive a Pap smear until age 21, regardless of sexual activity.

SCREENING GUIDELINES

According to the American College of Obstetricians and Gynecologists (ACOG) recommendations released December 2009:

- Routine annual screening Pap tests should begin at age 21; women between the ages of 21 and 29 should receive screening Pap tests every 2 yr.
- If three consecutive Pap smears and pelvic exams 1 yr apart are normal in women > 30 yr who have no risk factors, the screening interval can be lengthened to every 3 yr.
- Lengthening of interval is not recommended if the patient or her sexual partner has more than one other sexual partner, or a history of a recent abnormal Pap smear.
- A pelvic examination should be performed yearly.

MICROSCOPIC ANALYSIS

Cytologic analysis of cells taken from a Pap smear will indicate cervical dysplasia if there is:

- Clumping of chromatin.
- ↓ cytoplasm resulting in a higher nucleus-to-cytoplasm ratio.

CLASSIFICATION OF ABNORMALITIES

- Remember, Pap smear gives information about cervical cytology. Two different systems exist that describe the possible findings of a Pap smear:
  1. Modern classification system (cervical intraepithelial neoplasia [CIN]): Describes the degree of abnormality of the cells.
  2. Bethesda staging system (squamous intraepithelial lesion [SIL]) describes three things:
     - The adequacy of the Pap test performed.
     - The degree of abnormality.
     - A description of the cells.
- Table 24-1 correlates the Bethesda staging with the CIN staging. All the terms are possible results of a Pap smear.

FINDINGS AND WORKUP

- **Atypical squamous cells of undetermined significance (ASCUS):** Three options:
  1. Repeat Pap every 6 months until two consecutive negative smears.
  2. Perform colposcopy.
  3. Perform HPV testing. If positive, will need to proceed with colposcopy.
- **Atypical squamous cells, cannot exclude high-grade squamous intraepithelial lesion (ASC-H):** Colposcopy with indicated biopsy.
- **Atypical glandular cells of undetermined significance (AGUS):** Colposcopy and endometrial sampling + endocervical curettage (ECC).
- **Low-grade squamous intraepithelial lesion (LGSIL):** Colposcopy with (ECC) and biopsies.
- **High-grade squamous intraepithelial lesion (HGSIL):** Colposcopy with ECC and biopsies. If there is a discrepancy between the cytology and the biopsy, then an excisional procedure should be performed (LEEP-loop electrosurgical excision procedure or cold knife conization-CKC).
- Very complex, many algorithms. Protocols available online at www.asccp.org.

TABLE 24-1. Modern Classification System vs. Bethesda Staging System

	MODERN CLASSIFICATION SYSTEM (CIN)	BETHESDA STAGING
Squamous lesions	Normal	Normal Benign cellular changes
	Atypical cells, possible inflammatory	Reactive cellular changes ASCUS
	CIN I—mild dysplasia: Neoplastic cells confined to lower one-third of epithelium (60% spontaneously regress)	LSIL
	CIN II—moderate dysplasia: Involvement of two-thirds of epithelium (43% regress)	ASC-H HSIL
	CIN III—severe dysplasia (carcinoma in situ): Involvement up to the basement membrane of the epithelium (33% regress, 12% advance to invasive cancer)	HSIL
	Squamous cell carcinoma	Squamous cell carcinoma
Glandular lesions	Atypical glandular cells	AGUS Atypical glandular cells favor neoplastic Endocervical adenocarcinoma in situ Adenocarcinoma

AGUS, atypical glandular cells of undetermined significance; ASC-H, Atypical squamous cells, cannot exclude HSIL; ASCUS, atypical squamous cells of undetermined significance; CIN, cervical intraepithelial neoplasia; HSIL, high-grade squamous intraepithelial lesion; LSIL, low-grade squamous intraepithelial lesion.

FOLLOW-UP

- All treatment methods have a first-time success approaching 95%.
- A Pap smear should be performed every 4–6 months after treatment for at least 12 months.
- If any Pap smear returns abnormal, a coloscopy should be performed.

COLPOSCOPY WITH CERVICAL BIOPSY

A 45-year-old G4P4 African-American female's Pap smear returns with a report of ASCUS. Her Pap smears have always been normal in the past. What is the next best step to evaluate her cancer risk?

Answer: HPV DNA testing. If HPV DNA testing is "positive," indicating the presence of high-risk HPV DNA, then a colposcopy and biopsy should be performed.

Both colposcopy and biopsies are needed for a histologic diagnosis.

On biopsy, 5–17% of cases of ASCUS and 24–94% of ASC-H demonstrate CIN II–III.

DEFINITION

- A procedure that utilizes staining and a low-magnification microscope, mounted on a stand, for the viewing of the cervix, vagina, and vulva.
- Provides illuminated, magnified view, which aids in identifying lesions and biopsying suspicious areas to *obtain histologic diagnosis.*

INDICATIONS FOR A COLPOSCOPY

- Done after any abnormal Pap smear! Except with ASCUS, you have the option of repeating a Pap instead.
    - ASCUS with high-risk HPV subtypes.
    - ASC-H.
    - Atypical glandular cells.
    - LGSIL.
    - HGSIL.

Ninety percent of women with abnormal cytologic findings can be adequately evaluated with colposcopy.

PROCEDURE

1. Speculum is inserted for visualization of the cervix and the Pap smear is repeated.
2. **Acetic acid is applied.** After 30 sec, the acetic acid dehydrates cells and causes precipitation of nucleic proteins in the superficial layers. The neoplastic cells appear whiter because of a higher nucleus/cytoplasm ratio.
3. **Colposcopy:** Then a low-power microscope (colposcope) is used to look for dysplasia. Signs of dysplasia include whiteness and abnormal vessels. The transformation zone must be visualized in its entirety. If the TZ or the entire extent of the lesion is not entirely visualized, then the colposcopy is considered inadequate.
4. **Cervical biopsy:** Neoplastic and dysplastic areas are then biopsied under colposcopic guidance. Contraindications include acute pelvic inflammatory disease (PID) and cervicitis. Pregnancy is **not** a contraindication.
5. **ECC:** A curette is used to scrape the cervical canal to obtain endocervical cells for cytologic examination. An ECC is contraindicated in pregnancy.

What must be completely visualized for adequate colposcopic evaluation?
1. TZ.
2. Extent of lesion in its entirety.

INFORMATION PROVIDED BY COLPOSCOPY AND ECC

If biopsy results or ECC is positive for CIN II or III, then a cone biopsy or a LEEP should be performed for further diagnosis or treatment.

CONE BIOPSY AND LEEP

- **Cold knife cone biopsy:** A procedure performed in the operating room in which a cone-shaped biopsy is removed with a scalpel, including part of the endocervical canal. Requires use of general anesthesia. Done less often now.
- **LEEP:** A procedure performed in an office setting or in an operating room. A small wire loop with an electric current is used to excise the TZ and the endocervix. This is the cone biopsy specimen. Local anesthesia/analgesia is required.

INDICATIONS FOR CONE BIOPSY/LEEP

- Inadequate view of TZ on colposcopy.
- Positive ECC.
- ≥ 2 grade discrepancy between colposcopic biopsy and Pap.

- Treatment for with CIN 1–III, and CIS (carcinoma in situ).
- Treatment for adenocarcinoma-in-situ.
- When cancer cannot be excluded after colposcopy, biopsy, and ECC.

LEEP

LEEP can also be used to diagnose and treat CIN.

GUIDELINES FOR LEEP TREATMENT

- Never treat during pregnancy.
- Never treat without excluding invasive carcinoma.
- When treating, excise entire TZ.
- Always excise keratinizing lesions.

Evaluation of biopsy margins may be difficult with LEEP, because of thermal artifact.

CRYOTHERAPY

An outpatient procedure that uses a probe cooled with nitrous oxide (N_2O to $-70°F$) to ablate lesions.

INDICATIONS

Treatment of LSIL or HSIL only if it is a lesion completely visualized on colposcopic exam.

COMPLICATIONS AND SIDE EFFECTS

- Profuse, watery, vaginal discharge and failure of therapy for HSIL.
- Long-term complications include cervical stenosis and a small ↑ in preterm labor.

LASER THERAPY

- Light amplification by stimulated emission of radiation (LASER): A high-energy photon beam generates heat at impact and vaporizes tissue.
- Causes less tissue destruction of the TZ compared to other methods.
- Very expensive.

INDICATIONS

Excision or ablation of CIN.

PREVENTION OF CERVICAL DYSPLASIA

Gardasil

- Licensed in 2006 by the FDA as the first quadrivalent HPV vaccine.
- Administered as three doses: 0.5 mL intramuscularly given at intervals of 0, 2, and 6 months.
- Contains virus-like particles from four HPV genotypes: 6, 11, 16, and 18.

Cervarix

- Licensed in 2010 by the FDA, as the first bivalent HPV vaccine.
- Administered in three doses: .5 ml intramuscularly given at intervals of 0, 1, and 6 months.
- Contains virus-like particles from two HPV genotypes: 16 and 18.

SUCCESS RATE

Gardasil: Protects against 70% of cervical cancers and 90% of genital warts.
Cervarix: Protects against 75% of cervical cancers caused from types 16 and 18.

INDICATIONS

- Gardasil: Give to females age 9–26 yr; Cervarix: Give to females 10–25 yr.
- Routinely given at age 11–12.
- Pregnancy Class B; not recommended for pregnant women.
- Can be given to breast-feeding women.
- Efficacy for previously exposed individuals has not been established.

SIDE EFFECTS

- Pain
- Redness
- Allergic reaction

FOLLOW-UP

- Routine cervical cancer screening still necessary.
- The need for booster dose at 5 yr has not been established.

> What HPV genotypes are contained in the Gardasil vaccine?
> Answer: Types 6, 11, 16, 18

Cervical Cancer

Cervical cancer is the third most frequent malignancy of the female genital tract. Eighty percent of cervical cancers are squamous cell carcinomas. They are related to human papillomavirus (HPV) infection while adenocarcinomas comprise 20% and can be related to maternal diethylstilbestrol (DES) exposure. Cervical cancer is staged, clinically, not surgically. Treatment depends on the stage of disease. Women diagnosed while pregnant face unique considerations, but overall have similar survival rates as nonpregnant patients.

EPIDEMIOLOGY

AGE AFFECTED

- Peak incidence between ages 45 and 55.
- Fifteen percent of women develop it before age 30.
- Increasing percentage of women diagnosed before age 20 (perhaps due to early screening or changes in sexual patterns).

RACE PREVALENCE

- More prevalent in African-American women and urban Hispanic women than white women.
- African-American mortality rate is two times greater than whites.

SYMPTOMS

Symptoms of cervical cancer become evident when cervical lesions are of moderate size.

> A 50-year-old G3P3 woman feels well, but notices postcoital bleeding and some pain during intercourse. What is the next step?
> **Answer:** Speculum exam with a Pap smear or biopsy if a lesion is visible.

- Early stages:
  - None.
  - Irregular/prolonged vaginal bleeding/pink discharge.
  - Postcoital bleeding (brownish discharge).
- Middle stages:
  - Postvoid bleeding.
  - Dysuria/hematuria.
- Advanced stages:
  - Weight loss, loss of appetite.
  - Bloody, malodorous discharge.
  - Severe pain, due to spread to sacral plexus.
  - Leg swelling (secondary to blockage of lymphatics).

DIFFERENTIAL DIAGNOSIS

- Polyps, nabothian cysts.
- Papillary endocervicitis/papillomas/inflammation.
- Vaginal malignancies.
- Tuberculosis, syphilitic chancres, and granuloma inguinale can also cause cervical lesions.
- Infections.

Squamous Cell Cancer

- Accounts for 80–85% of cervical cancer.
- Associated with HPV infection.

TYPES

- Keratinizing.
- Nonkeratinizing: *Well-demarcated* tumor-stromal borders.
- Small cell carcinoma: small round spindle shape cells with poorly defined tumor borders.

Adenocarcinoma

- Accounts for **10–20%** of all invasive cervical cancers.
- Arises from columnar cells lining the endocervical canal and glands.
- **Early diagnosis is difficult; the false-negative rate with Pap smear is 80%.**
- May be associated with maternal DES exposure.

Mestasis of Cervical Cancer

A. By direct extension:
- Rectal.
- Intra-abdominal.
- Bladder.
- Endometrial.

B. By hematogenous spread:
- Breast.
- Lung.
- Bone.
- Liver.

A 55-year-old G1P1 female presents to clinic with a complaint of postcoital bleeding. The patient's Pap smear and follow-up colposcopy with biopsy confirm a diagnosis of squamous cell cervical carcinoma. What is the next best step in staging this patient's cervical cancer?

Answer: A computed tomography (CT) scan of the abdomen/pelvis and a chest x-ray to evaluate for metastases to lymph nodes. This is done prior to the clinical staging of the cancer.

Clinical staging of cervical cancer is important for prognosis and treatment (see Tables 25-1 and 25-2).

In keratinizing type of cervical cancer, cells create foci of keratinization with cornified "pearls" that can be visible.

Small-cell carcinoma: Small, round, or spindle-shaped cell with *poorly defined* tumor-stromal borders.

Adenocarcinoma of the cervix is relatively resistant to radio- and chemotherapy compared to squamous cell carcinoma.

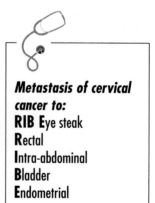

Metastasis of cervical cancer to:
RIB Eye steak
Rectal
Intra-abdominal
Bladder
Endometrial

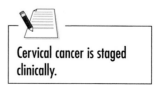

Cervical cancer is staged clinically.

TABLE 25-1. FIGO Staging, Revised 2009

STAGE 0—CARCINOMA IN SITU (CIN3)

STAGE I—CANCER CONFINED TO THE CERVIX ONLY

IA—Invasive cancer identified only microscopically. Gross lesions are stage IB.
  IA1—Invasion of stroma no greater than 3 mm in depth and no wider than 7 mm.
  IA2—Invasion of stroma greater than 3 mm and less than or equal to 5 mm in depth, but no wider than 7 mm.

IB—Clinically visible lesion confined to the cervix or lesions > IA.
  IB1—Lesion confined to cervix uteri ≤ 4 cm.
  IB2—Lesion confined to cervix > 4 cm.

STAGE II—CANCER EXTENDS BEYOND UTERUS, BUT NOT TO THE PELVIC SIDEWALL; INVOLVES THE UPPER VAGINA, BUT NOT THE LOWER THIRD

IIA—No parametrial involvement.
  IIA1—Clinically visible lesion < 4 cm.
  IIA2—Clinically visible lesion > 4 cm.

IIB—Parametrial involvement.

STAGE III—CANCER EXTENDED TO THE PELVIC SIDEWALL; TUMOR INVOLVES THE LOWER THIRD OF THE VAGINA; HYDRONEPHROSIS OR A NONFUNCTIONING KIDNEY

IIIA—No extension to the pelvic sidewall, but involves the lower third of the vagina.

IIIB—Extension to the pelvic sidewall; hydronephrosis or a nonfunctioning kidney.

STAGE IV—CANCER THAT HAS EXTENDED BEYOND THE TRUE PELVIS; INVOLVES EITHER THE MUCOSA OF THE BLADDER OR RECTUM OR BOTH

Stage IVA—Spread of cancer to adjacent pelvic organs (bladder/rectum).

Stage IVB—Spread of cancer to distant organs (outside of pelvis).

HIGH-YIELD FACTS

Cervical Cancer

TABLE 25-2. Grading of Cervical Carcinoma

GRADE	INVASIVE SQUAMOUS TUMOR	ADENOCARCINOMA
X	Cannot be assessed	
1	Well differentiated	▪ Small component of solid growth and nuclear atypia ▪ Mild to moderate
2	Moderately differentiated	Intermediate-grade differentiation
3	Poorly differentiated	▪ Solid pattern ▪ Severe nuclear atypia predominate
4	Undifferentiated	

MODES OF STAGING

- Pelvic and rectal exam (under anesthesia). It is important to palpate and inspect pelvis.
- Colposcopy, ECC, and biopsy.
- Hysteroscopy to evaluate the uterine lining.
- Chest x-ray.
- Liver function tests.
- Evaluate genitourinary tract via cystoscopy, intravenous pyelogram (IVP) or computed tomography (CT) with intravenous contrast dye.
- Evaluate lymph node enlargements or abnormalities with external CT-guided biopsies.
- Proctoscopy.

Radical hysterectomy requires removal of:
- Uterus
- Cervix
- Parametrial tissue
- Upper vagina

TREATMENT OF INVASIVE CERVICAL CANCER

- **Radical surgery:** Radical hysterectomy with lymph node dissection. Done only in patients with low-stage disease (IB–IIA).
- **Radiation therapy:** High-dose delivery to the cervix and vagina, and minimal dosing to the bladder and rectum:
  - External-beam whole pelvic radiation.
  - Transvaginal intracavitary cesium: Transvaginal applicators allow significantly larger doses of radiation to surface of cervix.

How does cervical cancer spread? Direct extension and lymphatic spread. Lymph nodes involved are external, internal, common iliac, and para-aortic nodes.

TREATMENT OF BULKY CENTRAL PELVIC DISEASE

- Radical hysterectomy with adjuvant or neoadjuvant radiation therapy.
- Tumor cytoreduction: Use of cytotoxic chemotherapy before definitive treatment with radiation or radical surgery.

HIGH-YIELD FACTS

Cervical Cancer

FOLLOW-UP OF CERVICAL CARCINOMA

- Patients are examined every 3 months for the first 2 yr, then every 6 months in yr 3–5, and yearly thereafter.
- An exam consists of a history, physical, and Pap.
- A chest x-ray and CT scan of abdomen are performed annually.

RECURRENT CERVICAL CARCINOMA

- Thirty percent of patients treated for cervical cancer will have a recurrence.
- Recurrence of cancer can occur anywhere, but occur mainly in the pelvis (vagina, cervix, or lateral pelvic wall).

SCREENING FOR RECURRENCE

Look for:

- Vaginal bleeding.
- Hematuria/dysuria.
- Constipation/melena.
- Pelvic and leg pain.
- Fistulas (in bladder or bowel).
- Sacral backache or pain in sciatic distribution.
- Costovertebral angle and flank pain.

CAUSE OF DEATH

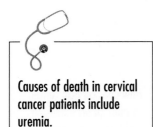

Leg pain following the distribution of the sciatic nerve or unilateral leg swelling is often an indication of pelvic recurrence.

Uremia is the major cause of death in cervical cancer (found in 50% of patients). **Excretory urogram** can identify periureteral compression by tumor.

TREATMENT

- Treatment of cervical cancer by stage:
  - **0–1:** Laser or cryotherapy (endocervix); loop electrosurgical excision procedure (LEEP) or cold knife cone biopsy (ectocervix); total abdominal hysterectomy (TAH; if completed childbearing), conization or cryo (if patient wants to retain uterus).
  - **1a–2a:** Radical hysterectomy or radiation, pelvic lymphadenectomy, para-aortic lymphadenectomy.
  - **2b–4b:** Chemotherapy (cisplatin) and radiation.
- General principles of treatment:
  - Patients may undergo definitive treatment only if disease is confined to pelvis.
  - Patients with local recurrence after radical hysterectomy are treated with **radiation.**
  - Patients previously treated with radiotherapy are treated only by **radical pelvic surgery.**
- Chemotherapy:
  - Response rates are higher with combination therapy.
  - Most combinations include platinum.
  - Response rates: 50–70% for 4–6 months of life.

Causes of death in cervical cancer patients include uremia.

Three percent of all invasive cervical cancers occur during pregnancy.

SYMPTOMS

- One-third of pregnant patients with cervical cancer are asymptomatic.
- Symptoms in pregnancy include vaginal bleeding and discharge.

SCREENING

- Cervical cytology should be performed at the initial obstetric visit (if > 21 years old).
- ASCUS and LGSIL in patients > 21 years old managed as in nonpregnant patient, although colposcopy may be deferred until 6 weeks postpartum.
- Atypical squamous cells with possible high-grade squamous intraepithelial lesion (ASC-H), high-grade squamous intraepithelial lesion (HGSIL), and atypical glandular cells (AGCs) require colposcopy with biopsy (endocervical curettage [ECC] contraindicated).
- If antepartum colposcopy is negative, repeat colposcopy at 6-week postpartum visit.
- Therapeutic conization is contraindicated during pregnancy. Diagnostic conization is reserved for patients in whom an invasive lesion is suspected but cannot be confirmed by biopsy *and* the results will alter the timing or mode of delivery. Otherwise, conization is performed postpartum. Cone biopsy, if necessary, should be performed in the second trimester. Complications are common including hemorrhage and preterm labor.
- Clinical staging unchanged, except magnetic resonance imaging (MRI) should replace CT scans.

TREATMENT

- Definitive treatment is incompatible with pregnancy continuation.
- Therapy should be influenced by **gestational age, tumor stage, and metastatic** evaluation. If the patient chooses to continue the pregnancy, therapy can be postponed until after delivery or the pregnancy can be terminated. A pregnancy can be terminated to begin treatment. Radiation cannot be given during pregnancy, only chemotherapy.
  - In early-stage disease a diagnostic CKC (cold-knife conization) can be done if the patient has a Stage IA1 cancer. If the stage is > Stage IA2, then after delivery, treatment can be instituted.
  - Second-trimester treatments can include platinum-based chemotherapies, which would allow prolongation of pregnancy for fetal maturity. A cold knife conization during pregnancy can lead to severe complications such as hemorrhage and loss of pregnancy.
  - Third-trimester treatments include radical hysterectomy and pelvic lymphadenectomy after high classic cesarean delivery.
  - Delays in treatment have not been reported to ↑ recurrence rates in stage I disease.

What is the basic treatment for *invasive* cervical cancer?
- If confined to cervix: Radical hysterectomy, pelvic lymphadenectomy, para-aortic lymphadenectomy
- If beyond cervix: Chemo and radiation

An ECC (endocervical curretting) is contraindicated in pregnancy.

DELIVERY

- Consideration of possible tumor hemorrhage and size/shape influence delivery method.
- Patients with small-volume stage IA tumors may be candidates for vaginal delivery.
- Episiotomies should be avoided due to case reports of cancer implantation at such sites.
- Patients with > Stage IA1 cancer, require a cesarean section for delivery, and then treatment.

PROGNOSIS

Limited data suggests **no difference** in prognosis of patients with cervical cancer diagnosed in pregnancy compared to nonpregnant patients.

ADENOCARCINOMA OF CERVIX

- Makes up 10–15% of cervical cancers.
- Affects women aged 16–27; median age—19 yr.
- Carcinomas mainly arise from the endocervix; lesions are "endophytic."
- Overall survival rate: 80%.
- Five-year survival rate for stage I disease: > 90%.

Women who took DES during pregnancy have a 1.35% ↑ relative risk of breast cancer.

SCREENING OF DES-EXPOSED WOMEN

- Annual Pap smear.
- Careful palpation of vaginal walls to rule out adenosis or masses.

TREATMENT

- Similar to treatment of squamous cell carcinoma of cervix.
- Preferred treatment is radical hysterectomy and pelvic lymph node dissection for stage IB or IIA.
- Vaginectomy if vagina is involved.

DISEASE RECURRENCE

- Most DES-related clear cell carcinomas recur after ≤ 3 yr of initial treatment.
- Pulmonary and supraclavicular nodal metastasis common; yearly screening chest x-ray recommended.

CHAPTER 26

Endometrial Hyperplasia and Endometrial Cancer

ENDOMETRIAL HYPERPLASIA

A precancerous condition. Types include:

- **Simple (cystic hyperplasia without atypia):**
  - Glandular and stromal proliferation.
  - One percent progress to cancer (most well differentiated).
- **Complex (adenomatous hyperplasia without atypia):**
  - Only glandular proliferation of the endometrium.
  - Three percent progress to cancer.
- **Atypical:**
  - Simple atypical (10% progress to cancer).
  - Complex atypical (29% progress to cancer).
  - Proliferation with **cytologic atypia.**

DIAGNOSIS OF ENDOMETRIAL HYPERPLASIA

- Endometrial **biopsy** (gold standard).
- Pap smear: If endometrial cells are found on a pap suspect endometrial pathology.
- Other procedures might pick it up:
  - Endocervical curettage (ECC).
  - Transvaginal ultrasound to evaluate the endometrial stripe in a postmenopausal woman.
- Hysterocopy with uterine curettage if endometrial biopsy is inadequate.

TREATMENT

- Simple hyperplasia with abnormal bleeding: Cyclical progestin therapy.
- Complex hyperplasia *or* simple atypical hyperplasia: Cyclical or continuous progestin therapy (or hysterectomy if uterine preservation is not desired).
- Complex atypical hyperplasia: Continuous high-dose progestin therapy if uterine preservation is desired; hysterectomy if uterine preservation is not desired.

EPIDEMIOLOGY OF ENDOMETRIAL CANCER

- Endometrial carcinoma is a malignancy arising from the lining of the uterus.
- It is the most common gynecologic malignancy in the United States, and is diagnosed in over 35,000 women annually. It is 1.3 times more common than ovarian cancer and twice as common as cervical cancer.
- Because endometrial cancer usually presents with obvious symptoms, it is most often diagnosed at an early stage.
- Lifetime risk is 3%.
- **Age at diagnosis:**
  - < 40 yr: 5%
  - 40–50 yr: 15%
  - > 50 yr: 80%
- Two types:
  - **Type I (most common):** An estrogen-dependent neoplasm that begins as proliferation of normal tissue. Over time, chronic proliferation becomes hyperplasia (abnormal tissue) and, eventually, neoplasia.
  - **Type II:** Unrelated to estrogen or hyperplasia. Tends to present with higher-grade or more aggressive tumors.

An endometrial thickness of < 5 mm in a postmenopausal woman with vaginal bleeding has a negative predictive value of 99% for endometrial cancer.

Atypical hyperplasia is more likely to progress to cancer in older women compared with younger women.

Women with Lynch syndrome (hereditary nonpolyposis colorectal cancer, or HNPCC) have a 40–60% lifetime risk of developing endometrial cancer, which is equal to their risk of developing colorectal cancer.

Any factor that lowers the level or time of exposure to estrogen ↓ the risk of endometrial cancer.

Side effects of progestins:
Weight gain
Edema
Thrombophlebitis
Headache
Hypertension

A 55-year-old G0P0 woman presents with a 2-month history of intermittent vaginal bleeding. She completed menopause 3 yr ago. She is obese and she has never been pregnant. What is the most likely diagnosis?
Answer: Endometrial cancer.

Endometrial cancer is the most common gynecologic cancer.

- **Abnormal bleeding** is present in 90% of cases:
  - Bleeding in postmenopausal women (classic).
  - Meno/metrorrhagia (in premenopausal cases).
- Abnormal Pap smear: 1–5% of cases. Pap smears are *not* diagnostic, but a finding of abnormal glandular cells of unknown significance (AGCUS) warrants further investigation.

DIFFERENTIAL DIAGNOSIS OF POSTMENOPAUSAL BLEEDING

A 59-year-old G2P2 postmenopausal woman comes in with 2 months of spotting in her underwear. She says that the bleeding is minimal but still requires wearing pads occasionally. She has no pain and still has regular sexual intercourse. She weighs 300 pounds. She is single and has no children. What is the next step?
Answer: Endometrial biopsy. The most likely diagnosis is endometrial cancer. Her risk factors are nulliparity, obesity, and prolonged estrogen exposure.

A postmenopausal woman has bleeding. What is next step? Endometrial biopsy.

DIFFERENTIAL DIAGNOSES

- Exogenous estrogens.
- Atrophic endometritis/vaginitis.
- Endometrial cancer.
- Endometrial/cervical polyps.
- Coagulopathy.
- Endometrial hyperplasia.

RISK FACTORS

- Endogenous unopposed estrogen (ie, polycystic ovarian syndrome [PCOS]).
- Estrogen-producing tumors (ie, granulosa cell tumors).
- Liver disease (a healthy liver metabolizes estrogen).
- Previous radiation (↑ sarcomas).
- Obesity (2–5 times ↑ risk).
- Early menarche/late menopause.
- Nulliparity (2–3 times ↑ risk; most likely when associated with anovulation).
- PCOS (chronic unopposed estrogen stimulation).
- Diabetes mellitus (2.8 times risk).
- Hypertension.
- Endometrial hyperplasia (highest risk is with complex atypia).
- Tamoxifen treatment for breast cancer (2–3 times ↑ risk).

Any factor that raises the level or time of exposure to estrogen increase the risk for endometrial cancer.

- Unopposed estrogen stimulation (eg, menopausal estrogen replacement: 4–8 times ↑ risk).
- Familial predisposition.
- Caucasian race.

PROTECTIVE FACTORS

- Regular ovulation.
- Combined oral contraceptives.
- Cigarette smoking.
- Multiparity.

DIAGNOSIS FOR POSTMENOPAUSAL BLEEDING

- Endometrial biopsy.
- D&C hysteroscopy, if endometrial biopsy, is inadequate.

ADDITIONAL WORKUP FOR ENDOMETRIAL CANCER

After diagnosis of endometrial cancer is made, the following should be performed to evaluate for possible metastasis:

- Physical exam.
- Pathology of the endometrial biopsy of D&C specimen.
- Chest x-ray.
- Complete metabolic panel, cbc, type and screen.
- Abdominal and pelvic computed tomography (CT).

> Hyperplasia without atypia has the lowest risk of progressing to cancer, and hyperplasia with atypia has the highest risk.

Histologic Subtypes

- **Endometrioid** (ciliated adenocarcinoma): 75–80%.
- **Papillary serous:** 5–10%:
  - **Poor prognosis.**
  - No history of elevated estrogen.
  - More common in blacks.
  - Acts like ovarian cancer.
  - Typically presents in late stage (stage IV).
- **Clear cell:** < 5%. Poor prognosis.
- **Sarcomas** (covered below).
- Poorly differentiated carcinomas (Poor prognosis).

STAGING OF ENDOMETRIAL CANCER

> Surgical staging is both diagnostic and therapeutic.

Endometrial cancer is staged surgically.

- The stage of an endometrial cancer is determined by:
  1. The spread of tumor in the uterus.
  2. The degree of myometrial invasion.
  3. The presence of extrauterine tumor spread.
- This assessment is accomplished through a surgical staging operation (similar to ovarian cancer). The staging of a patient's disease directs treatment and predicts outcome (see Table 26-1).

TABLE 26-1. **Staging of Endometrial Cancer FIGO Revised 2009**

STAGE	DESCRIPTION
*I: Tumor confined to the uterus	IA: No or less than half of myometrium
	IB: Invasion equal to or more than half of the myometrium
*II: Tumor invades cervical stroma, but does not extend beyond uterus**	
*III: Local and/or regional spread of the tumor	IIIA: Invasion of uterine serosa and/or adnexa
	IIIB: Invasion of vagina and/or parametrial involvement
	IIIC: Mets to pelvic/para-aortic lymph nodes
	IIIC1: Positive pelvic nodes
	IIIC2: Positive para-aortic lymph nodes with or without positive pelvic lymph nodes
*IV: Tumor invades bladder and/or bowel mucosa, and/or distant mets	IVA: Invasion of bladder and/or bowel mucosa
	IVB: Distant invasion, including intra-abdominal mets and/or inguinal lymph nodes

* Endocervical gland involvement is Stage I.

** Positive peritoneal cytology does not change the stage and is reported separately.

GRADING

Grading is determined by the tumor **histology**:

G1 Well differentiated   < 5% solid pattern
G2 Moderately differentiated 5–50% solid pattern
G3 Poorly differentiated   > 50% solid pattern

TREATMENT

Basic treatment for all stages (surgical staging is always the first step):

- Total abdominal hysterectomy (TAH).
- Bilateral salpingo-oophorectomy (BSO).
- Pelvic and para-aortic lymphadenectomy.
- Peritoneal washings for cytology ("loose or free cancer cells").

Grade is the most important prognostic indicator in endometrial cancer.

Grade 3 tumors usually *do not* have steroid hormone receptors, whereas grade 1 tumors usually do.

HIGH-YIELD FACTS

Endometrial Hyperplasia & Cancer

ADJUVANT THERAPY

After the above steps in treatment, adjuvant therapy depends on the stage.

Stages I–II   Adjuvant radiation therapy (includes internal and external radiation).

Stages III–IV   **External beam radiation**

Hormone therapy: Progestin therapy is often used as adjuvant hormonal therapy:
- If the cancer is progesterone receptor positive—70% have a 5-yr survival.
- If the cancer is progesterone receptor negative—15–20% have a 5-yr survival.

Adjuvant chemotherapy:
- Doxorubicin
- Cisplatin
- Carboplatin and paclitaxel (Taxol)

> **Side effects:**
> - Doxorubicin: Cardiotoxicity
> - Cisplatin: Nephrotoxicity

UTERINE SARCOMA

> A 53-year-old G1P1 postmenopausal woman presents with complaints of vaginal bleeding and pelvic pain. For the past 3 months, she has noticed that her abdomen has enlarged rapidly. What is the most likely diagnosis?
>
> **Answer:** Leiomyosarcoma.

- Uterine sarcoma is classified separately from endometrial cancer:
  - < 5% of uterine malignancies (a rare cancer).
  - Presents as a rapidly enlarging mass with bleeding.
  - < 1% of fibroids progress to cancer.
  - Poor prognosis.
- Risk factors are similar.
- Most cases are diagnosed with exploratory surgery for what was thought to be a uterine myoma (fibroid).

TYPES

A. Homologous (mesenchymal tissue that normally forms in the uterus).
B. Heterologous (foreign tissue to the uterus).

- **Leiomyosarcoma (LMS):**
  - Homologous.
  - One-third of uterine sarcomas.
  - Presents with rapidly growing pelvic mass +/– pain or vaginal bleeding.
- **Endometrial stromal sarcoma (ESS):**
  - Homologous.
  - Ten percent of uterine sarcomas.
  - Low-grade, indolent course.
  - Peak incidence in fifth decade.
  - Tumors contain estrogen and progesterone receptors which are sensitive to hormone therapy.

- **Carcinosarcoma (malignant mixed müllerian tumors):**
  - Heterologous.
  - Usually found in older patients (> 60).
  - Presents with postmenopausal bleeding and large uterus.
- **Undifferentiated sarcomas:** High-grade, aggressive tumors with poor prognosis.

DIAGNOSIS

- \> 10 mitosis/10 high-powered fields with cytologic atypia.
- Usually diagnosed from specimen sent after hysterectomy.
- Staged just like endometrial cancer.

TREATMENT

- Surgical (TAH/BSO, +/– lymphadenectomy, and peritoneal washings).
- Adjuvant therapy (chemotherapy) may decrease recurrence.
- Radiation may enhance local control after surgery. Unknown survival benefit.
- Multiagent chemotherapy is prescribed for metastatic sarcomas. Complete responses are rare.

Ovarian Cancer and Fallopian Tube Cancer

Ovarian cancer is a malignancy arising from the epithelial lining of the ovary or the cells of the ovary itself. As such, the two basic histological types of ovarian cancer are epithelial and nonepithelial. Ovarian cancer is the most deadly gynecologic malignancy because it is most often diagnosed at an advanced stage.

EPIDEMIOLOGY

- Second most common gynecologic malignancy.
- Fifth most common cancer for women.
- The deadliest gynecologic malignancy.
- Seventy percent of patients are diagnosed as stage III or IV.
- Lifetime risk is 1 in 70.
- Median age at diagnosis is 63 yr.

EPITHELIAL CELL OVARIAN CANCER

A 65-year-old G0 white female presents with a 4-month history of increasing waist size and a bloating sensation. She complains of occasional shortness of breath even at rest. She denies vaginal bleeding, nausea, or vomiting. She states that she has never been pregnant, and her pregnancy test today is negative. She doesn't understand why her pants are too small when she seems to be eating less. What is the suspected diagnosis?

Answer: Ovarian cancer. Initial steps in diagnosis: transvaginal ultrasound and CA-125. Definitive diagnosis: biopsy/surgery.

A 61-year-old G2P2 female is diagnosed with ovarian cancer after she presented with abdominal bloating. On pelvic ultrasound she is found to have 6 cm bilateral ovarian masses and ascites. What would the next step be in management?

Answer: Total abdominal hysterectomy (TAH) with bilateral salpingo-oophorectomy (BSO), omentectomy, and then chemotherapy with carboplatinum and paclitaxel. The patient will get serial CA-125 levels on follow-up examinations.

The majority of ovarian cancers are epithelial.

HISTOLOGIC SUBTYPES

Six subtypes arising from epithelial tissue:

- Serous: 50%
- Mucinous: 25%
- Endometrioid: 10%
- Clear cell: 6%
- Brenner: 4%
- Undifferentiated: 5%

Ovarian cancer is the deadliest gynecologic cancer because it is difficult to detect before dissemination. It is the second most common gynecologic cancer.

Seventy percent of cases of ovarian cancer are diagnosed at stage III or IV.

Epithelial cell ovarian cancer accounts for 85% of all ovarian cancers.

Omental caking is a fixed pelvic and upper abdominal mass when associated with ascites. It is pathognomonic for ovarian cancer.

Ovarian cancer typically spreads by exfoliation of cancerous cells into the peritoneal fluid.

CLINICAL REMINDER

- Initial stages are usually asymptomatic. Signs/symptoms are usually from metastasis to other organs.

SIGNS AND SYMPTOMS

- Pelvic mass/pain.
- Abdominal mass ("omental caking").
- Pleural effusion (dyspnea).
- Ascites.
- Ventral hernia (due to ↑ intra-abdominal pressure).
- Early satiety.
- Nausea/vomiting.
- Change in bowel habits.
- Widening of abdominal girth.

RISK FACTORS

- Early menarche, late menopause.
- Nulliparity.
- Late childbearing.
- Advanced age (50–70).
- Family history of ovarian cancer.
- Personal or family history of breast cancer.
- Caucasian race.
- Talcum powder, high-fat diet, fertility drugs (data inconclusive on these).

WORKUP

- CA-125:
  - A tumor marker that is elevated in 80% of cases.
  - It is useful in tracking the progression of the disease and the response to treatment.
  - It may be elevated in many premenopausal medical conditions.
  - It is not effective as a screening tool.

PROTECTIVE FACTORS

- Breast-feeding
- Oral contraceptives
- Multiparity
- Tubal ligation
- Hysterectomy

HEREDITARY OVARIAN CANCER SYNDROMES

Ten to fifteen percent of cases occur in association with genetically predisposed syndromes called **hereditary ovarian cancer (HOC) syndromes.** In these patients, ovarian cancer is diagnosed at a median age of 50 yr. There are three types:

1. **Breast-ovarian cancer syndrome:** Involves cancer of the breast and ovary and is linked to the mutation of BRCA-1 and BRCA-2 genes in 90% of HOC. BRCA is a tumor suppressor gene that is located on chromosome 17.

More than 5 yrs of OCP use ↓ risk of ovarian cancer by 25–50%. This protection lasts 15 yrs after discontinuation.

The serous type of epithelial ovarian cancer is the most common type of ovarian cancer and is bilateral 65% of the time.

Ovarian cancer spread is normally through the peritoneal fluid, which carries cancer cells to other abdominal structures.

Ovarian cancer metastasis to the umbilicus is "Sister Mary Joseph's nodule." This is a palpable nodule.

In a postmenopausal woman with a pelvic mass, CA-125 is much more specific for ovarian cancer compared to a premenopausal woman.

2. **Lynch II syndrome—hereditary nonpolyposis colon cancer (HNPCC):** Involves sites that may include breast, ovaries, uterus, and colon.

3. **Site-specific ovarian cancer:** Accounts for < 1% and has an extremely strong genetic link. Usually, two or more first-degree relatives have the disease.

OVARIAN CANCER WORKUP

- Unfortunately, ovarian cancer is often diagnosed after the disease has spread beyond the ovary (advanced stage).
- As with any pelvic mass, the first step of evaluation is ultrasound.
- Definitive identification of adnexal mass by laparoscopy/laparotomy follows.
- CA-125: Tumor marker for epithelial ovarian cancer (not very sensitive or specific).

SCREENING RECOMMENDATIONS

- Women with **standard risk** (< 2 first-degree relatives with ovarian cancer): No routine screening recommended. A first-degree relative is considered a mother, sister, or daughter.
- Women with **high risk** (> 2 first-degree relatives with ovarian cancer): Genetic testing and counseling.
- If high risk, perform:
  - Annual CA-125 (poor tool for screening).
  - Annual transvaginal ultrasound.
  - Annual pelvic exam.
  - Consider BRCA screening. Consider prophylactic oophorectomy if positive.

STAGING

Ovarian cancer is staged surgically (see Table 27-1). The staging surgery includes:

- Peritoneal washings (for cytology).
- TAH.
- BSO.
- Omentectomy.
- Pelvic and para-aortic lymphadenectomy.

TREATMENT

The purpose of surgery in patients with ovarian cancer is twofold:

1. To accurately stage the patient's disease.
2. To achieve "optimal cytoreduction" of the disease, which means removing all sites of primary or metastatic tumor > 1 cm in size. This kind of debulking surgery has been shown to improve survival in patients with *any* stage ovarian cancer.

Malignant conditions that cause ↑ CA-125:

- Endometrial cancer
- Lung cancer
- Breast cancer
- Pancreatic cancer

Benign conditions that cause ↑ CA-125:

- Endometriosis
- Pelvic inflammatory disease (PID)
- Leiomyoma
- Pregnancy
- Hemorrhagic ovarian cyst
- Liver disease

Large ovarian tumors can cause bowel obstruction and other gastrointestinal symptoms.

Before a staging surgery, a CT scan of the chest/abdomen/pelvis is helpful to evaluate the extent of the disease, including retroperitoneal lymph node enlargement and liver metastases.

Krukenberg tumors are ovarian tumors that are metastatic from another primary cancer, usually from the gastrointestinal tract.

TABLE 27-1. **Staging of Ovarian Cancer (FIGO)**

STAGE	DESCRIPTION
I: Tumor limited to ovaries	IA: One ovary, capsule intact
	IB: Both ovaries, capsules intact
	IC: Tumor on ovary surface, capsule ruptured, ascites with malignant cells, or positive peritoneal washings
II: Pelvic spread	IIA: Involvement of uterus/tubes
	IIB: Involvement of other pelvic structures
	IIC: IIA or IIB plus tumor on ovary surface, capsule ruptures, ascites with malignant cells, or positive peritoneal washings
III: Spread to the abdominal cavity	IIIA: Positive abdominal peritoneal washings (indicates microscopic seeding)
	IIIB: < 2 cm implants on abdominal peritoneal surface
	IIIC: > 2 cm implants on abdominal peritoneal surface and/ or positive retroperitoneal or inguinal nodes
IV: Distant metastasis	Parenchymal liver/spleen spread
	Pleural effusion, skin or supraclavicular nodes

POSTOP MANAGEMENT

- In selected patients, chemotherapy can improve survival and disease-free intervals.
- First-line chemotherapy: Paclitaxel and cisplatin *or* paclitaxel and carboplatin:

POOR PROGNOSTIC INDICATORS

- Short disease-free interval.
- Mucinous or clear cell tumor.
- Multiple disease sites.
- High/rising CA-125.

CA-125 is elevated in 80% of cases of ovarian cancer, but only in 50% of stage I cases. It is most useful as a tool to gauge progression/regression of disease.

NONEPITHELIAL OVARIAN CANCER

Account for 15% of ovarian cancers. Histologic types include:

- **Germ cell tumors:** 8% of all ovarian cancers; include teratomas, dysgerminomas, choriocarcinomas.
- **Sex-cord stromal tumors:** 1% of all ovarian cancers; include granulosa-theca cell tumors, Sertoli-Leydig tumors.

Surgical staging:
Ovarian, endometrial, vulva, and fallopian tube cancers
Clinical staging:
Cervical and vaginal

HIGH-YIELD FACTS

Ovarian & Fallopian Tube Cancer

Ovarian Germ Cell Tumors (GCTs)

Eight percent of ovarian cancers are GCTs. They are the primary cause of ovarian cancer in women < 30 years old. They arise from totipotential germ cells that normally are able to differentiate into the three germ cell tissues. Most are benign.

CLINICAL PRESENTATION

- Abdominal pain with rapidly enlarging palpable pelvic/abdominal mass.
- Acute abdomen.
- Fever.
- Vaginal bleeding.
- Usually found in children or young women.

DYSGERMINOMA

 A 7-year-old girl complains of abdominal pain, and a workup reveals an adnexal mass. She undergoes an exploratory laparotomy and an excisional biopsy. What is the most likely pathology?
Answer: Dysgerminoma.

- **Most common** (45% of malignant germ cell tumors); arises from undifferentiated totipotential germ cells.
- Affects *young* women (< 30 years old).
- Ten percent are bilateral.
- Twenty percent are associated with pregnancy.
- Very chemo and radiation sensitive.
- Lactic dehydrogenase (LDH) is the tumor marker (see Table 27-2).

ENDODERMAL SINUS TUMOR

- Arises from extraembryonic tissues (resembles a yolk sac).
- Ten percent of GCTs.
- Most aggressive GCT.
- Characteristic **Schiller-Duval bodies.**
- α-fetoprotein (AFP) is the tumor marker (see Table 27-2).

TERATOMA

- Contains tissue from ectoderm, mesoderm, and endoderm.
- Contains hair, teeth, skin, sebum, and bone.
- **Immature** (malignant teratoma): Haphazard tissue from the ectoderm, mesoderm, and endoderm.
- **Mature** solid and/or cystic (also called dermoid):
  - Ninety-five percent of teratomas.
  - Benign: Can lead to torsion > 5cm.
- **Struma ovarii:**
  - Benign teratoma.
  - Mostly thyroid tissue.
  - May cause hyperthyroidism.
- **Carcinoid:** Rare.

TABLE 27-2. Ovarian Tumors and Their Serum Markers

Ovarian Tumor	Serum Tumor Marker
Dysgerminoma	LDH
Endodermal sinus tumor	AFP
Embryonal and choriocarcinoma	β-hCG, AFP
Epithelial ovarian tumor	CA-125
Granulosa cell tumor	Inhibin
Sertoli-Leydig cell tumor	Testosterone

Schiller-Duval bodies ← } often a combo

AFP, α-fetoprotein; β-hCG, β-human chorionic gonadotropin, GCT, germ cell tumor; LDH, lactic dehydrogenase.

CHORIOCARCINOMA

- Rare nongestational choriocarcinoma; arises from cytotrophoblasts and syncytiotrophoblasts (extraembryonic tissues).
- Highly malignant.
- Affects women < 20 years old.
- **β-human chorionic gonadotropin (β-hCG)** is the tumor marker.

Know tumor markers cold for the wards.

EMBRYONAL CARCINOMA

- Rare; composed of primitive embryonal cells.
- Affects females age 4–28 yr.
- Tumors may cause **sexual precocity** or abnormal uterine bleeding.
- **β-hCG and AFP are the tumor markers** (see Table 27-2).

MIXED GCTs

- Ten percent of GCTs.
- Dysgerminoma and endodermal sinus tumor is the most common combination.
- **LDH, AFP,** and **β-hCG** may be elevated.

TREATMENT OF MALIGNANT GCTs

- Surgery: **Unilateral** salpingo-oophorectomy and complete surgical staging.
- Adjuvant chemotherapy: Recommended for all malignant GCTs except stage IA, grade I immature teratomas. Stage IA, grade 1 immature teratomas have a high cure rate with surgery alone. The BEP regimen is the standard of care:

Up to 80% survival with complete resection.

BEP Regimen	Side Effects
Bleomycin	Pulmonary fibrosis
Etoposide	Blood dyscrasias
CisPlatin	Nephrotoxicity (extreme nausea and vomiting)

Granulosa cell tumors are very chemosensitive.

PROGNOSIS OF OVARIAN GCTs

Prognosis is generally good because most are discovered *early*. Five-year survival is 85% for dysgerminomas, 75% for immature teratomas, and 65% for endodermal sinus tumors.

Ovarian Sex-Cord Stromal Tumors

- Arise from the sex cords and specialized stroma of the embryonic gonads (before they differentiate into ovaries or testes).
- Some of these tumors are functional tumors and secrete estrogen or testosterone.
- They behave as low-grade malignancies and usually affect older women.

GRANULOSA-THECA CELL TUMOR

- Secretes **estrogens**.
- Can present with **feminization, precocious puberty, menorrhagia,** or **postmenopausal bleeding.**
- Association with endometrial cancer in 5% of cases.
- Characteristic Call-Exner bodies (eosinophilic bodies surrounded by granulosa cells).
- Inhibin is the tumor marker.

SERTOLI-LEYDIG CELL TUMOR

- Secretes **testosterone**.
- Frequently presents with **virilization, hirsutism,** and **menstrual disorders.**
- Testosterone is the tumor marker.

TREATMENT OF OVARIAN SEX-CORD STROMAL TUMORS

- **Surgical:**
  - TAH-BSO in women who have completed childbearing.
  - **Unilateral** salpingo-oophorectomy in young women with low-stage/grade neoplasia.
- **Adjuvant therapy:** Chemotherapy and radiation are not commonly used in patients with stage I disease but is recommended for all patients with stage II–IV disease and those with recurrence.

FALLOPIAN TUBE CARCINOMA

- Fallopian tube carcinomas usually are adenocarcinomas.
- The most common histologic subtype is **papillary serous** (90%).
- They spread through the peritoneal fluid in a similar fashion to ovarian cancer.
- It is a very rare type of cancer that can affect any age.
- **Classic presenting triad:**
  - Pain
  - Vaginal bleeding
  - Watery vaginal discharge

- Many are diagnosed during a laparotomy for other indications.
- **Hydrops tubae perfluens** is the pathognomonic finding, defined as cramping pain relieved with watery discharge.

STAGING, TREATMENT, AND PROGNOSIS

All similar to ovarian cancer.

In any woman with postmenopausal bleeding or a profuse watery discharge, fallopian tube carcinoma should be considered.

CHAPTER 28

Vulvar Dysplasia, Vulvar Cancer, and Vaginal Cancer

Vulvar dysplasia describes precancerous lesions. Dysplasia simply describes cellular changes, characterized by changes in size, shape, hyperchromasia, and presence of mitotic figures.

VULVAR INTRAEPITHELIAL NEOPLASIA (VIN)

- Dysplastic lesions of the vulva that have potential to progress to carcinoma.
- Etiology is unknown, although human papillomavirus (HPV) has been implicated because of similarity in pathology and often concomitant presence of cervical intraepithelial neoplasia (CIN).

RISK FACTORS

- Like cervical cancer, vulvar cancer risk factors include HPV types 16, 18, 31, and 33, and the precancerous lesions are classified as intraepithelial neoplasia (termed VIN as opposed to CIN).
- HPV types 6 and 11 are commonly found in vulvar warts.
- HPV(human papillomavirus).
- History of vulvar skin disease.

PRESENTATION

Pruritus and/or irritation (recent or long-standing), raised white lesions.

- Pruritus and/or irritation (recent or long-standing).
- Raised white lesions.

DIAGNOSIS

- **Biopsy** (most important for diagnosis).
- Colposcopic exam (must include vulva, vaginal, cervix, perineal, and perianal).

STAGING

As in cervical dysplasia, VIN is based on degree of epithelial spread:

- VIN I: Involvement of less than one-half of epithelium.
- VIN II: Involvement of more than one-half of epithelium.
- VIN III: Full-thickness involvement (carcinoma-in-situ).

TREATMENT

VIN lesions are multifocal, thus requiring treatment of many areas. Treatment is according to the size of the lesion:

- Small, well-circumscribed VIN: Wide local excision.
- Multifocal lesions: Laser vaporization.
- Extensive (large) lesions: Skinning vulvectomy.

The most common complaint in vulvar cancer is itching and burning of the vulva.

A precursor to vulvar cancer can be:

- A lump or wart-like lesion
- Lichen sclerosis
- Lichen planus

Gardasil, the vaccine for HPV, protects against strains 6, 11, 16, and 18. Lower-numbered strains generally cause condylomas, whereas higher-numbered strains generally cause dysplasia and cancer with time.

HIGH-YIELD FACTS

Vulvar Dysplasia, Vulvar Cancer, and Vaginal Cancer

A 64-year-old G3P3 woman presents with vaginal itching. She has been to her dermatologist and tried numerous topical treatments without relief. She has a 1-cm white lesion on her labia that, upon palpation, begins to bleed. What is the first step in diagnosis? What other findings in her medical and social history might put her at ↑ risk for cancer?

Answer: The first step in diagnosis is biopsy! Other findings that might put her at ↑ risk for cancer include age, itching, and bleeding on exam.

- Most often found in women age 60–70.
- Unlike the cervix, the vulva does not have a transformation zone.
- Vulvar intraepithelial lesions are less likely than cervical intraepithelial lesions to become high grade or cancers.
- Vulvar cancer is the fourth most common gynecologic cancer (4–5% of all gynecologic cancers) and can arise as carcinoma of various types:
  - Squamous (90%).
  - Adenocarcinoma (Paget disease, Bartholin's gland).
  - Basal cell carcinoma.
  - Melanoma (4–5%).
  - Metastasis.
  - Sarcoma.
  - Verrucous carcinoma.
- The vulva includes the external genital structures. Vulvar cancers are not common cancers. Most are **squamous cell carcinoma**.

SIGNS AND SYMPTOMS

- Pruritus (most common).
- Ulceration.
- Mass (often exophytic).
- Bleeding.

RISK FACTORS

- Postmenopausal.
- Smoking.
- Immunodeficiency syndromes.
- Other risk factors:
  - Age
  - HPV
  - VIN
  - HIV
  - Vulvar skin disease (dystrophy)
  - Melanoma
  - Atypical moles

DIAGNOSIS

Biopsy of the suspicious lesion.

STAGING

See Table 28-1. Vulvar cancer is surgically staged.

Condyloma acuminata: Genital warts associated with HPV, which have a pearly, and plaque-like or cauliflower appearance. Vs. **Condyloma lata:** Genital warts in secondary syphilis, which are nonpainful, raised, grayish-white lesions.

Remember that a dark-pigmented lesion could be a melanoma, even in the vulvar region.

Most common site of vulvar dysplasia is labia majora.

Pruritus is the most common symptom of vulvar cancer. Always biopsy itchy, white lesions on exam.

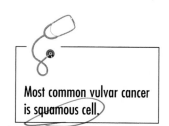
Most common vulvar cancer is squamous cell.

TABLE 28-1. Vulvar Cancer Staging, FIGO Revised 2009

STAGE I: TUMOR CONFINED TO THE VULVA
IA: Lesions < 2 cm in size, confined to the vulva or perineum, stromal invasion < 1.0 mm. No nodal invasion IB: Lesions > 2 cm in size or with stromal invasion > 1.0 mm, confined to the vulva or perineum. No nodal metastasis

STAGE II: TUMOR OF ANY SIZE WITH EXTENSION TO ADJACENT PERINEAL STRUCTURES (¹/₃ LOWER URETHRA, ¹/₃ LOWER VAGINA, ANUS); NEGATIVE NODES

STAGE III: TUMOR OF ANY SIZE WITH OR WITHOUT EXTENSION TO ADJACENT PERINEAL STRUCTURES (¹/₃ LOWER URETHRA, ¹/₃ LOWER VAGINA, ANUS) WITH POSITIVE INGUINO-FEMORAL LYMPH NODES
IIIA: (i) With lymph node metastasis (> 5 mm), or (ii) 1–2 lymph node metastasis(es) (< 5 mm), or IIIB: (i) With 2 or more lymph node metastases (> 5 mm), or (ii) 3 or more lymph node metastases (< 5 mm) IIIC: With positive nodes with extracapsular spread

STAGE IV: TUMOR INVADES OTHER REGIONAL (²/₃ UPPER URETHRA, ²/₃ UPPER VAGINA), OR DISTANT STRUCTURES
IVA : Tumor invades any of the following: (i) upper urethral and/or vaginal mucosa, bladder mucosa, rectal mucosa, or fixed to pelvic bone, or (ii) fixed or ulcerated inguino-femoral lymph nodes IVB: Any distant metastasis including pelvic lymph nodes

Clear cell adenocarcinoma of the vagina often correlates with in utero diethylstilbestrol exposure (DES); these patients often present young.

TREATMENT

- **Stages I–II:** Radical vulvectomy and lymphadenectomy (wide local excision is sometimes possible for certain small lesions < 1 cm).
- **Stages III–IV:** As above, plus removal of affected organs and adjunct radiation therapy.

TABLE 28-2. Staging of Vaginal Cancer

STAGE
I: Limited to vaginal mucosa
II: Beyond mucosa but not involving pelvic wall
III: Pelvic wall involvement
IV: Involvement of bladder, rectum, or distant mets

A 72-year-old G4P4 female presents to the office complaining of a "large ball" on the inside of the vagina. She notices that it bleeds on occasion. What is the next step in managing this patient?
Answer: Biopsy the lesion.

- Primary cancer arises in vagina.
- A rare gynecologic malignancy (2% of gynecologic cancers).
- Usually presents in **postmenopausal women.**
- Increased risk in premenopausal women exposed to DES in utero.
- Most common type is **squamous cell carcinoma** (other types are the same as vulvar cancer types).
- Having CIN or VIN is a risk factor for development of vaginal cancer.

Vulvar cancer: Surgically staged.
Vaginal cancer: Clinically staged.

SIGNS AND SYMPTOMS

- Ulcerated mass
- Exophytic mass
- Abnormal vaginal discharge
- Bleeding
- Asymptomatic
- Pain in advanced cases

DIAGNOSIS

Biopsy of suspicious lesion.

STAGING

See Table 28-2. Vaginal cancer is clinically staged. The stage of tumor is the most important predictor of prognosis.

TREATMENT

- **Stages I–II:** Surgical resection and radiation.
- **Stages III–IV:** Radiation only.

HIGH-YIELD FACTS

Vulvar Dysplasia, Vulvar Cancer, and Vaginal Cancer

Vulvar Disorders

Vulvar disorders encompass a wide range of conditions, from isolated local findings to systemic illnesses. A good understanding of the vulvar anatomy will help to identify these disorders. Vulvar dystrophies are a group of disorders characterized by various pruritic, white lesions of the vulva. Lesions must be biopsied to rule out malignancy.

VULVAR DYSTROPHIES

A 60-year-old G1P1 woman has a history of a raised, silver-colored rash but has new lesions on her vulvar region that are not responding to her previously effective ultraviolet (UV) treatment. She reports that she can't stop scratching them. Examination shows irritated, raised, white lesions. What next step will be most helpful in diagnosing this rash? Is this patient at ↑ risk for malignancy? What microscopic changes contribute to the white appearance?

Answer: The next step in diagnosing this rash is punch biopsy. An ↑ risk of vulvar carcinoma is associated with lichen planus and lichen sclerosus. The white appearance is secondary to lichenification.

Paget Disease of the Vulva

A 65-year-old G3P3 Caucasian woman who has been menopausal for 10 yr comes to her gynecologist for an itchy genital lesion. It has been present for almost 2 yr. On exam, it appears there is a red eczematous lesion on her vulva. She has a 10-yr history of breast cancer. How would you manage this solitary lesion? Is there a risk of recurrence after treatment?

Answer: Biopsy of the lesion reveals Paget disease of the vulva. Solitary lesions need wide local excision down to subcutaneous fat. Paget disease of the vulva is frequently associated with other cancers. Recurrence is fairly common; continue yearly screening.

PRESENTATION

- Pruritic, erythematous, eczematoid lesion.
- Postmenopausal Caucasian females.
- Can be associated with other underlying local invasive carcinomas or adenocarcinoma of the gastrointestinal (GI) tract or breast.

DIAGNOSIS

Direct biopsy of lesion. Will visualize paget cells under the microscope.

TREATMENT

- If solitary lesion without malignancy: Wide excision to subcutaneous fat.
- Recurrences are frequent after treatment.

Patients with Paget disease of the vulva will need to be followed annually with:

- Breast exams.
- Cytologic evaluation of the cervix and vulva.
- Screening for GI disease.

Patients with Paget disease are at increased risk of cancer.

Lichen Simplex Chronicus (LSC)

- LSC is a hypertrophic dystrophy caused by chronic irritation resulting in the raised, white, thickened lesions.
- It is a skin disorder characterized by chronic itching and scratching.
- Lesions may also appear red and irritated due to itching.
- Microscopic examination reveals acanthosis and hyperkeratosis.

Lichen Sclerosus

- An atrophic lesion characterized by paperlike appearance on both sides of the vulva and epidermal contracture leads to loss of vulvar architecture.
- Microscopic examination reveals epithelial thinning with a layer of homogenization below and inflammatory cells (see Figure 29-1). There is also loss of the rete ridges.

Lichen simplex chronicus carries ↑ risk of malignancy.

If an itch-scratch cycle is mentioned choose LSC!

Wickham striae are fine, white, lacy lesions, found in oral lichen planus (commonly on the gingiva).

HIGH-YIELD FACTS

Vulvar Disorders

FIGURE 29-1. Vulvar lichen sclerosus.

Notice the paper-thin appearance, bilateral distribution, and pale color, with a loss of architecture. In severe cases, contractures and fissures can occur in the posterior fourchette. (Reproduced, with permission, from DeCherney AH, Nathan L, Goodwin TM, et al. *Current Diagnosis & Treatment: Obstetrics & Gynecology*, 10th ed. New York: McGraw-Hill, 2007: 617.)

4 P's of lichen planus:
Pruritic
Planar
Purple
Polygonal

Lichen Planus

- An uncommon condition.
- There may be shiny, purple lesions visualized on the vulva.
- A recurrent rash due to inflammation.
- Most lesions are found in the inner vulva and the vagina.
- Skin becomes very thickened (hypertrophied) and may cause scarring.
- May present as vulvo-vaginal-gingival syndrome.

DIAGNOSIS OF VULVAR DYSTROPHIES

Keyes 3- to 5-mm punch biopsy of vulva.

TREATMENT OF VULVAR DYSTROPHIES

- Steroid cream (testosterone, clobetasol/temovate); oral steroids in severe cases.
- Diphenhydramine at night to prevent itching during sleep.
- Ultraviolet light for continued scratching.

PSORIASIS

- A common dermatologic condition characterized by red plaques covered by silver scales.
- Although it commonly occurs over the knees and/or elbows, lesions can be found on the vulva as well.
- Pruritus is variable.

TREATMENT

- Steroid cream—goal is to decrease scratching and rubbing.
- Topical vitamin D.

VESTIBULITIS

- Vulvar pain is a common gynecologic problem.
- Inflammation of the vestibular glands → tenderness, erythema, and pain associated with coitus (insertional dyspareunia and/or postcoital pain).
- Etiology is unknown.
- Although the affected area turns white with acetic acid under colposcopic examination, these lesions are not dysplastic.

DIAGNOSIS

Lightly touch the vulvar vestibule with a cotton-tipped applicator. The diagnosis is made if this touch produces severe pain.

TREATMENT

- Temporary sexual abstinence.
- Trichloroacetic acid.
- Xylocaine jelly for anesthesia.
- Surgery—if lesions are unresponsive to treatment, vestibulectomy is possible, though with risk of recurrence.

Before diagnosing vulvar dystrophy, always rule out more common diagnoses such as a contact dermatitis.

Bartholin's Abscess

A 35-year-old G0 woman calls to make an appointment for a tender nodule she found 3 days ago at the opening of the vagina on the right. She had some discomfort the other night during intercourse but didn't discover anything until yesterday morning. Now she says it's uncomfortable to walk. What is the most likely diagnosis?

Answer: Bartholin's abscess.

- The Bartholin's glands are two pea-sized glands, located at the 5 o'clock and 7 o'clock position.
- A normal gland cannot be palpated.
- Bartholin's abscesses occur when the main duct draining Bartholin's gland is occluded, which usually occurs due to infection.

TREATMENT

- Incision and drainage and marsupialization (suturing the edges of the incised cyst to prevent reocclusion) or
- Ward catheter (a catheter with an inflatable tip left in the gland for 10–14 days to aid healing).
- Inflammatory symptoms generally arise from infection and can be treated with antibiotics.
- Antibiotics and sitz baths may also be prescribed.

Sebaceous Cysts (Epidermoid Cyst)

- The most common vulvar cyst.
- Cysts are mainly asymptomatic.
- Occur beneath the labia majora (rarely minora) when pilosebaceous ducts become occluded.
- Besides the palpable, smooth mass, patients are generally asymptomatic.
- If expressed, yellow, thick, cheesy material is extruded.
- Most cysts do not require any treatment.
- If it becomes infected, it can be treated with incision and drainage.

Hidradenomas

A 30-year-old G3P3 overweight African-American woman presents with painful inflammation of her bikini line. She can't keep her skin dry. On exam, there are draining sinuses and scarring of the skin. What is the diagnosis?

Answer: Hidradenitis suppurativa is most commonly found in intertriginous areas of the body, such as the mons pubis, the genitocrural folds, buttocks, and axillae. Women are four times more likely than men to develop hidradenitis suppurativa.

The vestibular glands (Bartholin's glands) are located at the 5 and 7 o'clock positions of the inferolateral vestibule (area between the labia minora).

Bartholin's abscess tends to develop rapidly over 2–4 days. Symptoms include acute pain, dyspareunia, and pain with walking. They are usually unilateral and can rupture on their own in 5 days. The pain is improved after the cysts ruptures.

Bartholin's glands are analogous to the male Cowper's gland (bulbourethral gland). It secretes a thick, alkaline fluid during coitus.

Bartholin's gland cysts are often asymptomatic, unilateral, 1–8 cm in size, tense, and nonpainful.

HIGH-YIELD FACTS

Vulvar Disorders

> **Subcutaneous involvement surrounding the apocrine glands can evolve into thick, palpable sinus tracts that become draining fistulas.**

- This condition is a chronic infection of the apocrine glands, found in reproductive-age women. A foul smelling discharge may be present on exam.
- Hidradenomas (apocrine sweat gland cysts) also occur beneath the labia majora as a result of ductal occlusion.
- As the infection grows over time, scarring and pits can form.
- These cysts tend to be pruritic.
- Diagnosis is made by biopsy.
- Treatment: Topical steroid creams and long-term, oral antibiotics. Severe cases are also treated by excision of the infected skin.

Other Rare Cysts

- **Cyst of canal of Nuck**: A hydrocele (persistent processus vaginalis); contains peritoneal fluid.
- **Skene's duct cyst:**
  - Very rare and very small.
  - Ductal occlusion and cystic formation of the Skene's (paraurethral) glands occurs, and patients have discomfort.
- Treatment:
  - If asymptomatic, supportive treatment
  - If symptomatic, excision of cyst.

CHAPTER 30

Gestational Trophoblastic Disease

Gestational trophoblastic disease (GTD) is a general term that encompasses a spectrum of interrelated conditions originating from the placenta. In GTD, there is abnormal growth that continues beyond the end of pregnancy. These conditions include complete and partial hydatidiform moles, invasive moles, gestational choriocarcinomas, and placental site trophoblastic tumors.

DNA of complete mole is always a paternal.

DEFINITION

- GTD are entities arising from placental syncytiotrophoblasts and cytotrophoblasts. It refers to a spectrum of abnormalities of the trophoblast associated with pregnancy. They represent an aberrant fertilization event.
- The four tumors are:
    - Hydatidiform mole (complete or partial).
    - Persistent/invasive trophoblastic disease.
    - Choriocarcinoma.
    - Placental site trophoblastic tumor.

HYDATIDIFORM MOLE

Complete Mole

A 22-year-old G1P0 at 12 weeks by dates presents with vaginal bleeding and an enlarged-for-dates uterus on exam. Her blood pressure is 160/90, there are no fetal heart sounds, and an ultrasound shows a snowstorm pattern. After dilation and curettage (D&C), what would most likely be the karyotype?

Answer: 46,XX in a complete mole.

DNA of a partial mole is both maternal and paternal.

A placental (trophoblastic) tumor forms when a maternal ova devoid of deoxyribonucleic acid (DNA) "empty egg" is "fertilized" by the paternal sperm (see Figure 30-1):

FIGURE 30-1. Complete mole on ultrasonography.

KARYOTYPE

- Most have karyotype 46,XX, resulting from sperm penetration and subsequent DNA replication.
- Some have 46,XY, believed to be due to two paternal sperms simultaneously penetrating the ova.
- The BHCG value may be higher as compared to a partial mole.

EPIDEMIOLOGY

Incidence is 1 in 1,500 pregnancies in the United States, 1 in 200 in Mexico, 1 in 125 in Taiwan.

Partial Mole

- A mole with a fetus or fetal parts (see Figure 30-2).
- Women with partial (incomplete) molar pregnancies tend to present later than those with complete moles.

KARYOTYPE

Usually 69,XXY, and contains both maternal and paternal DNA.

EPIDEMIOLOGY

One in 50,000 pregnancies in the United States.

Invasive Mole

- A variant of hydatidiform mole that invades the myometrium or blood vessels.
- It is by definition, malignant trophoblastic disease and can spread to extrauterine sites. Twenty percent of patients will develop malignant sequelae after a complete hydatidiform mole.
- The treatment involves complete metastatic workup and appropriate malignant/metastatic therapy (see below). A D&C is not recommended for treatment, because of the increased risk of uterine perforation. Chemotherapy is the usual treatment.

The treatment for partial and complete molar pregnancy is prompt removal of intrauterine contents with D&C.

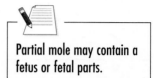

Partial mole may contain a fetus or fetal parts.

A young woman who passes grape-like vesicles from her vagina should be diagnosed with hydatidiform mole.

FIGURE 30-2. Partial mole on ultrasonography.

HISTOLOGY OF HYDATIDIFORM MOLE

- Trophoblastic proliferation.
- Hydropic degeneration (swollen villi).
- Lack/scarcity of blood vessels.

SIGNS AND SYMPTOMS

- The most common symptom is abnormal painless bleeding in the first trimester.
- Passage of villi (vesicles that look like grapes).
- Preeclampsia < 20 weeks.
- Uterus large for gestational age.
- High human chorionic gonadotropin (hCG) level for gestational age.

MEDICAL COMPLICATIONS OF MOLAR PREGNANCY

- Preeclampsia.
- Hyperemesis gravidarum.
- Hyperthyroidism!
- Anemia.
- Pulmonary trophoblastic embolization.

DIAGNOSIS

- Elevated hCG (usually > 100,000 mIU/mL). 15-25% theca lutein cysts visualized (secondary to the high BHCG levels).
- Absence of fetal heartbeat.
- Ultrasound: "Snowstorm" pattern.
- Pathologic specimen: Grapelike vesicles.
- Histologic specimen (see above).

TREATMENT OF COMPLETE OR PARTIAL MOLES

- Dilation and curettage (D&C) to evacuate and terminate pregnancy. Total abdominal hysterectomy (TAH) can be performed in women who have completed childbearing.
- Follow up with the workup to rule out invasive mole (malignancy):
    - Chest x-ray (CXR) to look for lung mets.
    - Liver function tests to look for liver mets.
- hCG monitoring: Weekly until negative for 3 weeks, then monthly until negative for 6 months; yearly for 1–3 yr. If the hCG level rises, does not fall, or falls and then rises again, the molar pregnancy is considered persistent/malignant.
- Contraception should be used during the 1-yr follow-up.
- Administer RhoGAM for RH negative patients.

METASTATIC WORKUP

- CXR, computed tomography (CT) of brain, lung, liver, kidneys.
- Labs: CBC, Comprehensive metabolic panel, clotting studies, and blood type, Rh, and antibody screen.

TREATMENT (FOR NONMETASTATIC MOLAR PREGNANCIES)

- Chemotherapy methotrexate or Actinomycin D (as many cycles as needed until hCG levels return to negative) or
- Total abdominal hysterectomy + chemotherapy (fewer cycles needed).
- Treatment for metastatic molar pregnancy is the same as for choriocarcinoma (see below).

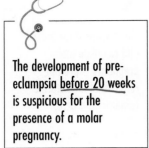

The development of pre-eclampsia before 20 weeks is suspicious for the presence of a molar pregnancy.

GTD secrete hCG, lactogen, and thyrotropin.

Twenty percent of complete moles will be malignant. < 5% of partial moles will be malignant.

Any of the following on exam indicates molar pregnancy:
- Passage of grapelike villi
- Preeclampsia early in pregnancy
- Snowstorm pattern on ultrasound

RECURRENCE RISK

One to two percent in subsequent pregnancy.

TREATMENT (METASTATIC MOLAR PREGNANIES)

Same as choriocarcinoma (see below).

CHORIOCARCINOMA

> A 31-year-old G2P2 woman, 5 months after a vaginal delivery reports to the ED complaining of nausea, vomiting, and abnormal vaginal bleeding. Her pregnancy test is positive. A D&C was performed and the histology revealed sheets of trophoblastic cells and no chorionic villi. What is her diagnosis? What is the next step in management?
>
> **Answer:** Diagnosis is Choriocarcinoma. The workup should be initiated to determine if there is metastatic or nonmetastic choriocarcinoma.

HISTOPATHOLOGY

Choriocarcinoma has characteristic sheets of trophoblasts with extensive hemorrhage and necrosis, and unlike the hydatidiform mole, choriocarcinoma has no villi. These tumors metastasize early. Common sites for metastasis include vagina, lung, liver, and brain.

EPIDEMIOLOGY

Incidence is about 1 in 16,000 pregnancies.

DIAGNOSIS

- Increasing or plateauing β-hCG levels.
- Absence of fetal heartbeat.
- Uterine size/date discrepancy.
- Specimen (sheets of trophoblasts, no chorionic villi).
- A full metastatic workup is required when choriocarcinoma is diagnosed.

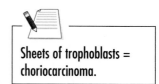

Nonmetastatic malignancy has almost a 100% remission rate following chemotherapy.

Sheets of trophoblasts = choriocarcinoma.

TREATMENT AND PROGNOSIS OF NONMETASTATIC CHORIOCARCINOMA

- Chemotherapy: Methotrexate or Actinomycin D (as many cycles as needed until hCG levels return to negative) or; give 1–2 additional cycles after first negative β-hCG.
- Total abdominal hysterectomy (TAH) + chemotherapy (fewer cycles needed).
- Remission rate is near 100%.

TREATMENT OF METASTATIC CHORIOCARCINOMA, METASTATIC INVASIVE MOLE, OR METASTATIC HYDATIDIFORM MOLE

- Treatment is determined by the patient's risk (high or low) or prognostic score.
- Low-risk patients (score < 7), can be treated with single-agent chemotherapy for 5 days and a hysterectomy.

- High-risk patients (score > 7), can be treated with multiagent chemotherapy, in addition to radiation.
- Chemotherapy is continued until after the hCG levels have negative. hCG levels are monitored for 1 yr after normalization. All patients are placed on reliable contraception during this time of monitoring.
- Serial β-hCG's are every 2 weeks until negative; then every 3 months, then monthly for 1 year. Give 1–2 additional cycles after first negative β-hCG.
- Risk of recurrence: < 1%.

PROGNOSTIC GROUP CLINICAL CLASSIFICATION

See Table 30-1 and Table 30-2.

TABLE 30-1. FIGO Prognostic Scoring System (2000)

RISK FACTOR	SCORE			
	0	**1**	**2**	**4**
Age (yr)	≤ 39	> 39		
Pregnancy	Hydatidiform mole	Abortion	Term	
Interval from pregnancy event to treatment (in months)	< 4	4–6	7–12	> 12
hCG (pre-treatment) (IU/mL)	< 1000	1000-10,000	10,000–100K	> 100K
Largest tumor size uterus (in cm)	3–4	5–6		
Site of metastases	Lung Vagina	Spleen Kidney	GI	Brain Liver
Number of metastasis	0	1–4	4–8	> 8
Prior chemotherapy agent	–	–	Single	Two or more drug agents

Scores are added to give the prognostic score.

TABLE 30-2 Treatment According to Score/Prognostic Factors

Low risk (score < 7)	Single-agent therapy (methotrexate)
High risk (score > 7)	Multiple-agent therapy (EMACO therapy—etoposide, MAC, and vincristine)

PLACENTAL SITE TROPHOBLASTIC TUMOR (PSTT)

- A rare form of GTD.
- Characterized by infiltration of the myometrium by intermediate trophoblasts, which stain positive for human placental lactogen. There are no chorionic villi present.
- Unlike other GTDs, hCG is only slightly elevated.

TREATMENT

- TAH: Prognosis is poor if there is tumor recurrence or metastasis.
- These tumors (most are cured by TAH) are not sensitive to chemotherapy.

CHAPTER 31

Sexually Transmitted Infections and Vaginitis

Each year approximately 1 million women in the United States experience an episode of symptomatic PID. PID affects 10% of women in reproductive years.

Rarely is a single organism responsible for PID, but always think of chlamydia and gonorrhea first (these are most common).

Requirement for a clinical diagnosis of PID:

1. Abdominal tenderness
2. Adnexal tenderness
3. Cervical motion tenderness

Positive lab tests are not necessary for diagnosis. PID is a clinical diagnosis.

Chandelier sign: When you touch the cervix, there is so much pain that the patient jumps to the chandelier.

Sexually transmitted infections (STIs), also known as venereal diseases or sexually transmitted infections, are a major source of morbidity. The group includes bacteria, viruses, parasites, and protozoan infections that are transmitted by close contact. Transmission occurs via mucous membranes of the vulva, vagina, penis, rectum, mouth, throat, respiratory tract, or eyes.

PELVIC INFLAMMATORY DISEASE (PID)

A sexually active 21-year-old G1P1 complains of lower abdominal pain and vaginal discharge for the past 10 days. Additionally, she reports nausea and vomiting. Her temperature is 101.4°F (38.6°C). Examination confirms cervical motion tenderness, uterine tenderness, and bilateral adnexal tenderness. You diagnose her with PID. What treatment should be given?

Answer: Inpatient cefoxitin/cefotetan + doxycycline. Criteria for hospital admission include vomiting and fever. *2nd gen cef + doxy*

DEFINITION

Inflammation of the female upper genital tract (uterus, tubes, ovaries, ligaments) caused by ascending infection from the vagina and cervix.

COMMON CAUSATIVE ORGANISMS

- *Neisseria gonorrhoeae.*
- *Chlamydia trachomatis.*
- *Escherichia coli.*
- *Streptococcus.*
- *Gardnerella vaginalis, Peptostreptococcus,* and *Bacteroides.*

DIAGNOSIS

Physical Exam
- Abdominal tenderness.
- Adnexal tenderness.
- Cervical motion tenderness.
- Oral temperature > 101°F (38.3°C).
- Purulent cervical or vaginal discharge.

Lab Results and Other Possible Exam Signs
- Gram stain of discharge with gram-negative diplococci.
- Presence of abundant white blood cells (WBCs) on microscopy of vaginal secretions.
- Pelvic abscess.
- Elevated WBC count, erythrocyte sedimentation rate (ESR), C-reactive protein (CRP).
- Culture evidence of *N gonorrhoeae* or *C trachomatis.*

Laparoscopy
- Reveals pus draining from the fallopian tubes; collected in the cul-de-sac.
- The "gold standard" for diagnosis, but it is usually employed only in cases unresponsive to medical treatment.
- Ten percent of women with acute PID will develop perihepatic inflammation, known as Fitz-Hugh–Curtis syndrome.

- "Violin string" adhesions can be seen at the liver capsule on laparoscopy with this syndrome.

RISK FACTORS

- Age < 35 years.
- Multiple sexual partners.
- New sex partner(s).
- Unprotected intercourse.
- Concomitant history of STD.
- Presence of intrauterine contraceptive device.
- Nulliparity.

CRITERIA FOR HOSPITALIZATION

- Pregnancy.
- Peritonitis.
- Gastrointestinal (GI) symptoms (nausea, vomiting).
- Abscess (tubo-ovarian or pelvic).
- Uncertain diagnosis.
- Surgical emergency cannot be excluded.
- Outpatient failure within 48 hr or unable to tolerate oral antibiotic treatment.
- Lack of compliance.
- Immunocompromised.
- High fever > 100.9°F (38.3°C).

TREATMENT

- **Inpatient:**
  - Cefoxitin/cefotetan + doxycycline (preferred for chlamydia).
  - Clindamycin + gentamicin (preferred for abscess).
- **Outpatient:**
  - Levofloxacin/ofloxacin + metronidazole.
  - Ceftriaxone/cefoxitin + doxycycline +/– metronidazole.
  - Sexual partners should also be treated empirically.

GONORRHEA

A 19-year-old G2P2 female presents with known exposure to gonorrhea 7 days prior. She reports an ↑ in vaginal discharge for the past day, but denies any other symptoms. On physical exam, you notice minimal vaginal discharge. You obtain a swab for gonorrhea culture. What is the next step?

Answer: Perform the culture and treat the patient empirically. Since she admits to a recent exposure to gonorrhea, there is no need to wait for the culture to come back. In women, asymptomatic infection is common and symptoms may not begin until 7–21 days after infection.

An infection of the urethra, cervix, pharynx, or anal canal, caused by the gram-negative diplococcus, *Neisseria gonorrhoeae*.

Criteria for hospitalization for PID—
GU PAP
GI symptoms
Uncertain diagnosis
Peritonitis
Abscess
Pregnancy

Gonorrhea of the throat is particularly difficult to treat. A swab at 72 hr after starting treatment is necessary; retreat if this swab is positive.

In what media does *Neisseria* gonorrhea grow? Thayer-Martin in CO_2-enriched environment.

Treat gonorrhea in a patient allergic to penicillin with specitinomycin.

There is a 50–90% chance of transmission after one exposure to gonorrhea.

Ten to fifteen percent of women with gonorrhea will progress to PID if untreated.

When treating gonorrhea, empirical treatment of chlamydial coinfection is also given.

Chlamydia is twice as common as gonorrhea.

Fitz-Hugh–Curtis perihepatitis presents as right upper quadrant pain, fever, nausea, and vomiting. It can be caused by gonorrhea or chlamydia.
- ↑ liver function tests
- "Violin string" adhesions visualized on laparoscopy

PRESENTATION

- Asymptomatic.
- **Dysuria.**
- **Endocervicitis.**
- **Vaginal discharge.**
- PID.

DIAGNOSIS

- Culture in Thayer-Martin agar.
- Gonozyme (enzyme immunoassay).
- DNA/polymerase chain reaction (PCR) amplification (gold standard).

TREATMENT

- Ceftriaxone 125 mg IM single dose or
- Cefixime 400 mg PO single dose or
- Ciprofloxacin 500 mg PO single dose or
- Ofloxacin 400 mg PO single dose or
- Levofloxacin 250 mg PO single dose.
- If coinfection with chlamydia is not ruled out:
  - Azithromycin 1 g PO single dose or
  - Doxycycline 100 mg PO bid × 7 days.
- Sexual partners should also be treated.

CHLAMYDIA

A 16-year-old G0P0 female presents with ↑ vaginal discharge 5 days after unprotected sexual intercourse. On physical exam, a mucopurulent cervicitis is noticed. *Chlamydia trachomatis* infection is suspected. What complications are prevented by treating this patient?

Answer: Complications for a *Chlamydia* infection include PID, Fitz-Hugh–Curtis syndrome, Reiter syndrome, trachoma-conjunctivitis, pelvic adhesions, and chronic pelvic pain.

Chlamydia is an infection of the genitourinary (GU) tract, GI tract, conjunctiva, nasopharynx, caused by *Chlamydia trachomatis*, an obligate intracellular bacteria.

PRESENTATION

- There are numerous serotypes of chlamydia.
- Serotypes A–K cause more localized GU manifestations.
- The L serotypes cause a systemic disease (lymphogranuloma venereum).

Serotypes A–K

Serotypes A–K of *C trachomatis* can have the following presentation:

- Asymptomatic.
- **Mucopurulent discharge.**
- **Cervicitis.**
- **Urethritis.**
- PID.

- Trachoma: Conjunctivitis resulting in eyelash hypercurvature and eventual blindness from corneal abrasions.
- Fitz-Hugh–Curtis syndrome.
- Reiter syndrome.

can't see, can't pee, can't climb a tree

Serotypes L1–L3

Serotypes L1–L3 of *C trachomatis* cause **lymphogranuloma venereum.** This is a systemic disease that can present in several forms:

- Primary lesion: Painless papule on genitals.
- Secondary stage: Inguinal lymphadenitis with fever, malaise, and loss of appetite.
- Tertiary stage: Rectovaginal fistulas, rectal strictures.

DIAGNOSIS

Nucleated amplification testing of the cervix (NAAT, PCR).

TREATMENT

- Doxycycline 100 mg bid × 7 days or azithromycin 1 g PO single dose.
- Lymphogranuloma venereum: Doxycycline 100 mg BID × 21 days.

A 22-year-old G1P1 woman has a positive rapid plasma reagin (RPR) with a titer of 1:4. What is the next step in the workup?

Answer: Order a specific serologic test, such as the fluorescent treponemal antibody absorption test (FTA-ABS) or microhemagglutination test for *Treponema pallidum* (MHA-TP). A false-positive RPR can be seen with certain viral infections (Epstein-Barr, hepatitis, varicella, measles), lymphoma, tuberculosis, malaria, endocarditis, connective tissue disease, and pregnancy.

Syphilis is an infection caused by the spirochete *Treponema pallidum*.

PRESENTATION

Syphilis has various stages of manifestation that present in different ways:

- **Primary syphilis: Painless hard chancre** of the vulva, vagina, or cervix (or even anus, tongue, or fingers), usually appearing 1 month after exposure. Spontaneous healing after 1–2 months.
- **Secondary syphilis: Generalized rash** (often macular or papular on the palms and soles of the feet), condyloma lata, mucous patches with lymphadenopathy, fever, malaise, usually **appearing 1–6 months after primary chancre.** Spontaneous regression after about 1 month.
- **Latent syphilis:** Asymptomatic disease with serologic proof of infection. Further classified as **early latent** if syphilis was acquired within the past year or **late latent** if acquired over a year prior.
- **Tertiary syphilis: Presents years later** with granulomas of the skin and bones (gummas), cardiovascular lesions (eg, aortic aneurysms), neurosyphilis (eg, tabes dorsalis, paresis, and meningovascular disease).

Reiter Syndrome
Classic triad of conjunctivitis, urethritis, and reactive arthritis:
Can't see, can't pee, can't climb a tree.

Use azithromycin rather than doxycycline for pregnant women with chlamydia. Doxycyline causes discoloration of the fetal teeth, if used during pregnancy.

Physicians often treat both gonorrhea and chlamydia even if diagnosing only one.

Syphilis is the most likely diagnosis for a woman with painless genital lesions who then later develops hand, foot, and mouth rashes.

DIAGNOSIS

- **Screening: nontreponemal tests** are RPR or Venereal Disease Research Laboratory test (VRDL). These are nonspecific and can give positive results for many conditions.
- **Treponemal tests:** FTA-ABS and MHA-TP are very specific diagnostic tests, performed if RPR/VDRL is positive, for confirmation.
- Visualization of spirochetes on darkfield microscopy is an additional test available.

TREATMENT

- **Benzathine penicillin G** for all stages, though in differing doses.
- Doxycycline.
- Treatment, during pregnancy, is only Benzathine Penicillin G. It crosses the placenta to prevent **congenital syphilis**. If a patient is allergic to penicillin, a desensitization must be done.

GENITAL HERPES

Penicillin G is the best treatment for syphilis.

Screening tests for syphilis:
- RPR
- VDRL

Confirmatory tests for syphilis:
- FTA-ABS
- MHA-TP

A 17-year-old G1P1 female presents to your office complaining of 5 days of vulvar pain and discomfort with urination. On physical exam, she has a large number of symmetrically placed ulcerated lesions on the vulva. What lab tests should be obtained?

Answer: Viral cultures or Tzanck smear to diagnose herpes simplex virus.

- Infection caused by herpes simplex virus type 2 (HSV-2) in 85% of cases, and by type 1 (HSV-1) in 15% of cases.
- HSV is a DNA virus.
- Eighty percent of adults have antibodies to HSV-2, most without history of infection.

PRESENTATION

Patients with herpes can be asymptomatic, but may present with the following:

- **Primary infection:** Malaise, myalgias, fever, vulvar burning, or vulvar pruritus, followed by **multiple painful genital vesicles** with an erythematous base that progress to painful ulcers, usually 1–3 weeks after exposure.
- **Recurrent infection:** Recurrence from viral stores in the sacral ganglia, resulting in a *milder version* of primary infection including vesicles.
- **Nonprimary first episode:** This is defined as **initial infection by HSV-2** in the presence of *preexisting antibodies to HSV-1* or vice versa. The preexisting antibodies to HSV-1 can make the presentation of HSV-2 milder.

COMPLICATIONS

- ↑ risk of cervical cancer
- ↑ risk of neonatal infection

DIAGNOSIS

- Gross examination of vulva for typical lesions.
- Cytologic smear—multinucleated giant cells (Tzanck test).

Pregnancy may give false-positive RPR.

Perform a viral culture on a painful vaginal/vulvar lesion. If the result is positive for genital herpes, treat with an antiviral medication.

Stress, illness, and immune deficiency are some factors that predispose to herpes recurrence.

- Viral cultures of fluid from an unroofed vesicle/ulcer.
- PCR.
- Western blot assay for antibodies against HSV.

TREATMENT

Treatment for HSV is palliative and not curative.

- **Primary outbreak:** Acyclovir 400 mg TID × 7–10 days; valtrex 500 mg BID for 7–10 days.
- **Recurrent infection:** Acyclovir 400 mg TID × 5 days; valtrex 500 mg daily for 7 days.
- **Pregnancy:** Acyclovir 400 mg BID; valtrex 500 mg daily beginning at 36 weeks of pregnancy.
- A vaccine is under development.
- Famciclovir is another antiviral that is dosed less frequently, and can be used in pregnancy.

Always biopsy an undiagnosed suspicious lesion in order to obtain a definitive diagnosis.

HUMAN IMMUNODEFICIENCY VIRUS (HIV) AND ACQUIRED IMMUNE DEFICIENCY SYNDROME (AIDS)

A 30-year-old G3P3 female presents for a follow-up visit after initial STD screening. Her test results include a positive enzyme-linked immunosorbent assay (ELISA) for HIV. What is the next step in the workup?
Answer: Order a Western blot to confirm antibodies against HIV.

Cesarean delivery is indicated for active herpes infection.

HIV is an RNA retrovirus that causes AIDS. The virus infects CD4 lymphocytes and other cells and causes ↓ cellular immunity.

Treatment of AIDS is palliative and not curative.

PRESENTATION

- **Initial infection:** Mononucleosis-like illness occurring weeks to months after exposure—fatigue, weight loss, lymphadenopathy, night sweats. This is followed by a long asymptomatic period lasting months to years.
- **AIDS:** Opportunistic infections, dementia, depression, Kaposi sarcoma, wasting.

RISK FACTORS

- Intravenous drug use.
- Blood transfusions between 1978 and 1985.
- Prostitution.
- Multiple sex partners/unprotected sex.
- Bisexual or homosexual partners.
- Vertical transmission.

DIAGNOSIS

- **ELISA:** Detects antibodies to HIV. It is sensitive but not as specific. This is a screening test.
- **Western blot:** Done for confirmation if ELISA is positive. It is very specific.
- **PCR:** An alternative means of testing if the Western blot is indeterminate. This is a confirmatory test.

- CD4 T-cell counts and plasma HIV-RNA viral load are measured to monitor patient's response to therapy.
- Highly active antiretroviral therapy (HAART) is used. It consists of varying combinations of nucleoside/nucleotide reverse transcriptase inhibitors, nonnucleoside reverse transcriptase inhibitors, and protease inhibitors.

HUMAN PAPILLOMAVIRUS (HPV)

> A 16-year-old G0P0 female presents complaining of painless growths on her vulva. On exam, numerous irregular, colored, raised lesions are noted. What test can help to make a definitive diagnosis?
>
> **Answer:** Condylomata acuminata can be diagnosed on physical exam. Biopsy can be done to confirm.

- Subtypes 6 and 11 are associated with genital warts (**condylomata acuminata**).
- Subtypes 16, 18, 31, and 33 are associated with cervical and penile cancer.

PRESENTATION

Warts of various sizes (sometimes described as cauliflower-like papules) on the external genitalia, perineum, anus, vagina, and cervix.

DIAGNOSIS

- Warts are diagnosed on physical exam. Biopsy can be done for confirmation.
- Cervical dysplasia caused by HPV infection is screened via Pap smear.

TREATMENT

- Condylomata acuminata are treated with cryosurgery, laser ablation, electrocautery, trichloroacetic acid, and aldara cream.
- See Chapter 24 for treatment of cervical dysplasia.

CHANCROID

> A 21-year-old G1P1 female presents with a painful genital ulcer on the vulva. On exam, there is an irregular deep, well-demarcated ulcer with a gray base along with inguinal lymphadenopathy. The culture and gram stain returns as chancroid. What is the causative organism?
>
> **Answer:** *Haemophilus ducreyi*, the diagnosis is confirmed with a culture in a special media, that requires special growth conditions.

PRESENTATION

- Chancroid presents as a soft, papule on external genitalia that becomes a painful ulcer (unlike syphilis, which is hard and painless) with a gray, nonindurated, base, with ragged edges.
- Inguinal lymphadenopathy, or bubo, also is possible.
- Incubation period is 1 week.

ETIOLOGY

Haemophilus ducreyi, a small gram-negative rod.

DIAGNOSIS

Gram stain of ulcer or inguinal node aspirate showing gram-negative rods in chains—"school of fish."

TREATMENT

Ceftriaxone, ciprofloxacin, or azithromycin.

PEDICULOSIS PUBIS (CRABS)

A 26-year-old female presents after unprotected sexual intercourse with intense genital pruritus. You suspect pediculosis pubis. How do you confirm the diagnosis?

Answer: By visualizing the mite *Phthirus pubis,* which has a crablike appearance under microscopy.

PRESENTATION

- Pruritus in the genital area from parasitic saliva.
- Ninety percent are commonly seen in the pubic hair.
- The incubation period is 1 month.

ETIOLOGY

Blood-sucking parasitic crab louse, *Phthirus pubis.* The louse is transmitted by close sexual contact.

DIAGNOSIS

- History of pruritus.
- Visualization of crabs or nits.

TREATMENT

- Pyrethrin, permethrin (Nix) cream, or lindane (Kwell) shampoo.
- Proper cleaning of clothing and bedding is also necessary.
- Lindane is contraindicated in pregnancy.
- Reevaluate after 7 days.

Distinguishing painful ulcerating genital lesions with vesicles:

- **Herpes**: Multiple painful ulcers, base red.
- **Chancroid**: 1–3 painful ulcers, base yellow gray.
- **Syphilis:** 1 painless ulcer, indurated.
- **Lymphogranuloma venereum:** 1 painless ulcer, not indurated. Chlamydia
- **Granuloma inguinale:** Ulcer, rolled, elevated, rough.

Lactobacillus, the normal flora in the vagina, creates an acidic environment that kills most other bacteria. Raising the pH allows other bacteria to survive.

A 25-year-old G2P2 female complains of a large amount of foul-smelling vaginal discharge. On physical exam, you notice a frothy, yellow-green discharge and multiple petechiae on the cervix. The wet mount of the discharge shows motile protozoa. What is the treatment of choice?

Answer: Metronidazole is the treatment of choice for trichomoniasis. In addition to the classic frothy, yellow-green malodorous discharge, petechiae are often seen on the cervix during exam (commonly called *strawberry cervix*).

HIGH-YIELD FACTS

Sexually Transmitted Infections and Vaginitis

TABLE 31-1. Vaginitis

	PHYSIOLOGIC (NORMAL)	BACTERIAL VAGINOSIS	CANDIDIASIS	TRICHOMONIASIS
Clinical complaints	None	**Malodorous discharge**, especially after menses, intercourse	**Pruritus, erythema, edema**, odorless discharge, dyspareunia	**Copious, frothy discharge**, malodorous, pruritus, urethritis
Quality of discharge	**Clear** or **white**, no odor, in vaginal vault	Homogenous **gray** or **white**, thin, sticky, adherent to vaginal walls	**White, "cottage cheese–like,"** adherent to vaginal walls	**Green** to **yellow**, sticky, "bubbly" or "frothy"
pH	3.8–4.2	**> 4.5**	4–4.5	**> 4.5**
Microscopic findings	Epithelial cells Normal bacteria include mostly *Lactobacillus*, with *Streptococcus*, *epidermidis*, *Streptococcus* as well as small amounts of colonic flora	Visualize with saline **Clue cells** (epithelial cells with bacteria attached to their surface) Bacteria include *Gardnerella (Haemophilus)* and/or *Mycoplasma*	In 10% KOH **Budding yeast** and pseudohyphae	In saline **Motile, flagellated, protozoa**
"Whiff" test	Negative (no smell)	**Positive** (fishy smell)	Negative	Positive or negative
Treatment		Oral or topical **metronidazole**; oral or topical **clindamycin**	Oral, topical, or suppository **imidazole** (or other various antifungals)	Oral **metronidazole** (*Note*: Metronidazole has potential disulfiram-like reaction and has a metallic taste)
Treat sexual partners?		Not necessary	Not necessary	**Yes**

DEFINITION

Inflammation of the vagina and cervix, often resulting in ↑ discharge and/or pruritus, and usually caused by an identifiable microbe (see Table 31-1). The only vaginitis that is sexually transmitted is trichomoniasis.

ETIOLOGY

- **Antibiotics:** Destabilize the normal balance of flora.
- **Douche:** Raises the pH.
- **Intercourse:** Raises the pH.
- **Foreign body:** Serves as a focus of infection and/or inflammation.
- There are several common organisms that cause vaginitis: *Gardnerella* (bacterial), *Candida*, and *Trichomonas*. The distinguishing features are described with the following characteristics.
  - **Clinical characteristics.**
  - **Quality of discharge.**
  - **pH:** Secretions applied to test strip of pH paper, reveal pH of discharge.
  - **"Whiff" test:** Combining vaginal secretions with 10% KOH: Amines released will give a fishy odor, indicating a positive test.
  - **Diagnosis** is based on microscopic findings.

If a woman has a strawberry field appearance of the cervix, what is the most likely diagnosis? *Trichomonas* vaginitis.

Clinical diagnosis depends on the examination of the vaginal secretions under the microscope and measurement of the vaginal pH.

The most common complaint of a patient with candidiasis (yeast infection) is itching.

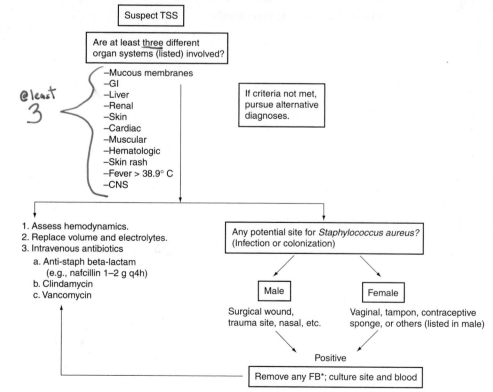

FIGURE 31-1. Toxic shock syndrome (TSS) workup.

(Modified, with permission, from Pearlman MD, Tintinalli JE, eds. *Emergency Care of the Woman.* New York: McGraw-Hill, 1998: 615.)

What is the most common infection with an IUD? *Actinomyces:* sulfa granules, gram positive + rod, (like fungi).

- A rare, acute illness characterized by multiple organ involvement, hypotension, a sunburn rash, and constitutional symptoms.
- Caused by the preformed *Staphylococcus aureus* toxin.
- Not a sexually transmitted infection.
- See Figure 31-1.

Breast Disease

Benign breast disease and breast lumps may be encountered after a physical exam or noted on imaging studies. The following will provide you with a basic guide in the initial evaluation of breast complaints.

BREAST ANATOMY

A 34-year-old G3P3 woman presents with 3 months of pain in her right breast. She reports that her mother had breast cancer at the age of 64, for which she received surgery and chemotherapy. Examination reveals a 2-cm cystic mass to the right of her areola, mobile, somewhat tender. Ultrasound (US) reveals a cystic structure, not complex in nature. Aspiration of the mass yields clear fluid and relieves her pain. The cyst resolves with aspiration. What is your next management step?

Answer: Reassure the patient that the mass is benign in nature. Continue routine clinical breast exams (CBE), annually.

The breasts:
- Large sebaceous glands located in the anterior chest wall; weigh 200–300 grams (in premenopausal yrs).
- Composed of 20% glandular tissue and 80% fat/connective tissue.
- Lymphatic drainage:
  - Drains to regional nodes in axilla and the clavicle.
- Blood supply:
  - Internal thoracic artery
  - Lateral thoracic artery
  - Posterior intercostal artery
  - Thoracoacromial artery

APPROACH TO BREAST COMPLAINTS

- Approach to complaints:
  - Biopsy, and take a history of complaint.
  - Record the location of the breast complaint.
  - Examine each breast systematically for at least 3 min.
  - Age: Document age of the patient—biggest risk factor for development of breast cancer.
  - Screening mammogram: Every 1–2 yr from the age of 40 to 49; after 50, annually.
  - Timing of complaints in relation to menstrual cycle.
- A breast self-examination (SBE) should be encouraged, and a yearly clinical breast examination (CBE), by a health care provider, is recommended. A SBE should begin at 18 years old and a CBE by a health care provider should begin at age 21. It should take 3–5 minutes to perform a CBE, by a health care provider.
- CBE:
  - Inspect for skin changes and breast asymmetry.
  - Exam in supine and sitting position.
  - Use systemic palpation method.
    - Use three middle fingers to palpate the breasts.
    - Apply pressure to the breast with the pads of the fingers.

Screening mammogram should be performed every 1–2 yr beginning at age 40–49, and annually at age 50. CBE should be performed by a health care provider annually.

Rule of 3s:
- 3 minute breast exam
- 3 middle fingers used for breast exam
- 3 palpation pressures during exam (superficial, intermittent, deep)

Two methods to perform a breast exam:
- Concentric pattern (circular)
- Vertical (lawnmower type)

- Flatten the breast against the chest wall during palpation.
- Apply gentle pressure to the nipple to look for a nipple discharge.
- Examine for lymph node enlargement in the axillary and supraclavicular area.

COMMON BREAST COMPLAINTS

Breast Mass

Breast mass workup.
- **History and physical exam:**
- **Imaging (ultrasound/MMG/MRI).**
- **Aspiration for fluid.**
- **Excisional biopsy (if needed).**
- If a patient palpates a breast mass that the clinician does not palpate, imaging studies should be ordered (see Figure 32-1). Re-examine and/or refer to a breast surgeon in 2–3 months if nothing is appreciated on clinical examination. Always report detection of a breast mass by its quadrant location (see Figure 32-1).
- Palpated masses should be aspirated or biopsied. US may help to localize deep masses and assist in aspiration and/or biopsy.
- Over the age of 40, **diagnostic mammogram** should be the initial imaging modality of choice for a breast lump. If a woman is < 40, evaluation of a breast mass should begin with US (ultrasound) the breast tissue is more dense.
- Ultrasound is the initial imaging modality in women < 40 years of age. US helps to differentiate a cystic versus a solid breast mass.
- Aspirate the mass if it is cystic.
- Aspiration:
  - If fluid is cloudy/bloody, → excisional biopsy and imaging.
  - If fluid is clear and resolution of cyst, then monitor.
  - If cyst remains after aspiration, then excisional biopsy.
- A palpable mass not detected on US or mammogram requires surgical referral for biopsy/excision.
- A solid, dominant, persistent mass requires a tissue diagnosis, by aspiration or biopsy.
- A nonpalpable mass, found on an imaging study, requires either following with further imaging or immediate biopsy, depending on how suspicious it appears on the image ("spiculated" masses are very suspicious).
- The **differential diagnoses** of benign breast masses:
  - **Fat necrosis** is usually a result of trauma to the breast with subsequent bleeding into the breast tissue. It is rare but often confused with cancer. The breast may contain a firm, tender, ill-defined mass that requires surgical excision.
  - **Fibroadenoma** is a common lesion seen in patients in the age range of 20–40. They are rubbery, firm, freely mobile, solid, and well circumscribed. Imaging with US can guide biopsy, and if the pathology returns fibroadenoma, it can be followed clinically.
  - **Phylloides tumors** usually occur in older women and are typically larger than fibroadenomas. They should be removed completely.
  - **Fibrocystic breast changes** are a pathologic diagnosis and should not be used to describe clinical findings. The classic symptoms include cyclic bilateral breast pain. The signs include ↑ engorgement, pain,

Examine lymph nodes:
- Supraclavicular
- Infraclavicular
- Medially
- Inferiorly
- Laterally (axillary line)

Suspicious findings (for a cancer) on exam:
- Fixed, hard, irregular mass
- Mass > 2 cm

Suspicious findings (for a cancer) on mammogram:
- Clusters of calcifications.
- ↑ breast density.
- Irregular margins of mass (spiculations).

Risk factors for breast cancer:
- Personal hx of breast cancer.
- Early menarche.
- Nulliparity.
- Alcohol intake.
- Obesity.
- Decreased physical activity.
- Use of prolonged HRT (> 5 yrs) during menopausal years.

and excessive nodularity. These lesions do not place the patient at ↑ risk for cancer but should be completely excised.

- **Atypical hyperplasia** is usually discovered after mammogram-directed biopsy. Complete excision of this mass is warranted, and these lesions ↑ the risk of future breast cancer *anywhere in the breasts* (not just at the site of the lesion).

Nipple Discharge

- This complaint may represent either **benign** or **malignant** breast disease.
- Bilateral milky discharge from multiple ducts is **galactorrhea** and may be normal, although it can be associated with hypothyroidism, prolactin-producing tumor, or medications.
  - Medications that can cause a nipple discharge include antipsychotics, antidepressants, gastrointestinal drugs, and some antihypertensives.
  - If galactorrhea persists more than 6 months from the time of breast-feeding, thyroid function tests and prolactin level are warranted.
- Nipple discharge that is spontaneous and bloody, from a single duct, persistent, and stains the clothes is more likely to be an **intraductal carcinoma or papilloma**—requires investigation with imaging and biopsy.
- Imaging begins with mammogram and US. Surgery referral for abnormal findings.
- **Differential diagnoses,** in addition to cancer, include the following:
  - **Intraductal papillomas**
  - **Duct ectasia**
  - **Galactorrhea**

Breast Pain

- History and physical exam, noting the cyclicity and duration of the pain. Inquire about menstrual history, hormone use, dietary habits (caffeine, tea, sodas, chocolate), and the presences of breast implants trauma.
  - **Cyclical** pain is bilateral in nature. Pain is ↑ during the luteal phase dissipating with menses onset. Fibrocystic breast changes and cyclical mastalgia may require more than just reassurance if the exam is negative.
  - **Noncyclical** pain is more likely unilateral, in the following instances: Large breasts, ductal ectasia, inflammatory breast cancer, pregnancy, and some medications.
- If clinical exam is negative and the pain is cyclical, reassurance is reasonable.
- If negative for masses, reassure patient.
- If positive for masses, order imaging studies.
- **Treatment** may consist of reducing intake of caffeine, treatment with nonsteriodal anti-inflammatory drugs (NSAIDs), acetaminophen, and a "support" bra.

Risk factors for hereditary breast cancer:
- Ashkenazi Jew
- Personal hx of breast/ ovarian cancer
- < 40 yrs old
- Two or more relatives with breast cancer (< 50 yrs)

Oral contraceptives commonly cause breast pain.

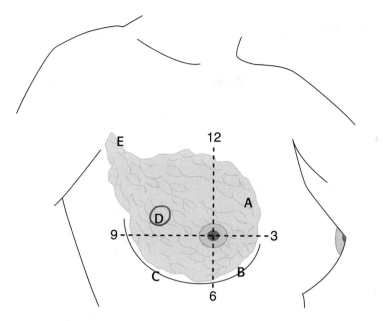

FIGURE 32-1. **Female Breast Quadrants**

A: UIQ (upper inner quadrant); B: LIQ (lower inner quadrant); C: LOQ (lower outer quadrant;
D: UUQ (upper outer quadrant), majority of breast cancers are detected in this quadrant;
E: Tail of Spence (outer portion of breast toward the axilla).

Breast Skin Changes

- On exam, the skin is inspected for any edema, erythema, or retraction.
- Ulceration, eczema, and redness around the nipple can be Paget disease. Mammogram and surgery referral is warranted.
- Erythema, tenderness, and a mass is suspicious for **inflammatory breast cancer** (also referred to as "peau d'orange"). Mammogram and surgery referral is warranted.
- Warmth, tenderness, induration, and erythema may also be mastitis or a breast abscess even in the nonlactating woman. If fluctuance is appreciated, a breast US and drainage with antibiotics are the treatment of choice.

CHAPTER 33

Women's Health Maintenance

Obstetricians/gynecologists must be aware of screening tests suggested for their patients. These tools are used for the prevention and/or early detection of serious medical conditions and diseases.

SCREENING TESTS

A 65-year-old, postmenopausal woman comes to your clinic for a well-woman exam. She has not seen a physician for several years. What screening and health maintenance tests will she need?

Answer: This patient will need a Pap smear, annual clinical breast exam, mammogram, colon cancer screening, cholesterol/lipid screening, fasting glucose, complete blood count (CBC), urinalysis, blood urea nitrogen (BUN), creatinine, hemoglobin, influenza vaccine, tetanus-diphtheria (Td) booster, and pneumococcal vaccine.

Pap Smear (ACOG, December 2009)

- Begin Pap testing at age 21. At ages 21–29, Pap test is every 2 years. After 30, Pap testing can be every 3 years.
- This applies to low-risk women. High-risk women require more frequent screening.

Breast Exams

- An annual clinical breast exam (CBE) should be performed, by a health care provider, on all women beginning at age 21.
- All females should perform breast self-exams once per month beginning at age 18 (eg, premenopausal women should examine their breasts one week after their menstrual period).

Mammography

- Screening begins at age 40. Order a mammogram every 1–2 yr.
- Annually beginning at age 50.

Colon Cancer Screening

- Begin screening at age 50 in low-risk patients. One of five screening options should be selected:
  1. Fecal occult blood testing (FOBT), followed by colonoscopy for positive results.
  2. Flexible sigmoidoscopy every 5 yr.
  3. FOBT with flexible sigmoidoscopy.
  4. Double-contrast barium enema every 5 yr.
  5. Colonoscopy every 10 yr.
- High-risk patients include those with inflammatory bowel disease, colonic polyps, colon cancer, or a family history of familial polyposis coli, colorectal cancer, or cancer predisposition syndrome. These patients should begin screening earlier and more frequently.

Laboratory Testing

THYROID-STIMULATING HORMONE (TSH)

- Screening begins at age 50, then every 5 yr.
- Periodic screening (age 19–64) if strong family history of thyroid disease or if autoimmune disease.

CHOLESTEROL

- Every 5 yr beginning at age 45.
- Every 3–5 yr between ages 65 and 75.
- Periodic screening if:
  - Familial lipid disorder.
  - Family history of premature coronary artery disease (CAD) (< 55 yr), diabetes mellitus (DM), or multiple coronary heart disease risk factors (tobacco, hypertension, obesity).
  - Elevated cholesterol.
  - History of parent or sibling with blood cholesterol ≥ 240 mg/dL.
  - History of sibling, parent, or grandparent with premature (< 55 yr) coronary artery disease.

FASTING GLUCOSE

- Test every 3 yr beginning at age 45.
- Screening can begin at a younger age or more frequent in a patient with risk factors:
  - Family history of DM (one first- or two second-degree relatives).
  - Obese.
  - History of gestational DM.
  - Hypertension.
  - High-risk ethnic group (Hispanic/African-American/Native American).
  - History of polycystic ovarian syndrome.
  - History of vascular disease.

TUBERCULOSIS (TB) SKIN TESTING

- Regular testing for teens.
- Human immunodeficiency virus (HIV): HIV-positive people should be tested regularly.
- Exposure to TB-infected person requires testing.
- Medically underserved/low-income populations.
- Immunocompromised persons.
- Intravenous (IV) drug user.
- Resident of a long-term care facility.
- Recent TB skin test converter.

SEXUALLY TRANSMITTED INFECTION TESTING

- History of multiple sexual partners.
- History of sex with a partner who has multiple sexual contacts.
- Persons whose partner has a sexually transmitted infection (STI).
- History of STI.
- Annual screening for all sexually active females under age 25.
- Women with developmental disabilities.
- Women who exchange sex for drugs or money.
- Women who use IV drugs.
- Women who are in a detention facility.

Routine screening for chlamydial and gonorrheal infection is recommended for all sexually active adolescents and high-risk females, even if they are asymptomatic. These tests are done simultaneously as the presence of one of these infections is a high risk for the presence of the other.

HIV Testing in Women

- Aged 13–65 years old annually.
- Seeking treatment for STIs.
- Who have more than one sexual partner.
- With a history of prostitution/IV drug abuse.
- With a history of sex with an HIV-positive partner.
- Whose partners are men who have sex with men (MSM).
- Who were transfused between 1978 and 1985.
- Who are in an area with high prevalence of HIV infection.
- With recurrent genital tract disease.
- Who have invasive cervical cancer.
- Who are pregnant or planning to become pregnant.
- Who are in a detention facility.

Bacteriuria Testing/Urinalysis

Periodically for women with DM and women who are age 65 or older.

IMMUNIZATIONS

- Td booster once between ages 11 and 18, then every 10 yr.
- Measles, mumps, rubella (MMR) for all nonimmune women.
- Hepatitis B vaccine once for those not previously immunized.
- Varicella vaccine, one series, for those not immunized.
- Hepatitis A vaccine if at high risk (such as chronic liver disease, illegal drug user, individuals traveling to endemic countries).
- Influenza vaccine annually for anyone wishing to reduce their chance of becoming ill. Also for high-risk conditions such as:
  - Resident of a chronic care facility.
  - Immunosuppression.
  - Hemoglobinopathy.
  - Diabetes.
  - Asthma.
  - Renal disease.
  - Cardiovascular disease.
  - Health care provider.
- Meningococcal vaccine before entering high school for those not immunized.
- Pneumococcal vaccine if age 65, or sooner for women with:
  - Sickle cell disease.
  - Asplenia.
  - Alcoholism/cirrhosis.
  - Influenza vaccine risk factors.
  - Revaccination after 5 yr in these groups.
- Human papillomavirus vaccine (HPV): One series for those age 9–26.
- Herpes zoster vaccine: Single dose in adults age 60 or older.

HEALTH EDUCATION

Good diet and exercise are crucial for leading a healthy life. There are many factors that determine each individual's diet and exercise requirements, which all must be considered by the physician.

Nutrition and Exercise

- The issues of nutrition and body weight should be emphasized during the three major transitional periods in a woman's life:
  1. Puberty
  2. Pregnancy
  3. Menopause
- One's body weight is determined by three major factors:
  1. Genetics and heredity, which control:
     - Resting metabolic rate.
     - Appetite.
     - Satiety.
     - Body fat distribution.
     - Predisposition to physical activity.
  2. Nutrition.
  3. Physical activity and exercise.

GOALS

- Maintain a healthy diet consisting of frequent small meals (ie, 4–6 instead of 2–3).
- Utilize the Food Guide Pyramid as a tool in making food choices in daily life. Persons should eat from the five food groups daily. The following are recommended:
  - Eat 6 oz of grains every day (whole bread, breads, crackers, rice or pasta).
  - Eat 2.5 cups of vegetables daily (eat more dark green vegetables).
  - Eat 2 cups of fruit daily (fresh, frozen, or canned). Limit fruit juices.
  - Drink 3 cups of milk daily (low fat or fat free for milk, yogurt, or other milk products).
  - Eat 5.5 oz of meat and beans daily (baked, broiled, or grilled).
- Adjust caloric intake for age and physical activity level:
  - As one ages, there is a ↓ in resting metabolic rate and loss of lean tissue.
  - Older women who are physically active are less likely to lose lean tissue and can maintain their weight with higher caloric intake.
- Physical activity during all stages of life should include exercise at moderate intensity for 30 min on most days of the week.

High-fat diets have adverse effects on lipid metabolism, insulin sensitivity, and body composition.

Exercise will ↑ the body's metabolic rate and prevent the storage of fat.

SUBSTANCE ABUSE

A 53-year-old G1P1 female presents to your office for a well-woman exam. When asked about alcohol use, she informs you that she drinks several glasses of wine every evening. How should you screen for alcoholism?

Answer: Using the CAGE questionnaire has been shown to be very effective in screening for problem drinking.

- Substance abuse is a serious condition that can affect every aspect of a patient's life. The role of an OB/GYN physician is to provide universal screening for substance abuse. This can be accomplished by direct questioning or via questionnaire.

CAGE Questionnaire for Alcoholism

C — Have you ever felt like you should **CUT BACK** on your drinking?

A — Have you ever been **ANNOYED** when people criticize your drinking?

G — Have you ever felt **GUILTY** about your drinking?

E — Have you ever needed a drink first thing in the morning to steady your nerves or "cure" a hangover **(EYE OPENER)**?

■ An example of screening would be the CAGE questionnaire. Two "yes" answers has a sensitivity of 93% and a specificity of 76% for alcoholism.

Alcohol

Women experience more accelerated and profound medical consequences of excessive alcohol than men (a phenomenon called *telescoping*):

■ Cirrhosis.
■ Peptic ulcers that require surgery.
■ Myopathy.
■ Cardiomyopathy.
■ Stroke.
■ Menstrual disorders.
■ Early menopause.
■ Stroke.
■ Malignancies.
■ When combined with cigarette smoking, it can cause oral and esophageal cancers.
■ Fetal alcohol syndrome:
  ■ Teratogenic effects are dose related.
  ■ Includes growth retardation, facial anomalies, and mental retardation.

Tobacco

■ Cigarette smoking is the most preventable cause of premature death and avoidable illness in the United States. It is important to apply the **5As** to screening women:
  ■ **A**sk about tobacco.
  ■ **A**dvise to quit.
  ■ **A**ssess willingness to quit.
  ■ **A**ssist in quit attempt.
  ■ **A**rrange for follow-up.
■ Linked to lung cancer, coronary artery disease (CAD), and respiratory diseases.
■ Most common factor in chronic obstructive pulmonary disease (COPD).
■ **Endocrine effects:** Smokers reach menopause earlier and have ↑ risk of osteoporosis.
■ **Obstetric effects:** Reduced fertility, ↑ rates of spontaneous abortion, premature delivery, low-birth-weight infants, fetal growth restriction, and placental abruption.
■ Children who grow up exposed to secondhand smoke have higher rates of respiratory and middle ear illness.

SEAT BELT USE

■ Deaths due to accidents are leading cause of death in females age 13–18.
■ Accidents cause more deaths than infectious diseases, pulmonary diseases, diabetes, and liver and kidney disease.

Alcohol:
■ Accounts for 100,000 deaths per year in the United States.
■ Excessive use for women is about one-half the quantity considered excessive for men.
■ When compared to men, women have relatively reduced activity of gastric alcohol dehydrogenase to begin alcohol metabolism and have less body water in which to distribute unmetabolized alcohol.

Lung cancer is the most common cause of cancer death in women. Related to 400,000 deaths/yr.

Accidents are the most common cause of death for adolescents.

- Motor vehicle accidents account for 50,000 deaths per yr and 4–5 million injuries per yr.
- Seat belts ↓ chance of death and serious injury by > 50%.

Improved and successful prevention of pregnancy and STIs by more adolescents requires counseling that includes:

- Encouragement to postpone sexual involvement.
- Provision of information about contraceptive options, including emergency contraception and side effects of various contraceptive methods.
- Education on safe sex practices.

Domestic Violence

- Domestic violence refers to a relationship in which an individual is victimized (physically, psychologically, or emotionally) by a current or past intimate partner.
- Each year in the United States, 2 million women are abused by someone they know.
- Every woman should be screened for domestic violence because it can occur with any woman, in any situation.

> Any injury during pregnancy, especially one to the abdomen or breasts, is suspicious for abuse.

RECOGNITION OF DOMESTIC VIOLENCE

- Injuries to the head, eyes, neck, torso, breasts, abdomen, and/or genitals.
- Bilateral or multiple injuries.
- A delay between the time of injury and the time at which treatment is sought.
- Inconsistencies between the patient's explanation of the injuries and the physician's clinical findings.
- A history of repeated trauma.
- The perpetrator may exhibit signs of control over the health care team, refusal to leave the patient's side to allow private conversation, and control of victim.
- The patient calls or visits frequently for general somatic complaints.
- **Pregnant women:**
  - Late entry into prenatal care, missed appointments, and multiple repeated complaints are often seen in abused pregnant women.
  - Pregnant women, in general, are at highest risk to experience domestic violence, during the pregnancy.

DIAGNOSIS (SEE TABLE 33-1)

Use screening questionnaire.

MEDICAL OBLIGATION TO VICTIMS

- Listen in a nonjudgmental fashion, and assure the patient that it is not her fault, nor does she deserve the abuse.
- Assess the safety of the patient and her children.

TABLE 33-1. Abuse Assessment Screen

1. Have you ever been emotionally or physically abused by your partner or someone important to you?
2. Within the past year, have you been hit, slapped, kicked, or otherwise physically hurt by someone?
3. Since you've been pregnant, have you been hit, slapped, kicked, or otherwise physically hurt by someone?
4. Within the past year, has anyone forced you to have sexual activities? Has anyone in the past forced you to have sexual activities?
5. Are you afraid of your partner or anyone you listed above?

- If the patient is ready to leave the abusive relationship, connect her with resources such as shelters, police, public agencies, and counselors.
- If the patient is not ready to leave, discuss a safety or exit plan and provide the patient with domestic violence information.
- Carefully document all subjective and objective findings. The records can be used in a legal case to establish abuse.

Sexual Assault

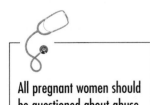

A 27-year-old G0P0 female presents to your office stating that she was raped the night before. What are her options if she desires emergency contraception?
Answer: (1) Plan B: 0.75 mg levonorgestrel q12h × 2 doses; (2) Oral: 2 tabs stat, then 2 tabs 12 hr later; (3) mifepristone (RU486) 600 mg × 1 dose.

Sexual abuse occurs in approximately two-thirds of relationships involving physical abuse.

- **Sexual assault** occurs when any sexual act is performed by one person on another without that person's consent.
- **Rape** is defined as sexual intercourse without the consent of one party, whether from force, threat of force, or incapacity to consent due to physical or mental condition.

Rape-Related Posttraumatic Stress Disorder (RR-PTSD)

A "rape-trauma" syndrome resulting from the psychological and emotional stress of being raped.

SIGNS AND SYMPTOMS

All pregnant women should be questioned about abuse during EACH trimester.

- **Acute phase:**
  - Eating and sleep disorders.
  - Vaginal itch, pain, and discharge.
  - Generalized physical complaints and pains (ie, chest pain, backaches, and pelvic pain).
  - Anxiety/depression.
- **Reorganization phase:**
  - Phobias
  - Flashbacks
  - Nightmares
  - Gynecologic complaints

MANAGEMENT

Physician's Medical Responsibilities
- Obtain complete medical and gynecologic history.
- Assess and treat physical injuries in the presence of a female chaperone (even if the health care provider is female).
- Obtain appropriate cultures; check bloodwork for STI's (HIV, syphilis, hepatitis B/C).
- Counsel patient and provide STI prophylaxis.
- Provide preventive therapy for unwanted pregnancy.
- Assess psychological and emotional status.
- Provide crisis intervention.
- Arrange for follow-up medical care and psychological counseling.

Physicians are not obligated to perform procedures if they are morally opposed. There is an obligation to refer patients as necessary.

Physician's Legal Responsibilities
- Obtain informed consent for treatment, collection of evidence, taking of photographs, and reporting of the incident to the authorities.
- Accurately record events.
- Accurately describe injuries.
- Collect appropriate samples and clothing.
- Maintain the chain of command.
- Label photographs, clothing, and specimens with the patient's name; seal and store safely.

The greatest danger for spousal abuse to occur involves a threat or an attempt to leave the relationship.

TREATMENT

- **Infection prophylaxis:** Gonorrhea, chlamydia, and trichomonal infections:
  - Ceftriaxone 125 mg IM + azithromycin 1 g PO in a single dose or
  - Doxycycline 100 mg PO BID × 7 days + metronidazole 2 g PO in a single dose.
- Offer the hepatitis B vaccine.
- Offer anti-virals for HIV prophylaxis.
- Administer Td toxoid when indicated.
- **Postcoital regimen:**
  - **Plan B (levonorgestrel):** Consists of two tablets, each 0.75 mg taken 12 hr apart. Failure rate is 1%.
  - **Combined estrogen-progestin pills:** Ovral (50 μg ethinyl estradiol, 0.5 mg norgestrel): 2 tabs PO STAT, then 2 more tabs 12 hr later; 75% effective.

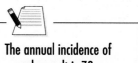

The annual incidence of sexual assault is 73 per 100,000 females.

Seventy-five percent of rape victims know their perpetrator.

Female Sexuality

It is important to consider every aspect of a woman's health, including her sexuality. Evaluation of sexual function should be a basic part of any well-woman exam.

Female Response Cycle

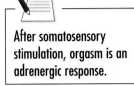

After somatosensory stimulation, orgasm is an adrenergic response.

Unlike men, women can experience multiple orgasms without a time lag in between.

- **Desire:** Begins in the brain with perception of erotogenic stimuli via the special senses or through fantasy.
- **Arousal:**
  - Clitoris becomes erect.
  - Labia minora become engorged.
  - Blood flow in the vaginal vault triples.
  - Upper two-thirds of the vagina dilate.
  - Lubricant is secreted from the vaginal surface.
  - Lower one-third of vagina thickens and dilates.
- **Plateau:**
  - The formation of transudate (lubrication) in the vagina continues in conjunction with genital congestion.
  - Occurs prior to orgasm.
- **Orgasm:** Rhythmic, involuntary, vaginal smooth muscle and pelvic contractions, leads to pleasurable cortical sensory phenomenon ("orgasm").

Sexuality: Fetus to Menopause

PRENATAL AND CHILDHOOD

It is normal for children under age 6 to be curious about their own or others' bodies.

- Sexual development begins prenatally when the fetus differentiates into a male or female.
- Sexual behavior, usually in the form of masturbation, is common in childhood.
- As children grow older, they are socialized into cultural emphasis on privacy and sexual inhibition in social situations.
- Between ages 7 and 8, most children engage in childhood sexual games, either same-gender or cross-gender play.

ADOLESCENCE

Gender identity and sexual preferences begin to solidify as puberty begins.

MENSTRUAL CYCLE

The menstrual cycle can affect sexuality (ie, in some women, there is a peak in sexual activity in the midfollicular phase).

PREGNANCY

Sexual intercourse should be avoided in high-risk pregnancies, such as placenta previa, placental abruption, preterm labor, and preterm ruptured membranes.

- For some women, intercourse is avoided during pregnancy due to fear of harming the baby or a self-perception of unattractiveness.
- Coitus is safe until 36 weeks in normal pregnancies.

POSTPARTUM

Women often experience sexual problems within the first 6 weeks of delivery, including:

- Perineal soreness.
- Excessive fatigue.
- Disinterest in sex.

This is secondary to changing hormone levels.

MENOPAUSE

- A ↓ in sexual activity is most frequently observed.
- Advancing age is associated with ↓ in:
  - Intercourse frequency.
  - Orgasmic frequency.
  - Enjoyment of sexual activity: Sexual enjoyment may also be ↓ with the ↑ duration of the relationship and with the partner's increasing age.
- ↓ sexual responsiveness may be reversible if caused by reduction in functioning of genital smooth muscle tissue.
- Psychosocially, middle-aged women often feel less sexually desirable.
- **Hormonal changes:** Low estrogen levels lead to less vaginal lubrication, thinner and less elastic vaginal lining, and depressive symptoms, resulting in ↓ sexual desire and well-being.

Sexual Dysfunction

It is important to first clarify whether the dysfunction reported is:

- Lifelong or acquired.
- Global (all partners) or situational.

EVALUATION STRATEGIES

- Look for possible etiologies:
  - Medical illnesses.
  - Menopausal status.
  - Medication use (antihypertensives, cardiovascular meds, antidepressants, etc.).
- Rule out other psychiatric/psychological causes:
  - Life discontent (stress, fatigue, relationship issues, traumatic sexual history, guilt).
  - Major depression.
  - Drug abuse.
  - Anxiety.
  - Obsessive-compulsive disorder.

MANAGEMENT STRATEGIES

- Medical illnesses need evaluation and specific treatment.
- Screen for and treat depression with psychotherapy or medication.
- Reduce dosages or change medications that may alter sexual interest (ie, switch to antidepressant formulations that have less of an impact on sexual function).
- Address menopause and hormonal deficiencies.

HIGH-YIELD FACTS

Female Sexuality

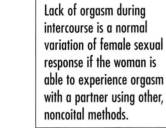

Sexual arousal disorders are accompanied by complaints of dyspareunia, lack of lubrication, or orgasmic difficulty.

Lack of orgasm during intercourse is a normal variation of female sexual response if the woman is able to experience orgasm with a partner using other, noncoital methods.

Sildenafil citrate (Viagra) and other vasodilators are currently undergoing clinical trials with women for sexual dysfunction treatment.

Exogenous administration of estrogen improves vaginal lubrication, atrophic conditions, hot flashes, headaches, and insomnia.

Menopause and Sexual Dysfunction

Menopause → vaginal atrophy and lack of adequate lubrication → painful intercourse → ↓ sexual desire.

FEMALE SEXUAL DYSFUNCTION DISORDERS

- **Hypoactive sexual desire disorder:** Persistent or recurrent absence or deficit of sexual fantasies and desire for sexual activity.
- **Sexual aversion disorder:** Persistent or recurrent aversion to and avoidance of genital contact with a sexual partner.
- **Sexual arousal disorder:**
  - Partial or total lack of physical response as indicated by lack of lubrication and vasocongestion of genitals.
  - Persistent lack of subjective sense of sexual excitement and pleasure during sex.
- **Female orgasmic disorder:** Persistent or recurrent delay in, or absence of, orgasm following a normal excitement phase.
- **Vaginismus:** Persistent involuntary spasm of the muscles of the outer third of the vagina, which interferes with sexual intercourse.

EVALUATION FOR A SEXUAL DYSFUNCTION DISORDER

- Take sexual experience into account. Women often become more orgasmic with experience.
- Physical factors that may interfere with neurovascular pelvic dysfunction (ie, surgeries, illnesses, or injuries).
- Psychological and interpersonal factors are very common (ie, growing up with messages that sex is shameful and for men only).
- Partner's lack of sexual skills.

TREATMENT FOR SEXUAL DYSFUNCTION

Treatment varies and in general involves the couple. Therapy should be instituted for both partners, in addition to the following:

- Treat the ↓ lubrication with the application of lubricants, such as KY Jelly or Astroglide.
- Menopausal symptoms may respond to oral or topical estrogen.
- For lifelong, generalized orgasmic disorder, there is rarely a physical cause. Treat with masturbation programs and/or sex therapy.

SEXUAL PAIN DISORDERS

- **Dyspareunia:** Recurrent genital pain before, during, or after intercourse.
  - **Evaluation:** Differentiate between physical disorder, vaginismus, lack of lubrication.
  - **Management:**
    - If due to vaginal scarring/stenosis due to history of episiotomy or vaginal surgery, vaginal stretching with dilators and massage.
    - If postmenopausal, vaginal estrogen cream to improve vaginal pliability.
    - Low-dose tricyclic antidepressants may be helpful.
    - Pelvic floor physical therapy (Kegel exercises).
    - Coital position changes.
- **Vaginismus:** Recurrent involuntary spasm of the outer third of the vagina (perineal and levator ani muscles), interfering with or preventing coitus.

- **Evaluation:**
  - Obtain history.
  - Rule out organic causes (ie, vaginitis, endometriosis, pelvic inflammatory disease, irritable bowel syndrome, urethral syndrome, interstitial cystitis, etc.).
  - Examine the pelvis for involuntary spasm.
  - Rule out physical disorder or other psychiatric disorder.
- **Management:**
  - Treat organic causes.
  - Psychotherapy.
  - Provide reassurance.
  - Physical therapy (ie, Kegel exercises, muscle relaxation massage, and gradual vaginal dilatation). The woman controls the pace and duration.

Many antidepressants worsen the sexual response by increasing the availability of serotonin and decreasing dopamine.

Estrogen use, in a postmenopausal female, improves sexual desire.

Ethics

Physicians in all fields of medicine encounter difficult ethical decisions. Understanding the various aspects of forensic medicine may not make these decisions easier but will likely cause the physician to more closely consider the outcomes of the decision being made.

It is the physician's responsibility to:

- Determine the patient's preferences.
- Honor the patient's wishes, when the patient can no longer speak for herself.

> A 35-year-old G2P2 female is scheduled for major surgery. She would like to delineate preferences for her care, in the event that she is unable to speak for herself. What options does she have?
>
> **Answer:** She can either write a living will (dictates her preferences) or appoint someone as her durable power of attorney to make decisions on her behalf.

- **Advance directives (living will and durable power of attorney for health care)** allow patients to voice their preferences regarding treatment if faced with a potentially terminal illness.
- In a **living will**, a competent, adult patient may, in advance, formulate and provide a valid consent to the withholding/withdrawal of life-support systems in the event that injury or illness renders that individual incompetent to make such a decision.
- In a **durable power of attorney for health care**, a patient appoints someone to act as a surrogate decision maker when the patient cannot participate in the consent process.
- The patient's legal spouse is the *de facto* durable power of attorney for health care if no other is appointed; the spouse cannot defy the conditions of a living will or make decisions if another person has been appointed durable power of attorney.

If a married person has a living will or has appointed another person to be a durable power of attorney, the spouse can not defy the conditions.

Any treatment that serves to prolong life without reversing the underlying medical condition.

The ethical responsibility of the physician is:

- To identify his or her own opinions on the issue at hand.
- To be honest and fair to their patients when they seek advice or services in this area.
- To explain his or her personal views to the patient and how those views may influence the service or advice being provided.

HIGH-YIELD FACTS

Ethics

A legal document that requires a physician to obtain consent for treatment rendered, an operation performed, or many diagnostic procedures.

Informed consent requires the following conditions be met:

1. Must be **voluntary.**
2. **Information:**
   - **Risks and benefits** of the procedure are discussed.
   - **Alternatives** to procedure are discussed.
   - **Consequences** of not undergoing the procedure are discussed.
   - Physician must be willing to **discuss the procedure** and answer any questions the patient has.
3. The patient must be **competent.**

EXCEPTIONS

The following are certain cases in which informed consent need not be obtained:

1. Lifesaving medical emergency.
2. Suicide prevention.
3. Normally, minors must have consent obtained from their parents. However, minors may give their own consent for certain treatments, such as alcohol detox and treatment for venereal diseases.

The information disclosed to a physician during his or her relationship with the patient is confidential. The physician should not reveal information or communications without the express consent of the patient, unless required to do so by law.

Exceptions

- A patient threatens to inflict serious bodily harm to herself or another person.
- Communicable diseases (ie, HIV).
- Gunshot wounds.
- Knife wounds.

MINORS

- When minors request confidential services, physicians should encourage minors to involve their parents.
- Where the law does not require otherwise, the physician should permit a competent minor to consent to medical care and should **not** notify the parents without the patient's consent.
- If the physician feels that without parental involvement and guidance the minor will face a serious health threat, and there is reason to believe that the parents will be helpful, disclosing the problem to the parents is equally justified.

CHAPTER 36

Menopause

Menopause signifies the depletion of oocytes and manifests as the absence of menses. The changes in female hormones can have significant morbidity for a woman. A variety of symptoms can occur, that can require medical treatment. The treatment may have adverse effects in some women, so its use should be considered carefully.

DEFINITIONS

- **Menopause** is the permanent cessation of menstruation caused by failure of ovarian estrogen production, in the presence of elevated gonadotropin levels (diagnosed after 6–12 months of amenorrhea).
- Menopause is preceded by the **climacteric** or **perimenopausal period**, the multiyear transition from optimal menstrual condition to menopause.
- The **postmenopausal period** is the time after menopause.
- See Figure 36-1.

FACTORS AFFECTING AGE OF ONSET

- Genetics.
- Smoking (↓ age by 3 yr).
- Chemo/radiation therapy.

PHYSIOLOGY DURING THE PERIMENOPAUSAL PERIOD

Oocytes Die

- Women's immature eggs, or **oocytes, begin to die** precipitously (via apoptosis) and become <u>resistant to follicle-stimulating hormone</u> **(FSH)**, the pituitary hormone that causes their maturation.

Final Menstrual Period (FMP)

Stages:	-5	-4	-3	-2	-1	0	+1	+2
Terminology:	Reproductive			Menopausal Transition			Postmenopause	
	Early	Peak	Late	Early	Late*		Early*	Late
				Perimenopause				
Duration of Stage:	variable			variable		(a) 1 yr	(b) 4 yrs	until demise
Menstrual Cycles:	variable to regular	regular		variable cycle length (>7 days different from normal)	≥2 skipped cycles and an interval of amenorrhea (≥60 days)	Amen. x 12 mos	none	
Endocrine:	normal FSH		↑ FSH	↑ FSH			↑ FSH	

*Stages most likely to be characterized by vasomotor symptoms   ↑ = elevated

FIGURE 36-1. The STRAW staging system.

(Reproduced, with permission, from Soules MR et al. Executive Summary: Stages of Reproductive Aging Workshop [STRAW]. *Fertil Steril* 2001;76[5]: 874–878.)

- Menopause is characterized by an elevated FSH due to:
  1. ↓ inhibin (inhibin inhibits FSH secretion; it is produced in smaller amounts by the fewer oocytes).
  2. Resistant oocytes require more FSH to successfully mature, triggering greater FSH release.

Ovulation Becomes Less Frequent

Women **ovulate less frequently**: Initially 1–2 fewer times per year, and eventually, just before menopause, only once every 3–4 months. This is due to a **shortened follicular phase**. The length of the luteal phase does not change.

Estrogen Levels Fall

> A 51-year-old female G4P4 complains of new onset of pain with intercourse and occasional vaginal itching that started in the past 6 months. Workup for sexually transmitted infections (STIs) is negative, and on wet mount you note very few epithelial cells consistent with atrophic vaginitis. What is the major hormonal change implicated in these symptoms?
>
> **Answer:** There is a decline in estrogen that causes atrophic vaginitis.

- **Estrogen (estradiol-17β) levels begin to decline**, resulting in **hot flashes** (which may also be due to ↑ luteinizing hormone [LH]).
- There is a major reduction in ovarian estrogen production at 6 months before menopause.
- Hot flashes can occur for 2 yr after the onset of estrogen deficiency begins and can last up to 10 or more years.
- Hot flashes usually occur on the face, neck, and upper chest and last a few minutes, followed by intense diaphoresis. Women often complain of sleep disruption, because of the diaphoresis.

PHYSIOLOGY DURING THE MENOPAUSAL PERIOD

- ↓ in estradiol level.
- **FSH and LH levels rise** secondary to absence of negative feedback.
- Androstenedione is aromatized peripherally to estrone (less potent than estradiol), which is the major estrogen in postmenopausal women.
- Androstenedione and testosterone levels fall. These two hormones are produced by the ovary.
- The most **important physiologic change** that occurs with menopause is the **decline of estradiol-17β** levels that occurs with the cessation of follicular maturation. Table 36-1 lists the organ systems affected by the ↓ estradiol levels.

FSH levels double to 20 mIU/mL in perimenopause and increase to 40 in menopause.

Oligo/anovulation leads to abnormal bleeding in perimenopause.

When menopause occurs after age 55, it is considered late menopause.

Premature ovarian failure is defined as menopause occurring before age 40.

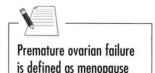

HIGH-YIELD FACTS

Menopause

A 50-year-old G1P1 female complains of hot flashes for 3 months during the day and night sweats so bad she has to change her shirt. On further questioning, she reports that she has ↑ irritability and a lack of libido for that same period of time. What is this woman's problem and what treatment could you offer her?

Answer: This woman is experiencing menopause. If her symptoms are distressing, she could be offered hormone replacement therapy to alleviate some of her symptoms.

Hormone replacement therapy (HRT) or estrogen replacement therapy (ERT) has been shown to counteract some of the side effects of estrogen loss listed in Table 36-1.

TABLE 36-1. Physiologic Effects of Menopause

ORGAN SYSTEM	EFFECT OF DECREASED ESTRADIOL	AVAILABLE TREATMENT
Cardiovascular	↑ LDL, ↓ HDL. After two decades of menopause, the risk of myocardial infarction (MI) and coronary artery disease is equal to that in men.	
Bone	Osteoporosis. Estrogen receptors found on many cells mediating trabecular bone maintenance (ie, ↓ osteoblast activity, ↑ osteoclast activity) due to ↓ estrogen levels.	▪ HRT/ERT becoming second line ▪ Calcitonin ▪ Raloxifene ▪ Etidronate (a bisphosphonate osteoclast inhibitor) ▪ Exercise ▪ Calcium supplementation ▪ 50% reduction in death from hip fracture with normal estrogen levels
Vaginal mucous membranes	Dryness and atrophy, with resulting dyspareunia, atrophic vaginitis.	HRT/ERT pill or cream
Genitourinary	Loss of urethral tone, dysuria.	HRT/ERT
Psychiatric	Lability, depression.	+/– HRT/ERT, antidepressants
Neurologic	Preliminary studies indicate there may be a link between low levels of estradiol and Alzheimer disease.	HRT/ERT
Hair and skin	Skin: Less elastic, more wrinkled. Hair: Male growth patterns.	HRT/ERT pill or cream

ERT, estrogen replacement therapy; HDL, high-density lipoprotein; HRT, hormone replacement therapy; LDL, low-density lipoprotein.

HIGH-YIELD FACTS

Menopause

Estrogen Replacement Therapy (ERT)

ERT—estrogen alone: Indicated in women status post hysterectomy.

Hormone Replacement Therapy (HRT)

- HRT—estrogen + progesterone: The progesterone component is needed to protect the endometrium from constant stimulation and resultant ↑ in endometrial cancer. It is indicated for women who still have their uterus.
- The Women's Health Initiative (WHI) and the Heart and Estrogen/Progestin Replacement Study (HERS) have prompted great changes in the understanding and recommendations of HRT.
- Cardiovascular: HRT does not seem to protect against cardiovascular disease. In fact, it could make it worse.
- Osteoporosis: Controversial because they protect against osteoporosis but there are other medications, such as bisphosphonates and raloxifene, that can do the same thing.
- Breast cancer: Seen to ↑ the risk of breast cancer.

INDICATIONS FOR HRT IN MENOPAUSE

- Presence of hot flashes.
- Prevention of atrophic vaginitis.

RECOMMENDATIONS

- Short-term therapy (< 5 yr) is acceptable for menopausal symptom relief. Prescribe the lowest dose that relieves the symptoms. Order a mammogram before initiating therapy and yearly thereafter.
- Osteoporosis can be prevented with HRT; however, other medications are as effective and can be used as first-line therapy.
- HRT should not be used to prevent cardiovascular disease.

RISKS OF HRT/ERT

- ↑ risk of breast cancer.
- ↑ incidence in endometrial cancer (ERT only).
- Thromboembolism, myocardial infarction (MI), stroke.
- Cholecystitis/cholelithiasis.

CONTRAINDICATIONS TO HRT/ERT

- Unexplained vaginal bleeding.
- Breast carcinoma (relative contraindication, not absolute).
- Metastatic endometrial carcinoma/ovarian carcinoma.
- Liver disease.
- History of thromboembolic disease.
- History of MI or stroke.
- May worsen hypertension or migraines.

Although HRT recommendations changed with the WHI study, there are many flaws in the design. Recommendations will likely change in the near future.

Menopause wreaks HAVOC:

Hot flashes
Atrophy of the
Vagina
Osteoporosis
Coronary artery disease

Estrogen creates a hypercoagulable state due to ↑ production of hepatic coagulation factors.

Pelvic Relaxation

With aging and ↑ pelvic pressure, there is a risk that the pelvic musculature will no longer be able to keep pelvic organs in their proper position. Prolapse can occur in various organs and is usually associated with a sensation of ↑ pressure. Diagnosis must be made examining the patient when supine and standing. When prolapse becomes symptomatic, treatment is warranted with surgery or a pessary device.

ANATOMY OF PELVIC FLOOR SUPPORT

The pelvic diaphragm is made up of the levator ani and coccygeal muscles.

Several crucial structures make up the support of the female pelvic floor. Disturbance of any of the following can result in prolapse:

- Bony structure.
- Cardinal broad and round ligaments.
- Endopelvic fascia.
- Pelvic diaphragm.
- Urogenital diaphragm.
- Perineum.

PROLAPSE

A 57-year-old G8P8 overweight woman (250 lbs) who has had three children comes to your office complaining of pressure and a bulge in her vagina that is worse when coughing, and has a recent onset of dyspareunia. What is your next step in management of this patient?

Answer: Perform a complete pelvic exam to assess for prolapse. Examine the patient in both the <u>supine</u> and <u>standing</u> position to help determine the severity of the prolapse.

Prolapse is the failure of pelvic musculature to maintain the pelvic organs in their normal position. There are several types.

TYPES

In general, think of prolapse as either limited to the upper vagina, to the introitus, or protruding through the vagina.

Prolapses can be classified according to the location of the protruding structure: anterior, apical, and posterior.

- **Anterior:**
  - Cystocele (bladder)
  - Cystourethrocele
- **Apical:**
  - Uterocele
  - Vaginal prolapse
- **Posterior:**
  - Rectocele: See Figure 37-1
  - Enterocele (intestine): See Figure 37-1

HIGH-YIELD FACTS

Pelvic Relaxation

368

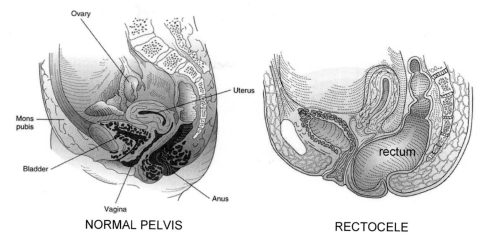

FIGURE 37-1. Types of prolapse.

(Reproduced, with permission, from Pernoll ML. *Benson & Pernoll's Handbook of Obstetrics and Gynecology*, 10th ed. New York: McGraw-Hill, 2001: 807–808.)

GRADING (BADEN-WALKER CLASSIFICATION)

Organ displacement:

To the level of the ischial spines:	Grade I
Between ischial spines and introitus:	Grade II
Up to introitus:	Grade III
Past introitus:	Grade IV

RISK FACTORS

Many conditions can cause prolapse: Disturbing the anatomical supports (childbirth), disrupting the innervations, or increasing abdominal pressure. Examples include:

- ↑ abdominal pressure: Obesity, cough (eg, chronic obstructive pulmonary disease), heavy lifting.
- Loss of levator ani function: Postpartum.
- Transection of supporting tissue: Postsurgical.
- Loss of innervation: Amyotrophic lateral sclerosis (ALS), paralysis, multiple sclerosis.
- Loss of connective tissue: Spina bifida, myelomeningocele.
- Atrophy of supporting tissues: Aging, especially after menopause.

SIGNS AND SYMPTOMS

- Feeling of "pressure."
- Organ protrusion, especially upon exertion.
- Incontinence.
- Groin pain.
- Dyspareunia.
- Spotting.
- Splinting to defecate.

Symptom alleviation/exacerbation is often related to pelvic effort (ie, better when prone, better in the morning, worse with standing, worse in evening).

Risk factors for developing prolapse:
- Advancing age
- Chronic obstruction
- Constipation
- Genetic predisposition
- Menopause
- Parity
- Prior surgery
- Pulmonary disease
- Tumor/mass

Remember to examine the patient in **both** the supine and standing positions.

Pessaries are especially useful in the elderly population or when surgery is contraindicated.

Complications of pelvic organ prolapse:
- Urinary retention
- Constipation
- Urinary tract infections
- Ulcerations
- Vaginal bleeding

DIAGNOSIS

- Diagnosis is made by direct visualization of prolapsed organ during complete pelvic examination.
- Patient should be **examined in the supine and standing position**.

TREATMENT

Nonsurgical

- **Asymptomatic prolapse:**
  - Usually requires **follow-up**, but no immediate intervention needed.
  - Pelvic-strengthening exercises (ie, **Kegel** maneuvers) and/or hormone/estrogen replacement therapy may be beneficial.
- **Symptomatic prolapse:** Can be treated with a pessary or surgically. A **pessary** is an object (prosthetic) placed in the upper vagina designed to help maintain support of the pelvic organs. Types include:
  - Smith-Hodge (oval ring).
  - Doughnut (ring).
  - Inflatable.
  - Gehrung (U-shaped).

Surgical

- Indications for surgery: Childbearing is completed and/or symptoms are interfering with patient's functioning and does not respond to nonsurgical treatment.
- There are several types of surgical repairs for each type of prolapse. New, minimally invasive techniques are being developed.
  - **Cystocele:**
    - **Anterior colporrhaphy:** Bladder buttress base sutures proximal to the bladder neck.
    - **Kelly plication** (anterior vaginal repair): Endopelvic fascial reinforcement via vaginal approach.
  - **Rectocele: Posterior repair**—posterior vaginal wall reinforcement with levator ani muscles via vaginal approach.
  - **Enterocele: Moschovitz repair**—approximation of endopelvic fascia and uterosacral ligaments via abdominal approach to prevent an enterocele. Similar transvaginal repair exists.
  - **Uterine prolapse: Hysterectomy**—a uterine prolapse often occurs in conjunction with another prolapse, so combined repairs are usually performed.
  - **LeFort procedure/colpoclesis:** Surgical obliteration of the vaginal canal in a female who is NOT sexually active. This procedure can be performed with any type of prolapse.

Urinary Incontinence

Urinary incontinence is an involuntary loss of urine that can be due to a variety of conditions. It can cause social embarrassment. Cystometrics and Urodynamic studies can help to differentiate between the different types of urinary incontinence. Distinguishing between the types of incontinence is important because management is drastically different.

Causes of urinary
incontinence —
This **U**rine **F**low is **S**o
Outrageous

Total
Urge
Functional
Stress
Overflow

DEFINITION

Involuntary loss of urine that is a symptom of a pathological condition. Incontinence can be due to reversible or irreversible (but treatable) causes. It inhibits the patient socially.

CAUSES

Reversible

- Delirium, infection, atrophic vaginitis, drug side effects, psychiatric illness, excessive urine production, restricted patient mobility, and stool impaction are *reversible* causes of urinary incontinence.
- It is helpful to explore these easily correctable causes before moving on to the more expensive and invasive workup for the irreversible causes.

Irreversible

STRESS INCONTINENCE

- Loss of urine (usually **small amount**) only with ↑ **intra-abdominal pressure** (ie, with coughing, laughing, exercise).
- Caused by **urethral hypermotility** and/or **sphincter dysfunction** that maintains enough closing pressure at rest but not with exertion.

URGE INCONTINENCE

Total incontinence is
continuous urinary and/or
fecal leakage due to a
fistulous tract. This occurs
as a result from:
- Prior pelvic surgery
- Obstetric trauma
- Radiation

A 52-year-old G4P4 active female complains of sudden urgency to go to the bathroom followed by loss before she makes it to the bathroom. The urges are not precipitated by laughing or coughing, nor is she constantly leaking throughout the day. What is the underlying cause of her incontinence?

Answer: This woman has an urge incontinence that is caused by unopposed detrusor muscle contraction.

- Sudden feeling of **urgency** followed by **emptying** of bladder.
- Caused by unopposed detrusor contraction.

OVERFLOW INCONTINENCE

- Constant dribbling +/– urgency with inability to completely empty the bladder.
- Caused by detrusor underactivity (due to a neuropathy) or urethral obstruction.

MIXED INCONTINENCE

Combinations of above.

HISTORY

Ask about aforementioned symptoms, medications, medical history (diabetes mellitus, neuropathies).

PHYSICAL

- Pelvic exam: Check for cystoceles, urethroceles, atrophic changes, and Q-tip test.
- Rectal exam: Check for impaction and rectocele; assess sphincter tone.
- Neurological exam: Assess for neuropathy.

LABS

Urinalysis and culture to rule out urinary tract infection.

Q-TIP TEST

- A cotton swab is placed in the urethra. The change in angle between the Q-tip and the woman's body is measured upon straining.
- Normal upward change is < 30 degrees, and a **positive test** is one with **> 30-degree change.**
- **A positive test indicates stress incontinence.**

CYSTOMETRY

- Cystometry provides measurements of the relationship of pressure and volume in the bladder.
- Catheters that measure pressures are placed in the bladder and rectum, while a second catheter in the bladder supplies water to cause bladder filling.
- Measurements include post **residual volume, volumes at which an urge to void occurs, bladder compliance, flow rates,** and **capacity.**
- **Diagnoses:** Stress, urge, and overflow incontinence.

URODYNAMIC STUDIES

- A set of studies that evaluate lower urinary tract function.
- Studies may include **cystometry** (see above), **bladder filling tests, cystoscopy, uroflowmetry,** and **leak-point pressure tests.**
- Can help diagnose and differentiate between types of incontinence.

Functional incontinence: A person can recognize the need to urinate, but cannot make it to the bathroom because of immobility.

Q-tip test: ↑ upward motion of the Q-tip is caused by loss of support from the urethrovesicular junction, indicating stress incontinence.

Stress incontinence treated with α-adrenergic agonists and surgical repair.

Stress Incontinence

- **Kegel exercises** strengthen urethral muscles.
- **Estrogen therapy.**
- α-adrenergic agonists (eg, phenylpropanolamine, pseudoephedrine).

A suburethral sling is the treatment for stress incontinence.

Urge incontinence treated with medications, timed voiding, and dietary changes.

- Surgical repair.
  - Burch is the gold standard.
  - Suburethral slings are more popular due to ease of placement.

Urge Incontinence

- **Medications:**
  - Anticholinergics.
  - Calcium channel blockers.
  - Tricyclic antidepressants.
- **Timed voiding:** Patient is advised to urinate in prescribed hourly intervals before the bladder fills.
- Surgery is rarely used to treat urge incontinence.
- Avoid stimulants and diuretics (ie, alcoholic beverages, coffee, carbonated beverages).

Overflow Incontinence

- **Due to obstruction:** Relieve obstruction.
- Due to detrusor underactivity: Treat possible neurological causes—diabetes mellitus, B_{12} deficiency.

Total Incontinence

Surgical repair for fistulas.

Medical Student Information of Interest

▶ Opportunities

▶ Web Sites of Interest

AMA-MSS Councils

The Medical student section of the AMA (AMA-MSS) has several councils for which it seeks medical students.

Application involves a current curriculum vitae, an essay on why you want to be a member of an AMA Council, which Council(s) you prefer, what you consider to be your major strengths and qualifications for the position, and what benefits you feel are likely to result from your participation.

- Council on Constitution and Bylaws
- Council on Ethical and Judicial Affairs
- Council on Legislation
- Council on Long Range Planning and Development
- Council on Medical Education
- Council on Medical Service
- Council on Scientific Affairs

AMA-MSS Committee Application

Medical students are sought to serve on the following AMA-MSS committees:

- Committee on Computers and Technology (formerly Computer Projects Committee)
- Committee on Long Range Planning
- Legislative Affairs Committee
- Minority Issues Committee
- Ad Hoc Committee on Community Service and Advocacy
- Ad Hoc Committee on Membership Recruitment and Retention
- Ad Hoc Committee on MSS Programs and Activities
- Ad Hoc Committee on Scientific Issues Committee (CSI)
- Ad Hoc Committee on International Health and Policy

All applications must be completed and submitted with a CV to American Medical Association, Department of Medical Student Services, 515 North State Street, Chicago, IL 60610. Fax: (312) 464-5845.

AMA POLITICAL ACTION COMMITTEE (AMPAC)

AMPAC is a bipartisan group that serves to advance the interest of medicine within Congress, specifically by supporting candidates for office that are friendly to medicine. They also provide numerous programs to educate physicians, medical students, and their families on political activism. The Board directs the programs and activities of this extremely important political action committee. Adding medical students to the leadership of this group will provide for better medical student representation within the group, as well as greater student involvement in this important process. Terms are for two years.

ACOG.org

ACOG.org is the official Web site for the American Congress of Obstetricians and Gynecologists. The Web site has several items of interest to medical students, including a career guide for medical students interested in the specialty.

Medical student membership in ACOG

- ACOG publications
- Reduced meeting fees
- Entry into their member-only Web site
- Updates in the specialty

JOIN AMWA (American Medical Women's Association)

Become a medical student life member of AMWA. Membership benefits include:
- Networking opportunities at the national and local levels—60 physicians branches and 120 student branches
- Continuing Medical Education (CME) programs
- Leadership and mentoring opportunities
- Professional and personal development programs
- AMWA's legislative network
- AMWA's Annual, Interim, and Regional Meetings offering career and personal development curricula
- Gender Equity Information Line to assist you with concerns on sexual harassment, gender bias, racial discrimination, and other matters
- Women's Health Advocacy

- Subscription to the *Journal of the American Medical Women's Association* (JAMWA), a quarterly peer-reviewed scientific publication
- AMWA Connections, a bimonthly newsletter keeping you connected to your colleagues
- Women's health projects and innovative "Train-the-Trainer" programs
- Discounts for AMWA publications such as *The Women's Complete Healthbook*, *The Women's Complete Wellness Book*, and *Developing a Child Care Program*
- Advanced access and reduced fees to AMWA's Career Development Institute
- Members-Only sections on the AMWA Web site

ms4c.org

Medical Students for Choice (MSFC) is dedicated to ensuring that women receive comprehensive reproductive health care, including abortion. One of the greatest obstacles to safe, legal abortion is the absence of trained providers. The more than 6,000 medical students and residents of <ms4c.org> are committed to ensuring that medical practitioners are prepared to provide their patients with the full range of reproductive health care choices.

www.ama-assn.org

- FREIDA Online—computer access to graduate training program data (members receive up to 30 free mailing labels)
- Airline discounts for travel to residency interviews (graduating seniors only)

- USP Drug Information for the Health Care Professional (free 1998 benefit for three and four multiyear membership options)
- Discounts up to 35% in AMA's Medical Student Catalog
- PaperChase—discounted online subscription to MEDLINE searches (free access after 5 P.M.)
- Policy Promotion Grants for chapter and community projects
- Educational loans consolidation

medscape.com

This site's medical student section includes features such as "today's headlines," a medical student discussion forum to vent and exchange study tips, a weekly "focus" story from a med student's perspective, free tools for your palm pilot, test-taking skills, study tips, and a "clerkshop clues" section that summarizes the latest advances relevant to OB/GYN, Medicine, Surgery, and other clerkships.

CLASSIFIED

Opportunities

Index

Gonorrhea, 156, 164, 173, 325–326, 343
  in pregnancy, 164
  routine screening for, 343
Granuloma inguinale, 325, 331
Granulosa-theca cell tumor, 300
Gravidity, 43

H

Haemophilus ducreyi, 330–331
Hashimoto's thyroiditis, 116
Health education, 344–345
  nutrition and exercise, 345
Heart and Estrogen/Progestin Replacement Study (HERS), 365
Heartburn during pregnancy, 61
HELLP syndrome, 124, 133
Hematologic changes, 36–37, 97
  postpartum, 97
  during pregnancy, 36–37
    blood volume, 36
    coagulation, 37
    immunology, 36
    iron, 36
Hemolytic diseaes of the newborn (HDN), 141
Hemorrhoids during pregnancy, 61
Hemostasis, postdelivery, 81
Hepatitis, 156
Hepatitis A vaccine, 344
Hepatitis B virus, in pregnancy, 165
Hereditary nonpolyposis colorectal cancer (HNPCC), 286, 296
Herpes simplex virus (HSV), 156, 164, 173, 325, 328–329
  genital herpes, 328–329
  in pregnancy, 164, 173
Herpes zoster vaccine, 344
Hidradenomas, 313–314
Hilar (Leydig) cell tumors, 235, 236
Hirsutism, 232, 233
  idiopathic, 233, 236
HIV. *See* Human immunodeficiency virus

Hormone replacement therapy (HRT), 364, 365
Hot flashes, 363
Human chorionic gonadotropin (hCG), 26–27, 53, 186
  overview, 26
  pregnancy test using, 26–27
    plasma hCG, 27
    urine hCG, 27
  in screening for congenital abnormalities, 53
Human immunodeficiency virus (HIV), 156, 165, 329–330, 344
  laboratory testing for, 344
  in pregnancy, 165
Human papillomavirus (HPV), 166, 260, 270, 275–276, 304, 330, 344
  in pregnancy, 165
  vaccine, 344
Hydatidiform mole, 316–319
  complete, 316–317
  invasive, 317
  partial, 317
Hydronephrosis, 120
Hydrops tubae perfluens, 301
11β-Hydroxylase deficiency, 234
17α-Hydroxylase deficiency, 222–223, 224
21-Hydroxylase deficiency, 233–234, 236
Hyperandrogenism, 231–236
  adrenal etiologies, 233–234
    congenital adrenal hyperplasia (CAH), 233–234
    Cushing syndrome and Cushing disease, 233
  androgens, sources of, 232
    adrenal production, 232
    ovarian production, 232
  definitions, 232
  hirsutism, idiopathic, 233
  history, 235
  ovarian etiologies, 234–235
    luteoma of pregnancy, 235
    polycystic ovarian syndrome (PCOS), 234
    stromal hyperthecosis, 234
    theca lutein cysts, 235

physical exam, 235–236
studies, 236
treatment, 236
Hyperemesis gravidarum, 137
Hypoestrogenic amenorrhea, 226
Hypergonadotropic hypogonadism (gonadal dysgenesis), 222, 227
Hyperhomocysteinemia, 124
Hyperplasia with atypia, 247, 338
Hyperprolactinemia, 218, 237–239
  definitions, 238
  etiology, 238–239
  prolactinoma, 238–239
Hypertension, chronic, 117–118
Hypertensive diseases of pregnancy, 130–133
  eclampsia, 133
  gestational, 130
  management of, 132
  preeclampsia, 130–131
  preexisting or chronic, 130
  superimposed preeclampsia, 131
Hyperthyroidism, 115–116
Hypertrichosis, 232
Hypoactive sexual desire disorder, 354
Hypothalamic-pituitary disorders, 223
Hypothyroidism, 109, 116
  postpartum, 109
  in pregnancy, 116
Hysterectomy, 204, 247, 370
Hysterosalpingogram, 218, 219
Hysteroscopy, 218, 244

I

Immune system in the developing embryo, fetus, and newborn, 156
Immunizations, 63, 344
  during pregnancy, 63
Imperforate hymen, 224
Implanon, postpartum use of, 103
Implantation, 31
In vitro fertilization (IVF) and embryo transfer, 220

Indomethacin, 143
Induced abortion, 178–180
  assessment of patient, 179
  methods, 179
    pharmacologic agents, 179
    surgical method, 180
  therapeutic, indications for, 179
Infant care, postpartum, 104
Infertility, 215–220
  assisted reproductive technologies (ART), 219–220
    artificial insemination with donor sperm, 220
    definition, 220
    gamete intrafallopian transfer (GIFT), 220
    in vitro fertilization (IVF) and embryo transfer, 220
    intracytoplasmic sperm injection (ICSI), 220
    intrauterine insemination, 220
    zygote intrafallopian transfer (ZIFT), 220
  definition, 216
  female factors affecting, 216
  male factors affecting, 216
  types, 216
  workup, 216–219
    male factor, 216–217
    ovulatory factor, 217–218
    tubal factor, 219
    uterine factors, 218–219
Inflammatory breast cancer (peau d'orange), 339
Influenza
  in pregnancy, 157–158
  vaccine, 158, 344
Informed consent, 359
Inhibin A, 53
Insemination, intrauterine, 220
Intracytoplasmic sperm injection (ICSI), 220
Intrauterine device, 103, 200–201
  Copper T, 200, 201
  postpartum use of, 103
Intrauterine insemination, 220
Irving method (tubal occlusion), 203
Ischial spines, 22

J

Jarisch-Herxheimer reaction, 163

K

Kallmann syndrome, 223
Karyotyping, 58
Kegel exercises, 354, 355, 370, 373
Kell isoimmunization, 142
Kelly plication, 370
Kidneys, during pregnancy, 38
Klebsiella, 100
Kleihauer-Betke test, 99, 140, 146
Kroener method (tubal occlusion), 203
Krukenberg's tumor, 296

L

Labor
  abnormal labor patterns, 86–87
    dystocia, 86–87
  abnormalities of third stage, 152–154
    early postpartum hemorrhage (PPH), 152–153
    placental attachment disorders, 153–154
    uterine inversion, 154
  assessment of patient in, 69
    history, 69
    vaginal exam (VE), 69
  Bishop score, 72
  cardinal movements of, 77–79
    descent, 77, 78
    engagement, 77, 78
    expulsion, 79
    extension, 77, 78
    external rotation (restitution), 78, 79
    flexion, 77, 78
    internal rotation, 77, 78
  cervical exam, 71–72
    consistency, 72
    dilation, 71
    effacement, 71
    position, 72
    station, 71

cesarean delivery, 90–91
  basic types, 90
  indications, 90–91
delivery, normal spontaneous vertex vaginal, 79–81
  episiotomy, 81
  head, delivery of, 79
  infant, delivery of, 79–80
  inspection, 80
  nuchal cord, checking for, 79
  perineal lacerations, 80
  placenta, delivery of, 80
  postdelivery hemostasis, 81
  shoulders, delivery of, 79
fetal heart rate patterns, 82–86
  beat-to-beat variability (BTBV), 86
  decelerations, 83–85
  definitions, important, 83
  fetal tachycardia, 85
  long-term variability (LTV), 86
  short-term variability (STV), 86
fetus, assessment of, 73–77
  Leopold maneuvers, 73–74
  malpresentations, 75–77
  normal presentation, 74
induction of, 88–90
  confirmation of fetal maturity, 89
  contraindications, 89
  indications, 88–89
  methods, 89
management of patients in, 81–82
  maternal vital signs, 82
  oral intake, 82
  vaginal exams, 81
monitoring during, 82
  fetal heart rate (FHR), 82
  uterine contractions, 82
operative vaginal delivery, 91–92
  forceps delivery, 91
  vacuum delivery, 92
pain control during, 92–94
  general anesthesia, 94
  intravenous analgesia and sedation, 92–93